Generative Machine Learning Models in Medical Image Computing

Le Zhang • Chen Chen • Zeju Li • Greg Slabaugh
Editors

Generative Machine Learning Models in Medical Image Computing

Springer

Editors
Le Zhang
School of Engineering
University of Birmingham
Birmingham, UK

Zeju Li
Oxford University
Oxford, UK

Chen Chen
University of Sheffield
Sheffield, UK

Greg Slabaugh
Queen Mary University of London
London, UK

ISBN 978-3-031-80964-4 ISBN 978-3-031-80965-1 (eBook)
https://doi.org/10.1007/978-3-031-80965-1

This Springer imprint is published by the registered company Springer Nature Switzerland AG
The registered company address is: Gewerbestrasse 11, 6330 Cham, Switzerland

Preface

The advancement of machine learning, especially deep learning, has dramatically transformed various domains, and medical image computing is no exception. Over recent years, generative models have emerged as a powerful tool, capable of synthesizing high-quality medical images and augmenting the analysis, diagnosis, and understanding of complex medical data. This book, *Generative Machine Learning Models in Medical Image Computing*, aims to provide a comprehensive overview of the latest generative techniques, applications, and challenges in the field, addressing critical issues ranging from data augmentation to image reconstruction and disease modeling.

Generative models in medical imaging hold tremendous potential to impact traditional imaging tasks such as segmentation, classification, and localization by producing synthetic data that enhances model training, helps overcome data scarcity, and supports various downstream applications. Unlike conventional methods, generative approaches enable a more nuanced understanding of data variations and complexities, including modeling rare diseases and generating patient-specific data. The contributions in this book showcase how these models can generate synthetic images across different medical modalities, including MRI, CT, ultrasound, and histopathology images, advancing the field of medical image synthesis and transformation.

This book is organized into several parts, each covering a significant aspect of generative models in medical imaging:

Part I: Segmentation introduces innovative approaches to data synthesis for segmentation tasks, addressing the challenge of generating annotated datasets and evaluating their use in real-world scenarios.

Part II: Detection and Classification discusses advanced generative techniques for disease detection and classification, exploring methods like vision-language pre-training and synthetic data generation for training robust detection models.

Part III: Image Super-resolution and Reconstruction focuses on how generative models enhance image resolution and reconstruct high-quality images from low-resolution data, contributing to improved diagnostic accuracy and patient outcomes.

Part IV: Various Applications delves into diverse applications of generative models, including cardiac anatomy modeling, text-to-image synthesis, and anatomical structure synthesis, providing insights into both technical challenges and clinical implications.

As editors, we are excited to bring together contributions from leading researchers in this field, aiming to showcase the breadth and depth of generative modeling techniques in medical image computing. This book serves as both an educational resource for newcomers and a reference for seasoned researchers, clinicians, and developers interested in the intersection of generative machine learning and medical imaging.

We hope this volume inspires further innovation and collaboration across disciplines, ultimately contributing to the betterment of healthcare through computational advancements.

Birmingham, UK — Le Zhang
Sheffield, UK — Chen Chen
Oxford, UK — Zeju Li
London, UK — Greg Slabaugh

Contents

Part I
Segmentation

Chapter 1
Synthesis of Annotated Data for Medical Image Segmentation

Virginia Fernandez, Pedro Borges, Mark Graham, Walter Hugo Lopez Pinaya, Tom Vercauteren, and Jorge Cardoso

Abstract In the past decade, the advances in deep learning technologies have enabled their application to medical image segmentation, showing great potential. Nonetheless, the scarcity of available labelled data can result in a lack of model generalisability. This is especially true for supervised methods requiring annotated data. Data augmentation can be used to partially alleviate data scarcity when training deep learning models. In particular, the use of deep learning-based generative modelling, which allows for the sampling of synthetic data from the modelled data distribution, has shown its potential for data augmentation in the past years. In this work, we address the topic of generative modelling to generate images and annotations, going over brainSPADE, a 2D and 3D generative model of healthy and pathological segmentations and corresponding multi-modal images for brain MRI, and how the synthetic data it produces can be applied to a range of segmentation tasks to mitigate the effects of data scarcity or domain shift.

1.1 Introduction

In the past decade, deep neural networks (DNNs) and, in particular, convolutional neural networks (CNNs) have revolutionised the field of medical imaging segmentation, quickly becoming state-of-the art (SotA) [19], as they allow for the segmentation of a wide range of regions of interest in a variety of imaging modalities [1]. Unfortunately, these methods require large, representative datasets to be trained on, the lack of which results in underperforming or biased networks [19, 24], or networks trained on constrained tasks (e.g. one type of imaging modality). Whereas in computer vision, available datasets like ImageNet comprise tens of thousands, even millions of images, most medical imaging datasets fall behind these numbers by a large margin. This is because they have to be acquired with costly equipment that requires trained personnel, take longer to acquire and that, because

V. Fernandez (✉) · P. Borges · M. Graham · W. H. L. Pinaya · T. Vercauteren · J. Cardoso
King's College London, London, UK
e-mail: virginia.fernandez@kcl.ac.uk

L. Zhang et al. (eds.), *Generative Machine Learning Models in Medical Image Computing*, https://doi.org/10.1007/978-3-031-80965-1_1

they constitute Protected Health Information (PHI), they are subject to tight data regulations which makes them harder to share across institutions. Moreover, the process of labelling, especially in the case of segmentations, is extremely time-consuming when done manually, which often restricts annotations to a specific task (e.g. tumour, multiple sclerosis lesions, etc.).

Some techniques have been used to improve DNN models and make them more robust to domain shifts and more generalisable: examples are multi-task learning [6, 10], domain adaptation [17] or randomisation [2], either within specific tasks, modalities and anatomies or at the core of holistic models [33]. Another way to address these generalisability issues is to perform data augmentation. Initially, the latter was constrained to applying user-defined transformations on images (such as affine or contrast transformations). its platforms allowing for the randomisation and combination of such transforms, such as MONAI [8], these transformations remain a powerful tool to avoid model over-fitting.

Despite its usefulness, this type of augmentation does not tackle some directions of variability that might be useful for model generalisability (e.g. motion, presence of pathologies etc.) or data completion (e.g. missing modalities). In recent years, this type of image-based augmentation has been coupled to novel methods implementing a more dataset-driven augmentation capable of capturing the variability of the data distribution; a promising way to do so is to synthesise new images using deep learning (DL) generative models.

Generative models learn the input data distribution and are stochastic, thus providing a potential infinity of images via sampling. Unsupervised deep neural networks such as variational auto-encoders (VAEs), generative adversarial networks (GANs) and, notably, the state-of-the-art (SotA) diffusion models are examples of DL-based generative models that have revolutionised the computer vision and medical imaging deep learning fields over the past years. Examples of highly photorealistic generative models in computer vision are Style-GAN [27] or Stable Diffusion [39], based on GANs and diffusion models respectively. In medical imaging, numerous publications have shown the potential of these models to tackle data scarcity [28, 29] in various imaging modalities, tasks and anatomies, improving downstream algorithms [29].

Most SotA segmentation algorithms, like nnU-Net [20], are supervised methods, therefore requiring annotations. Whereas many generative models, nowadays, are designed with some conditioning that can constitute an annotation for, e.g. a class token for a classification task, in the field of segmentation, obtaining (image, annotation) pairs is a more challenging task because the segmentation associated to a potential synthetic image might not necessarily be at the user's disposal.

This chapter tackles synthetic data generation for brain magnetic resonance imaging (MRI) segmentation. It is based on our 2022 and 2024 papers *"Can segmentation models be trained with fully synthetically generated data?"* [13] and *"A 3D Generative Model of Pathological Multi-modal MR Images and Segmentations"* [15]. In the next section, we will cover the main relevant architectures we used and other relevant previous and posterior works published in the field of generative modelling for medical imaging.

1.2 Related Works

1.2.1 Main DL Generative Models and Their Use in Medical Imaging

In 2014, Kingma et al. [30] proposed a deep neural network called the **"variational auto-encoder"** (VAE). In a VAE, an encoder processes the image into a latent space representation, which can be linear or spatial and then decoded back into the input image. VAEs are optmisied by maximising the evidence lower bound (ELBO), which results in the need to minimise the distance between reconstructed and input images via an $\mathcal{L}_1$ or $\mathcal{L}_2$ loss, and the distance between the latent space distribution and a prior for that latent, which, in a simplified scenario [30], can be set up to be a Gaussian $\mathcal{N}(0, \mathbf{I})$, via the use of the Kullback-Leibler divergence (D_{KL}). The generative power of VAEs is constrained due to the inherent blurring caused by the reconstruction loss [16]. Many papers have explored variations of VAEs, to sharpen its results or use different priors that fit the data more accurately.

Generative adversarial networks (GANs) were first proposed by Goodfellow et al. in 2016 [16]. GANs comprise two networks: a generator, which produces an image from a noise sample, and a discriminator, which needs to learn to distinguish real images from synthetic ones. GANs are trained using an adversarial loss, which pushes the discriminator to better classify real and synthetic images as such, and the generator causes the discriminator to fail to distinguish synthetic images from real ones. Since the first GAN implementation, numerous works have proposed modifications of the generator or the discriminator, particularly to improve the training stability of the adversarial game. An example are Patch-GAN discriminators [21]; which, instead of predicting whether a whole image is real or fake, they do it on a patch basis. GANs can also be coupled to VAEs in a VAE-GAN architecture [32]. GANs have been widely used in computer vision, resulting in SotA models such as StyleGAN [26] or Pix2PixHD [21]. In medical imaging, they are at the core of numerous papers about synthesis tasks [22]. An example of GAN success is *medigan*, a pre-trained medical imaging GAN models library that can be used to augment datasets in a variety of tasks [35].

In [18], Ho et al. proposed a deep learning-based **diffusion model**, revolutionising the field of image synthesis. Diffusion models learn the input data distribution by adding incremental amounts of noise to an image x_0 over T time-steps and then learning the reverse step-by-step denoising process back to the original image. Although the objective can be derived using different theoretical approaches, [18] uses Bayes' rule similarly to how VAEs are optimised. A U-Net architecture [40] predicts the noise ϵ_t that is added between time-steps t and $t-1$, which needs to match, via an $\mathcal{L}_1$ loss, a Gaussian noise sample $\mathcal{N}(0, \mathbf{I})$. Due to their stability during training and their capability to produce extremely photorealistic images, diffusion models are currently SotA, with notable examples being Stable Diffusion [39] or DALL-E 2 [38]. A disadvantage of diffusion models is that inference takes a long time, requiring iterating over the T time steps to produce an image.

Alternative schedulers such as DDIM can shorten this inference time [44], even though the sampling time is still far from that of a GAN. Another problem with diffusion models, especially when applied to medical imaging, where many images are volumetric, is that GPU memory and computing time are required to increase considerably with image size. Rombach et al. [39] proposed operating a diffusion model in the latent space of an autoencoder network in a latent diffusion model or LDM. Over the last years, the potential of this type of network has been shown in medical imaging: RoentGEN [5] is a text-to-image diffusion model trained on more than 100,000 images and capable of producing diverse and high-quality X-ray images. Khader et al. [29] showed how diffusion models can tackle data scarcity in many tasks, outperforming GANs on many occasions.

VAEs, GANs, and diffusion models are only three of the main generative models, but they are not the only ones. Another successful architecture with generative potential is transformers [47].

1.2.2 Semantic Conditioning

As briefly mentioned in the introduction, synthetic data can supplement real datasets for downstream tasks, but corresponding labels are required for many SotA DL-based algorithms. Conditioned generative modelling can be implemented via many methods, such as special normalisation blocks [12] or cross-attention [47]. This conditioning allows the user to guide the synthesis process so that images belong to specific classes or follow a continuous variable. In [37], Pinaya et al. used cross-attention blocks to condition brain MRI synthesis on age or ventricle size. X-ray synthesis is conditioned on radiological reports in the previously mentioned RoentGEN model [5]. Class, continuous variable, or text conditioning typically makes it possible to pair generated images with annotations input by the user, which makes it possible to train supervised DL algorithms for classification or regression tasks.

Supervised segmentation requires spatial categorical or probabilistic masks to accompany the data. Conditioning on them is referred to as *semantic conditioning*. Because segmentations have an image format, generic image-to-image translation architectures, such as pix2pixHD [21] can go from segmentations to images. Image-conditioning methods, such as concatenation, can also guide the synthesis process [11]. Another approach is to use special normalisation blocks: in [36], Park et al. proposed a semantic-specific normalisation method that yields images with high correspondence to the input map. This normalisation is implemented via a convolutional block called SPADE, which is embedded in multiple layers of a GAN. Generative models using SPADE allow for style and content disentanglement in the synthesis process and have shown potential for semantic synthesis in medical imaging, for example in cardiac MRI or ultrasound imaging synthesis [43, 45].

These methods allow for the provision of paired images and segmentations. Nonetheless, real segmentations are still required, which, in some cases and as pointed out in the introduction, can be hard to obtain as they rely on human annotators. In the brain, where its complex anatomy is challenging to model and where pathologies cover a wide range of shapes and emplacements, thus limiting the efficacy of pseudo-lesion synthesis methods [48], there is potential for a model capable of producing anatomically accurate semantic maps of healthy and pathological regions, along with their corresponding images.

In this chapter, we revise the contributions from [13] and [15], namely:

- Generation of 2D and 3D healthy and pathological brain semantic maps
- Generation of corresponding multi-modal 2D and 3D MRI images
- Application of synthetic dataset pairs to downstream segmentation tasks

1.3 Methods

Our pipelines for [13] and [15] consist of a label generator implemented via a latent diffusion model, and an image generator based on the SPADE VAE-GAN from [36] we named "brainSPADE". The pipelines differ mainly on the spatial dimensions used ([13] uses a 2D approach and [15] is 3D) and the fact that, in [15], conditioning was incorporated in the label generator to allow for the same model to produce healthy labels or labels containing either tumours or white matter hyperintensities (WMH).

1.3.1 Data

Subsets of the Southall and Brent Revisited (SABRE) V3 datasets [23], Alzheimer's Neuroimaging Disease Initiative (ADNI)[1] and Brain Tumour Segmentation (BraTS) 2021 challenge [34] were used to train the models in both works. For testing, a set of unseen sites from BraTS we will name "$\text{BraTS}_{\text{test}}$" was used, along with subsets of the Open Access Series of Imaging Studies (OASIS) [31] and the Autism Brain Imaging Data Exchange (ABIDE) [9] datasets. Images were registered to the ICBM T1 1mm isotropic template using ANTsPy (https://github.com/ANTsX/ANTsPy). Probabilistic labels of cerebrospinal fluid (CSF), grey matter (GM), white matter (WM), deep grey matter (DGM) and brainstem (BT) were obtained using GIF [3]. For SABRE and ADNI, manually labelled WMH labels were provided along with the datasets; similarly, labels of non-enhancing tumour core (NE

[1] The ADNI was launched in 2003 as a public-private partnership, led by Principal Investigator Michael W. Weiner, MD. The primary goal of ADNI has been to test whether serial MRI, positron emission tomography (PET), other biological markers, and clinical and neuropsychological assessment can be combined to measure the progression of mild cognitive impairment (MCI) and early Alzheimer's disease (AD). For up-to-date information, see www.adni-info.org.

Table 1.1 Summary of the datasets used in both 2D (second column) and 3D papers (third and fourth columns). Spatial resolution and used lesions are provided, as well as the modalities and number of training and test subjects used in the different publications. *N/A: dataset not used*

		3D	
	2D	1 mm^3	2 mm^3
Resolution	192 × 256	160 × 176 × 112	96 × 128 × 96
Lesions	Oedema, tumour	WMH, oedema, NE tumour, GD-tumour	
Skull-stripped	Yes	Yes	Yes
SABRE	T1, FLAIR	T1, FLAIR, T2	T1, FLAIR, T2
	Training: 200	Training: 630	Training: 630
	Test: 25	Test: 30	Test: 30
ADNI	T1, FLAIR	T1, FLAIR	T1, FLAIR
	Training: 38[a]	Training: 66[a]	Training: 66[a]
	Test: N/A	N/A	N/A
BRATS	T1, FLAIR	T1, FLAIR, T2	T1, FLAIR, T2
	Training: 128	Training: 103	Training: 103
	Test: 30+5	Test: 30	Test: 30
ABIDE ("near-OoD")	T1	N/A	N/A
	Test: 25+5		
OASIS ("far-OoD")	FLAIR	N/A	N/A
	Test: 25+5		

[a] ADNI was used to train the image generators, but not the label generators

tumour), peritumoral oedema (oedema) and GD-enhancing (GD-tumour) tumour were provided with BraTS. The last two layers were merged in [13] and left separate in [15]. The healthy labels were overlaid with the lesions when available. Since BraTS images are skull-stripped, we performed skull-stripping on the other images during training to ensure consistent model behaviour. Table 1.1 summarises the resolutions, lesions, number of subjects per dataset and modalities used.

For the 2D paper, [13], 2D axial slices were taken from all datasets. The label generator of healthy maps was trained on around 7000 192 × 256 slices from SABRE, whereas the label generator of semantic maps, including tumours, was trained on around 8000 BraTS slices. The image generator was trained on around 3000 segmentation slices and their corresponding images from ADNI, BraTS and SABRE, with an even distribution between the three datasets.

For the 3D paper [15], 2 mm^3 and 1 mm^3 isotropic volumes were used to train two different brainSPADE (label+image generator) models. 2 mm^3 isotropic 96 × 128 × 96 volumes were obtained via resampling. For the 1mm^3 sets, volumes had to be cropped to fit into GPU, resulting in 160 × 176 × 112 volumes.

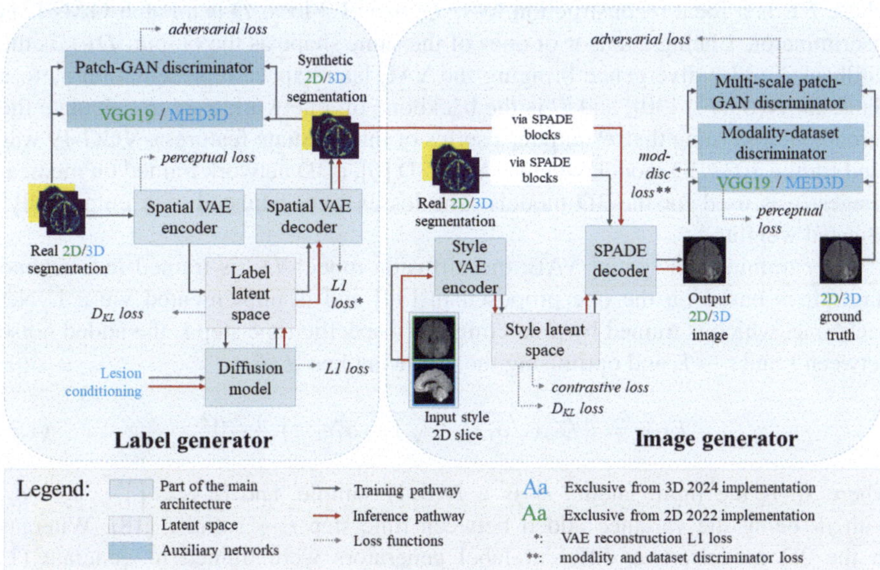

Fig. 1.1 Architecture of brainSPADE model, with highlighted differences between 2D and 3D, and training and inference pathways

1.3.2 brainSPADE Model

A diagram depicting the main brainSPADE pipeline, along with the difference between the 2022 2D (brainSPADE2D) and 2024 3D (brainSPADE3D) versions, is depicted in Fig. 1.1. brainSPADE consists of a latent diffusion model that synthesises semantic maps and an image generator that produces images matching the content of the input semantic map and the contrast of the input style image.

1.3.2.1 Label Generator

The label generator is a latent diffusion model comprising a spatial VAE that encodes the images into a latent space and then reconstructs it. A diffusion model operates within this latent space. These are trained in two stages.

For the **spatial VAE**, the 2D and 3D models differ in their number of downsamplings, resulting in latent spaces of $3 \times 48 \times 64$, $8 \times 24 \times 32 \times 24$ and $8 \times 20 \times 22 \times 14$ respectively (the first element being the number of latent channels). Given a 2D or 3D input segmentation map s, the network reconstructs it into $\hat{s}$ and is trained via the following loss:

$$\mathcal{L}_{VAE} = \lambda_{FL} FL(s, \hat{s}) + \lambda_{adv} \mathcal{L}_2(\mathcal{D}(\hat{s}), \mathbf{1}) + \lambda_{KL} D_{KL}(z_s, \mathcal{N}(0, \mathbf{I})) + \lambda_{perc} \mathcal{L}_2(\mathcal{P}(s), \widehat{\mathcal{P}(s)}) \quad (1.1)$$

where FL is a focal reconstruction loss, $\mathcal{L}_2$ is an L2 loss, $\mathcal{D}$ is a Patch-GAN [21] discriminator, $\mathbf{1}$ being a tensor of ones of the same shape as the output, D_{KL} is the Kullback-Leibler divergence bringing the VAE latent space representation z_s to a Gaussian $\mathcal{N}(0, (I))$ [30], and $\mathcal{P}$ is the backbone of a network used to calculate the perceptual loss (note that $\mathcal{P}$ outputs a series of intermediate features). VGG-19 was used for the 2022 2D model, whereas MED3D [6], a 3D network trained on medical images, was used for the 3D models. The losses were adjusted with empirically-adjusted weights λ.

After training the spatial VAE, the diffusion model $\mathcal{D}_m$ is trained in a second stage. It is based on the one proposed in [39] and is implemented via a U-Net backbone, which is trained by predicting, for a specific time step t, the added noise between t and $t-1$, and optimising the following loss $\mathcal{L}_{DM}$:

$$\mathcal{L}_{DM} = ||\mathcal{D}_m(\sqrt{\overline{\alpha_t}}x_0 + \sqrt{1-\overline{\alpha_t}}\epsilon_t, t) - \epsilon_t||^2 \tag{1.2}$$

where x_0 is the input latent[2] ϵ_t is a $\mathcal{N}(0, \mathbf{I})$ sample, and $\overline{\alpha_t} = \prod_{i=1}^{t} 1 - \beta_t$, with β_t being the variance added between time step $t-1$ and t [18]. Whereas in the 2D models, two different label generators were trained to generate (1) healthy segmentation maps (CSF, GM, WM, DGM, BT) and (2) segmentation maps including tumour layers (CSF, GM, WM, DGM, BT + tumour); the 3D work used cross-attention conditioning to control which lesions were present in the generated semantic volumes, resulting in a single label generator. This conditioning takes in an additional argument dc_{jl} per subject j and lesion type l (WMH, NE tumour, GD-tumour and oedema):

$$dc_{jl} = \frac{\sum_{n=1}^{N} s_{jln}}{max_j \sum_{n=1}^{N} s_{jln}} \tag{1.3}$$

where s_{jl} is the semantic map corresponding to that subject and lesion, and N is the number of voxels and s_{jln} is a specific voxel in the map.

1.3.2.2 Image Generator

The image generator is based on the SPADE VAE-GAN network [36]. The input to the VAE encoder is a 2D image slice containing the desired output contrast. This slice is encoded into a linear latent vector, or "style code", which is then decoded into an image. Each decoder comprises a convolutional block that uses a SPADE normalisation block, which takes in the activations and the input semantic map, resized to match the shape of the activations.

[2] In the case of the 1mm^3 model, the latent space had to be padded with zeros so that it is divisible by 2^{N_D}, where N_D is the number of downsamplings in the U-Net, resulting in a latent space of $8 \times 24 \times 24 \times 16$.

Although it is technically possible to use unpaired semantic maps and style slices, making SPADE able to disentangle style and content, it is done implicitly during training, as nothing prevents the encoder from retaining semantic information. To enforce disentanglement, [13] proposes to use unpaired styles and segmentations during training. Both in brainSPADE2D and brainSPADE3D, the encoder network is a 2D network taking in axial and sagittal slices, respectively, retrieved from the same subject from which the training (semantic map, ground truth) pair is. On the other hand, to make sure slices belonging to the same dataset and modality cluster together (and not, for instance, slices belonging to e.g. the same anatomical region), thereby aligning with the MRI contrast characteristics of the data, we implemented a "modality and dataset discriminator loss" $\mathcal{L}_{mod-dat}$ [13]:

$$\mathcal{L}_{mod-dat} = \lambda_{mod}\text{BCE}(C(\hat{i}), mod_i) + \lambda_{dat}\text{BCE}(C(\hat{i}), dat_i) \tag{1.4}$$

where $\hat{i}$ is the image generated from semantic map s_i and input style image i_s, BCE is the binary cross-entropy loss, λ_{mod} and λ_{dat} are loss weights and mod_i and dat_i are the one-hot encoded modality (T1 or FLAIR—and T2 in the case of [15]) and dataset (SABRE, BraTS or ADNI) of the input style image. Operator C is a two-tail classifier using the backbone of Densenet-121, that classifies both the modality and the dataset of the input 2D image. C was pre-trained on the training dataset, yielding an accuracy of ~90% for modality and ~80% for dataset.

In addition, a contrastive loss [7], named "slice consistency loss," is added in [13], and is implemented to enforce that the style codes remain invariant to spatial deformations, to ensure that only the contrast is picked up by the encoder:

$$\mathcal{L}_{cont} = \text{cosim}(\mathcal{E}(i_s), \mathcal{E}(\mathcal{T}(i_s))) \tag{1.5}$$

where *cosim* is the cosine similarity, $\mathcal{E}$ is the style encoder, and $\mathcal{T}$ is a random affine augmentation transform (including rotation, shearing and scaling).

The network is trained on these two losses, in addition to the original losses from [36], namely adversarial loss $\mathcal{L}_{adv}$, perceptual loss $\mathcal{L}_{perc}$, KLD loss $\mathcal{L}_{KLD}$ and the discriminator regulariser feature loss $\mathcal{L}_{feat}$, bringing the total loss $\mathcal{L}_{IG}$ to:

$$\mathcal{L}_{IG} = \lambda_{adv}\mathcal{L}_{adv} + \lambda_{feat}\mathcal{L}_{feat} + \lambda_{KLD}\mathcal{L}_{KLD} + \lambda_{perc}\mathcal{L}_{perc} + \lambda_{cont}\mathcal{L}_{cont} \tag{1.6}$$

$$+\lambda_{mod-dat}\mathcal{L}_{mod-dat} \tag{1.7}$$

where $\mathcal{L}_{adv} = \sum_{d=1}^{N_D} \text{Hinge}(\mathcal{D}_d(\hat{i}), \mathbf{1})$, with *Hinge* being the Hinge criterion [36] and $D_i, i \in \{1, \ldots, N_D\}$ being N_D multi-scale Patch-GAN discriminators; $\mathcal{L}_{feat} = \sum_{d=1}^{N_D} \sum_{f=1}^{F} \mathcal{L}_2(\mathcal{D}_d^f(\hat{i}), \mathcal{D}_d^f(i))$, with $f_j, j \in \{1, \ldots, F\}$ being intermediate features of each discriminator; $L_{KLD} = D_{KL}(\mathcal{E}(i_s), \mathcal{N}(0, \mathbf{I}))$, the KL divergence between the result from forwarding the style slice i_s through the VAE encoder $\mathcal{E}$; and $\mathcal{L}_{perc} = \mathcal{L}_2(\mathcal{P}(i), \mathcal{P}(\hat{i}))$, a perceptual loss identical to that from Eq. 1.1 using VGG-19. Weights λ for each loss are adjusted empirically. Note that, whereas $\mathcal{L}_{mod-dat}$

proved effective in [13], it was discarded in [15] as no significant improvement was observed with it, keeping $\lambda_{mod} = \lambda_{dat} = 0$ in the 3D approach.

We also replaced categorical semantic maps by probabilistic maps, where each voxel i has a depth of S semantic channels, and $\sum_{c=1}^{S} i_c = 1.0$, something that has been linked to increased image sharpness [41].

Due to the extensive memory requirements of 3D modelling for the 1mm^3 3D model, a patch-based approach was used for the image generator: patches of size 64 in the axial dimension were drawn from the semantic volumes during training. A sliding-window approach obtained $160 \times 176 \times 112$ images in inference. Further implementation details can be checked in each paper and their corresponding codebases.[3]

1.3.2.3 Inference

On inference, the only real data required by brainSPADE is the input style slice for the image generator, which is the desired contrast of the output image. On the 3D model, the lesion conditioning dc_{jl} can be specified or randomised to produce a semantic map with a specific phenotype. The lesion map is generated first and then forwarded, along with the style slice, to the image generator, which produces the images (or patches in the case of the $1\,\text{mm}^3$ 3D model). The inference pathway is shown in Fig. 1.1. Example images from brainSPADE2D and brainSPADE3D can be seen in Figs. 1.2 and 1.3 (figure drawn from [15]). The incorporation of conditioning in brainSPADE3D not only allows to generate different phenotypes with the same semantic model; Fig. 1.3 shows that the label generator can extrapolate to unseen phenotypes (WMH + tumour).

1.3.3 Segmentation Experiments

The main goal of a semantic map and image generator is to help train downstream segmentation models, either by supplementing real datasets or training only on synthetic data. For this, we used nnU-Net [20] ("2D", nnU-Net v1 in [13], "3D-full resolution", nnU-Net v2 in [15]), an automated, SotA segmentation method that ensures reproducibility. Only the number of epochs was modified to ensure convergence. Dice score was used to evaluate the performance of every model, in addition to accuracy, precision and recall for the binary segmentation tasks. Statistical significance was assessed via two-sided independent t-tests or signed Wilcoxon tests. The metrics calculation of 2D and 3D segmentation models was

[3] Code is available at https://github.com/virginiafdez/brainSPADE_RELEASE (2022 paper) and https://github.com/virginiafdez/brainSPADE3D_rel (2024 paper).

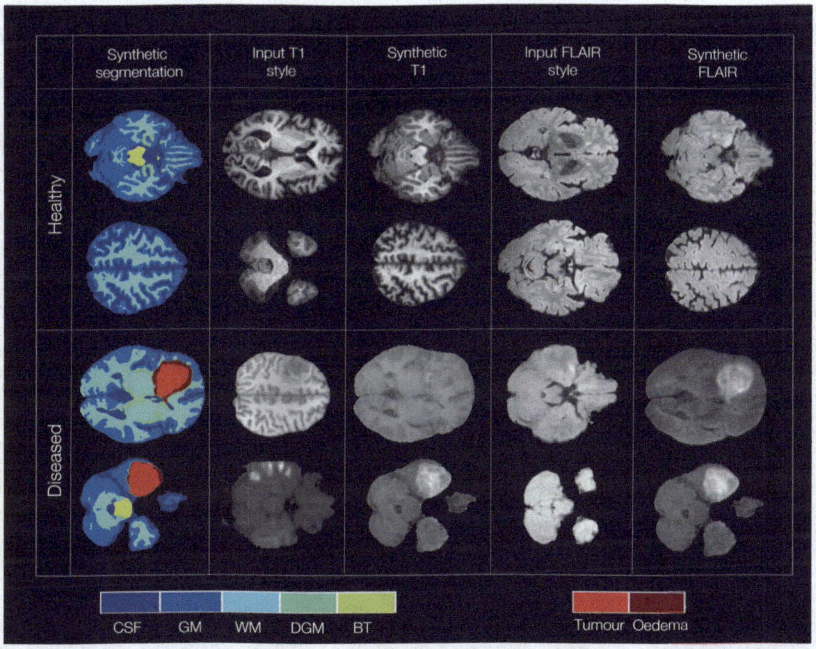

Fig. 1.2 Example label, T1 and FLAIR slices generated using the 2022 2D brainSPADE model. The top case used the healthy label generator, whereas the bottom one used the tumour label generator

always performed in 3D; for 2D networks, test volumes are forwarded slice by slice, and the resulting segmentations are reassembled back into 3D predictions. Computing the Dice in 3D allows calculated Dice scores not to be affected by a potential low ground truth voxel count of the regions to segment on some slices.

1.4 Experiments and Results

In both works, the central experiments focus on the following questions: (1) *can synthetic data be used to supplement existing datasets to train deep learning-based MRI segmentation algorithms?* (2) *can synthetic data be used as a standalone training set in the same tasks?* In this chapter, we focus on segmentation experiments. Additional quality metrics computation for labels and images (such as MSE or SSIM), are available in the papers [13, 15].

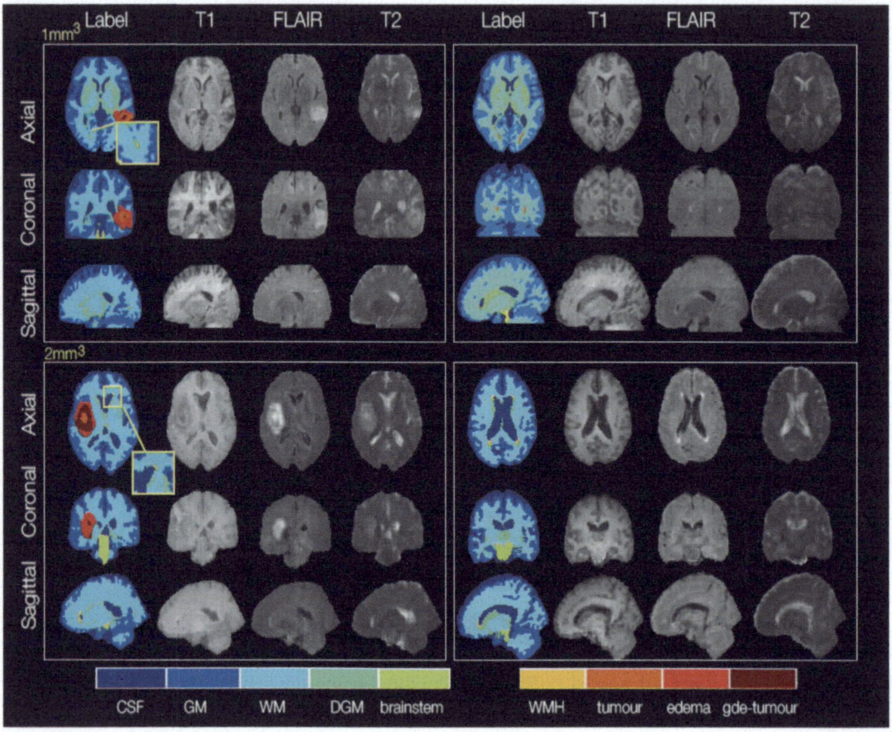

Fig. 1.3 Example axial, coronal and sagittal label, T1, FLAIR and T2 slices from images generated using the 3D 1mm^3 and 2mm^3 isotropic brainSPADE3D models. Two examples are shown for each case; the left cases were generated using > 0 tumour and WMH conditioning, whereas the right cases used only WMH conditioning. This figure was originally published in [15]

1.4.1 Segmenting Healthy Regions with Synthetic Data

brainSPADE2D and brainSPADE3D compare the performances of a nnU-Net segmentation model trained on real T1 images R_{id} to that of a model trained on synthetic T1 images S_{id}, to segment healthy regions (CSF, GM, WM—and DGM and brainstem for brainSPADE3D models). For the 2D model (brainSPADE2D), $\sim$7000 images (equivalent to the slices from SABRE used to train it) were used to train R_{id}, whereas 20,000 synthetic T1 images and labels were used to train S_{id}. In the case of both 3D models, 500 real and synthetic label and T1 volume pairs were used to train R_{id} and S_{id}, respectively. The resulting models were tested on 25 (brainSPADE2D) and 30 (brainSPADE3D) T1 SABRE volumes (see Sect. 1.3.3 for further information on testing). Results are reported in Table 1.2. R_{id} models worked significantly better in all three cases. In most cases, though, a comparable performance is achieved by models trained solely on synthetic data, showcasing the potential of synthetic data. The main difference is found for the deep grey

Table 1.2 Results obtained on the segmentation of CSF, GM, WM, DGM and brainstem for models trained on real 2D, 1mm^3 and 2mm^3 isotropic 3D T1 volumes and labels R_{id} and synthetic counterparts S_{id}. For each R_{id}-S_{id} pair, * indicates significantly better performance

	CSF	GM	WM	DGM	Brainstem	
2D model[a]	R_{id}	$0.953_{0.008}$*	$0.952_{0.006}$*	$0.965_{0.005}$*	N/A	N/A
	S_{id}	$0.919_{0.023}$	$0.925_{0.008}$	$0.945_{0.006}$	N/A	N/A
3D model (1 mm^3)[b]	R_{id}	$0.957_{0.005}$*	$0.959_{0.003}$*	$0.971_{0.003}$*	$0.875_{0.015}$*	$0.958_{0.021}$*
	S_{id}	$0.884_{0.014}$	$0.912_{0.009}$	$0.936_{0.005}$	$0.684_{0.034}$	$0.874_{0.036}$
3D model (2 mm^3)[b]	R_{id}	$0.947_{0.057}$*	$0.958_{0.046}$*	$0.968_{0.039}$*	$0.887_{0.065}$*	$0.962_{0.024}$*
	S_{id}	$0.869_{0.057}$	$0.895_{0.052}$	$0.931_{0.047}$	$0.703_{0.100}$	$0.905_{0.025}$

[a] Values obtained from [13] (table 1)
[b] Values obtained from [15] (table 3)

matter in the case of the 3D models (in the 2022 brainSPADE paper, DGM was included under the grey matter category). DGM is, indeed, an anatomically complex structure, with intensities spanning the WM-GM range. Whereas the probabilistic maps used to train the generative models take this uncertainty into account, splitting the label value into WM, GM and DGM channels, nnU-Net takes in categoricals (obtained by giving the voxel the value of the most probable label), which can result in noisy ground truth labels that differ from the synthetic ones, which have undergone smoothing due to the presence of a VAE within the label generator.

1.4.2 Addressing Out-of-Distribution Data with Synthetic Image and Label Pairs

This experiment was only performed in the 2022 brainSPADE2D work [13]. It attempts to study whether, given that SPADE is designed to extract contrast information from any given image, it can help bridge the gap between test sets belonging to a different distribution from that available for training (so-called "in-distribution" or "id"). In this task, 25 T1 volumes from the ABIDE dataset and 25 FLAIR volumes from the OASIS dataset (see Table 1.1), both unseen by the generative model, are used. The acquisition modality is the same in the first case, making it a "near" out-of-distribution ("n-OD"). In contrast, we are dealing with an entirely different modality and dataset in the second, so we consider it a "far" out-of-distribution ("f-OD").

Two synthetic datasets of 20,000 labels and respective T1 and FLAIR slices are generated using brainSPADE, and random slices from the "f-OD" and "n-OD" test sets as input styles to the image generator encoder. These datasets train segmentation models S_{n-OD} and S_{f-OD} to segment CSF, WM and GM. Aside from the 25 test subjects available for each case, the remaining subjects (see Table 1.1) were used to train reference models R_{n-OD} and R_{f-OD}. We tested all trained models, and the in-distribution models R_{id} and S_{id} from Sect. 1.4.1, on the 25 test

Table 1.3 Dice scores obtained on near (n-OD) and far (f-OD) out-of-distribution data by models trained on real in-distribution data from Sect. 1.4.1 R_{id} and S_{id} and models trained on synthetic and real n-OD and f-OD data. * indicates significantly better performance (p-value < 0.05) and ** indicates significantly better performance than every model besides R_{*-OD}

	n-OD			f-OD		
Model	CSF	GM	WM	CSF	GM	WM
R_{id}	$0.782_{0.002}$	$0.774_{0.019}$	$0.652_{0.036}$	$0.711_{0.042}$	$0.531_{0.033}$	$0.447_{0.180}$
S_{id}	$0.825_{0.023}$	$0.881_{0.008}$	$0.873_{0.007}$	$0.736_{0.054}$	$0.592_{0.033}$	$0.433_{0.178}$
S_{*-OD}	$0.841_{0.017}$**	$0.895_{0.010}$**	$0.891_{0.007}$**	$0.792_{0.034}$**	$0.784_{0.027}$**	$0.809_{0.031}$**
R_{*-OD}	$0.914_{0.022}$*	$0.971_{0.011}$*	$0.973_{0.009}$*	$0.830_{0.050}$*	$0.826_{0.047}$*	$0.862_{0.038}$*

volumes from each dataset. Results, collected from table 2 in [13], are available in Table 1.3. Whereas the reference models trained on real out-of-distribution data R_{*-OD} perform better than any other, models S_{n-OD} and S_{f-OD} (S_{*-OD}) perform significantly better than segmentation models trained on synthetic or real in-distribution data, showcasing the potential of brainSPADE2D to address domain shift.

1.4.3 *Lesion Segmentation*

Unlike neurotypical tissues like CSF, white or grey matter, brain lesions have more uncertain locations, shape and texture across subjects. Therefore, the potential for synthetic data is greater in this case, as it can fill the gaps within existing lesion datasets. The 2022 paper explores this in the context of tumour segmentation by combining a small dataset containing real lesions and manually segmented labels with a synthetic one. The 2024 paper addresses the benefits of generative models capable of extrapolating to unseen phenotypes to make models robust to the presence of unexpected lesions.

1.4.3.1 Tumour Segmentation Using Synthetic Data (2D)

This experiment from [13] addresses binary tumour segmentation when little data is available. A model R_{les} is trained on five subjects—1064 2D T1, FLAIR and tumour masks triplets—from the test set from BraTS, $\text{BraTS}_{\text{test}}$ (see Sect. 1.3.1). On the other hand, 20,000 synthetic T1, FLAIR and label triplets are generated using slices from $\text{BraTS}_{\text{test}}$ as style. These are used to train model S_{les}. The real and synthetic datasets are combined together and used to train hybrid model H_{les}. The models were tested on 30 $\text{BraTS}_{\text{test}}$ subjects, resulting in Dice, precision and recall measures available in the boxplots from Fig. 1.4. Whereas the model trained on synthetic data achieved lower performance overall than the model trained on

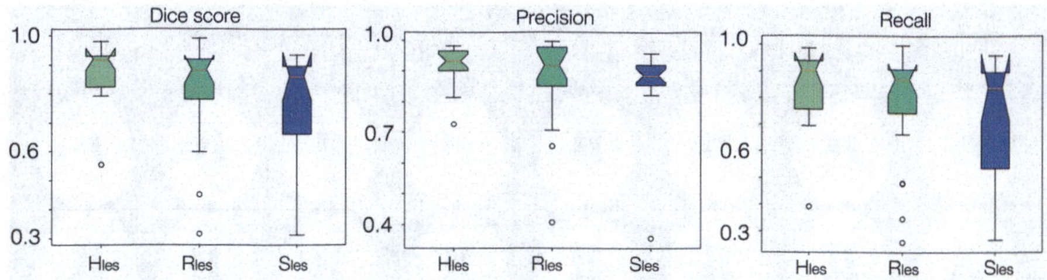

Fig. 1.4 Dice scores, precision and recall values obtained on the test set for H_{les}, R_{les} and S_{les} segmentation models on binary tumour segmentation. The values used for this plot are taken from table 3 in [13]

a small real dataset, H_{les} performed significantly better than every other model, showcasing the benefits of adding synthetic data to a small, labelled dataset.

1.4.3.2 WMH Segmentation in the Presence of Tumours

The 2024 brainSPADE3D paper shows that, when a model is trained on curated data containing only the lesion of interest (in this example, WMH), segmentation models fail when presented with test images that contain other lesions with overlapping features, such as similar intensities (e.g. peritumoral oedema). To show this, due to the absence of ground truth WMH masks in $\text{BraTS}_{\text{test}}$, a metric accounting for the tumour voxels mislabeled as WMH by the model, $\text{FP}_{\text{tumour}}$ is proposed:

$$FP_{tum} = \frac{N_{s_{tum} \cap s_{pred-wmh}}}{N_{s_{tum}}} \tag{1.8}$$

where s_{tum} is the ground truth tumour mask, $s_{pred-wmh}$ is the predicted WMH mask, $N_{s_{tum} \cap s_{pred-wmh}}$ is the number of voxels in the intersection between the two, and $N_{s_{tum}}$ is the number of tumour voxels.

As evidenced by Fig. 1.6 (which values have been extracted from table 4 in [15]) and visual examples in Fig. 1.5, a model trained on 500 real FLAIR volumes from SABRE, and corresponding WMH lesion segmentations, $M_{R_{100}S_0}$, achieves a Dice of 0.728 in a hold-out test of 30 SABRE volumes, as well as good precision and recall values. Nonetheless, when tested on $\text{BraTS}_{\text{test}}$, FP_{tum} is 0.325, showing a considerable mislabelling of tumours as WMH. As discussed in Sect. 1.3.2.3, the 3D label generators make it possible to extrapolate to unseen phenotypes (WMH + tumours). Using this feature, a synthetic dataset combining both lesions can be generated, resulting in 500 FLAIR volumes containing tumours and WMH, and corresponding WMH segmentations. When testing a model trained on this dataset, $SM_{R_0S_{100}}$, FP_{tum} decreases to 0.001, as can be seen in Fig. 1.6 (which values have been extracted from table 4 in [15]). However, as discussed in the previous experiment, an under-segmentation of WMH leads to a significant drop

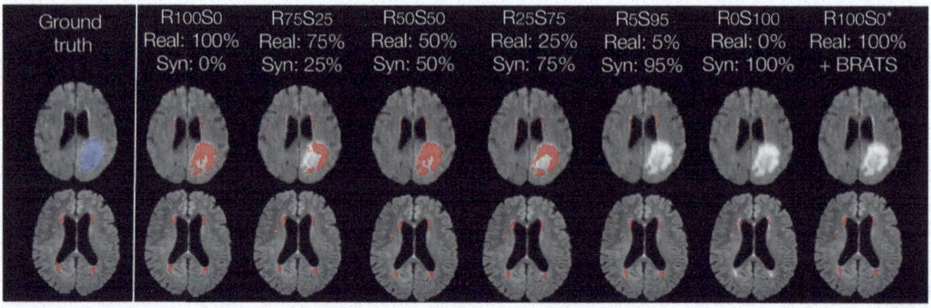

Fig. 1.5 This figure was originally published in [15] (except for the name of models, which have been changed for consistency across the chapter). The top row shows predictions made for $\text{BraTS}_{\text{test}}$. Note that the ground truth here depicts the tumour mask, which should not be segmented. The bottom row shows predictions made for SABRE. From left to right, the percentage of synthetic data increases, except for the last column, which shows results for model $R_{100}S_0$*, trained on real BraTS and SABRE subjects. The values used to plot this graph were taken from table 4 in [15]

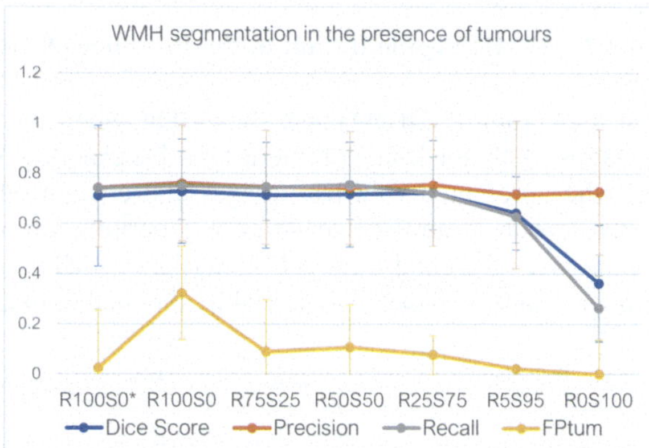

Fig. 1.6 Dice scores, precisions, recalls and FP_{tum} values obtained using different proportions of real and synthetic datasets. R100S0* refers to the model trained on real SABRE and BraTS volumes (leaving the WMH segmentations empty for BraTS)

in the Dice score to 0.362. Combination of both datasets, though, using different percentages, leads to a good compromise, resulting in high Dice scores and FP_{tum} values significantly lower than those obtained by $M_{R_{100}S_0}$. With only 5% of real data within the dataset, the Dice goes up to 0.642, keeping FP_{tum} under 0.03. This experiment also shows that training a model on a set of real BraTS volumes and empty labels, along with the SABRE volumes and their WMH segmentations, results in a model that associates BraTS contrast or the presence of tumours to an absence of WMH, which is not correct, emphasizing on the need for synthetic data in these scenarios. This last model achieves good Dice and FP_{tum} metrics, but visual examples from Fig. 1.5 show that segmentation is failing for this model, labelled "R100S0*" in the figures.

1.5 Discussion

brainSPADE is an example of how generative models can provide a variety of annotations and corresponding multi-modal images, which can be used to supplement or replace real datasets, maintaining comparable performance to them. brainSPADE2D [13] proposed a 2D model and showed that synthetic data could address domain shift and alleviate notably scarce datasets in the context of binary tumour segmentation. brainSPADE3D [15] made the model 3D, enabling, conditioning on multiple lesions, allowing the model to extrapolate to unseen data. Whereas a loss of fidelity is evidenced in 3D by comparing the images from Figs. 1.3 and 1.2, likely due to the increased computational cost and reduction of data availability when going from slices to full models, 3D modelling allows to condition the label generation process on more anatomically meaningful variables, such as the presence of lesions and their size, age or ventricular size, as shown by Pinaya et al. in [37].

The problem of image fidelity and loss of detail in 3D can be mitigated using more extensive datasets and models with more capacity [25]. In the previously cited example, the proposed high-resolution generative model was trained on the UK BIOBANK, a dataset encompassing 100,000 images, whereas brainSPADE3D was trained with 100 times less. More recent publications, such as the work by Khader et al. [29], show how generative models can generate high-fidelity 3D images in various anatomical regions and imaging modalities.

The boom of diffusion models in the past year has increased publications that apply generative models in medical imaging. Recently published works have shown that these models can promisingly produce labels and images simultaneously. The authors use diffusion models in [42] to produce polyp segmentation masks and corresponding endoscopic images. Likewise, Usman Akbar et al. [46] apply the same approach to BraTS images, generating multi-modal images and corresponding tumour segmentations. In a comprehensive study involving multiple segmentation baselines and generative models, the authors show that synthetic images can improve the performance of segmentation models and replace real data without severely compromising performance. Although these works remain constrained to a specific task, they show how combining images and labels can alleviate data scarcity in medical image segmentation. Our work shows how making generative models encompass more data, including different phenotypes or semantic regions, can further increase the generalisability of DL-based generative models.

An advantage of synthetic datasets and generative models is that, theoretically, they do not hold sensitive information, and thus, they can be shared, breaching the silos discussed in the introduction. However, the question of whether this is true has also been addressed by numerous works in the past few years; diffusion models, for instance, are more prone to memorise the training data distribution than their GAN counterparts [4], thus being more at risk of breaching the privacy of training datasets. Progress in the field of generative modelling should be accompanied by an assessment of how privacy-preserving these models are, including, if possible, solutions to prevent memorisation [4, 14].

1.6 Conclusion

In this chapter, we have outlined the potential of deep learning-based generative models to perform dataset-level data augmentation and address data scarcity in the context of medical imaging segmentation, mainly when these models can generate annotations to go along with the data. As an example, we discuss brainSPADE, a two-stage label and multi-modal image generator of healthy and pathological regions, first implemented in 2D in [13], then in 3D [15]. Through the experiments proposed in the papers we covered, we have shown how synthetic data can be used to train segmentation models or support small real datasets, reinforcing the potential of generative models. We hope that the work and ideas in this chapter shed some light on current state-of-the-art methods in this rapidly evolving field while paving the way for further developments.

Acknowledgments This work was supported by the UK Engineering and Physical Sciences Research Council (EPSRC) for the King's College London Smart Medical Imaging Centre for Doctoral Training. During their involvement in this work, M.J. Cardoso, Walter Hugo Lopez Pinaya, Pedro Borges, Mark S. Graham were funded by the Wellcome Flagship Programme (WT213038/Z/18/Z). M.J. Cardoso and T. Vercauteren were also funded by the Wellcome / EPSRC CME (WT203148/Z/16/Z).

We gratefully acknowledge NVIDIA Corporation for donating the GPUs used for this work.

Data were provided, in part, by OASIS-3: Longitudinal Multimodal Neuroimaging: Principal Investigators: T. Benzinger, D. Marcus, J. Morris; NIH P30 AG066444, P50 AG00561, P30 NS09857781, P01 AG026276, P01 AG003991, R01 AG043434, UL1 TR000448, R01 EB009352. AV-45 doses were provided by Avid Radiopharmaceuticals, a wholly-owned subsidiary of Eli Lilly.

Competing Interests Dr. Tom Vercauteren is co-founder and shareholder of Hypervision Surgical Ltd whose interests are unrelated to this work.

References

1. Antonelli M, Reinke A, Bakas S, Farahani K, Kopp-Schneider A, Landman BA, Litjens G, Menze B, Ronneberger O, Summers RM, van Ginneken B, Bilello M, Bilic P, Christ PF, Do RKG, Gollub MJ, Heckers SH, Huisman H, Jarnagin WR, McHugo MK, Napel S, Pernicka JSG, Rhode K, Tobon-Gomez C, Vorontsov E, Meakin JA, Ourselin S, Wiesenfarth M, Arbeláez P, Bae B, Chen S, Daza L, Feng J, He B, Isensee F, Ji Y, Jia F, Kim I, Maier-Hein K, Merhof D, Pai A, Park B, Perslev M, Rezaiifar R, Rippel O, Sarasua I, Shen W, Son J, Wachinger C, Wang L, Wang Y, Xia Y, Xu D, Xu Z, Zheng Y, Simpson AL, Maier-Hein L, Cardoso MJ (2022) The medical segmentation decathlon. Nat Commun **13**(1):1–13. https://doi.org/10.1038/s41467-022-30695-9. https://www.nature.com/articles/s41467-022-30695-9
2. Billot B, Greve DN, Puonti O, Thielscher A, Van Leemput K, Fischl B, Dalca AV, Iglesias JE (2023) Synthseg: segmentation of brain MRI scans of any contrast and resolution without retraining. Med Image Anal 86:102789. https://doi.org/10.1016/j.media.2023.102789. https://www.sciencedirect.com/science/article/pii/S1361841523000506

3. Cardoso MJ, Wolz R, Modat M, Fox NC, Rueckert D, Ourselin S (2012) Geodesic information flows. In: Medical image computing and computer-assisted intervention: MICCAI international conference on medical image computing and computer-assisted intervention, vol 15, (Pt 2), pp. 262–270. https://doi.org/10.1007/978-3-642-33418-4_33
4. Carlini N, Hayes J, Nasr M, Jagielski M, Sehwag V, Tramèr F, Zurich E, Balle B, Ippolito D, Wallace E, Berkeley U (2027) Extracting training data from diffusion models. In: Proceedings of the 32nd USENIX security symposium. https://www.usenix.org/conference/usenixsecurity23/presentation/carlini
5. Chambon P, Bluethgen C, Delbrouck JB, Van der Sluijs R, Połacin M, Chaves JMZ, Abraham TM, Purohit S, Langlotz CP, Chaudhari A (2022) RoentGen: vision-language foundation model for chest x-ray generation. http://arxiv.org/abs/2211.12737
6. Chen S, Ma K, Zheng Y (2019) Med3D: transfer learning for 3D medical image analysis. https://arxiv.org/abs/1904.00625v4
7. Chen T, Kornblith S, Norouzi M, Hinton G (2020) A simple framework for contrastive learning of visual representations. In: 37th international conference on machine learning, ICML 2020, PartF16814:1575–1585. https://arxiv.org/abs/2002.05709v3
8. Consortium M (2020) MONAI: medical open network for AI. https://doi.org/10.5281/ZENODO.6114127. https://zenodo.org/record/6114127
9. Di Martino A, Yan CG, Li Q, Denio E, Castellanos FX, Alaerts K, Anderson JS, Assaf M, Bookheimer SY, Dapretto M, Deen B, Delmonte S, Dinstein I, Ertl-Wagner B, Fair DA, Gallagher L, Kennedy DP, Keown CL, Keysers C, Lainhart JE, Lord C, Luna B, Menon V, Minshew NJ, Monk CS, Mueller S, Müller RA, Nebel MB, Nigg JT, O'Hearn K, Pelphrey KA, Peltier SJ, Rudie JD, Sunaert S, Thioux M, Tyszka JM, Uddin LQ, Verhoeven JS, Wenderoth N, Wiggins JL, Mostofsky SH, Milham MP (2014) The autism brain imaging data exchange: towards a large-scale evaluation of the intrinsic brain architecture in autism. Mol Psychiatr 19:659–667. https://doi.org/10.1038/mp.2013.78
10. Dorent R, Booth T, Li W, Sudre CH, Kafiabadi S, Cardoso J, Ourselin S, Vercauteren T (2021) Learning joint segmentation of tissues and brain lesions from task-specific hetero-modal domain-shifted datasets. Med Image Anal 67:101862. https://doi.org/10.1016/J.MEDIA.2020.101862
11. Dorjsembe Z, Pao HK, Odonchimed S, Xiao F (2023) Conditional diffusion models for semantic 3D brain MRI synthesis. http://arxiv.org/abs/2305.18453
12. Dumoulin V, Shlens J, Kudlur M (2016) A learned representation for artistic style. In: 5th international conference on learning representations, ICLR 2017 - conference track proceedings. https://arxiv.org/abs/1610.07629v5
13. Fernandez V, Pinaya WHL, Borges P, Tudosiu PD, Graham MS, Vercauteren T, Cardoso MJ (2022) Can segmentation models be trained with fully synthetically generated data? In: Zhao C, Svoboda D, Wolterink JM, Escobar M (eds) Simulation and synthesis in medical imaging. Springer, Cham, pp 79–90
14. Fernandez V, Sanchez P, Pinaya WHL, Jacenków G, Tsaftaris SA, Cardoso J (2023) Privacy distillation: reducing re-identification risk of multimodal diffusion models. https://arxiv.org/abs/2306.01322v1
15. Fernandez V, Pinaya WHL, Borges P, Graham MS, Vercauteren T, Cardoso MJ (2024) A 3D generative model of pathological multi-modal MR images and segmentations. Lecture notes in computer science (including subseries lecture notes in artificial intelligence and lecture notes in bioinformatics), vol. 14533, pp. 132–142. https://doi.org/10.1007/978-3-031-53767-7_13/FIGURES/3. https://link.springer.com/chapter/10.1007/978-3-031-53767-7_13
16. Goodfellow IJ, Pouget-Abadie J, Mirza M, Xu B, Warde-Farley D, Ozair S, Courville A, Bengio Y (2014) Generative adversarial nets (NIPS'14). In: Proceedings of the 27th international conference on neural information processing systems, vol. 2. MIT Press, Cambridge, pp 2672–2680
17. Guan H, Liu M (2022) Domain adaptation for medical image analysis: a survey. IEEE Trans Biomed Eng 69:1173–1185

18. Ho J, Jain A, Abbeel P (2020) Denoising diffusion probabilistic models. In: Advances in neural information processing systems 2020-Decem. https://arxiv.org/abs/2006.11239v2
19. Goodfellow I, Bengio Y (2015) Deep learning book. https://doi.org/10.1016/B978-0-12-391420-0.09987-X. arXiv:1011.1669v3
20. Isensee F, Jaeger PF, Kohl SAA, Petersen J, Maier-Hein KH (2021) nnU-net: a self-configuring method for deep learning-based biomedical image segmentation. Nat Methods 18(2):203–211. https://doi.org/10.1038/s41592-020-01008-z
21. Isola P, Zhu JY, Zhou T, Efros AA (2016) Image-to-image translation with conditional adversarial networks. In: Proceedings - 30th IEEE conference on computer vision and pattern recognition, CVPR 2017, pp. 5967–5976. https://doi.org/10.1109/CVPR.2017.632. https://arxiv.org/abs/1611.07004v3
22. Jeong JJ, Tariq A, Adejumo T, Trivedi H, Gichoya JW, Banerjee I (2022) Systematic review of generative adversarial networks (GANs) for medical image classification and segmentation. J Digit Imag 35(2):137. https://doi.org/10.1007/S10278-021-00556-W. /pmc/articles/PMC8921387//pmc/articles/PMC8921387/?report=abstracthttps://www.ncbi.nlm.nih.gov/pmc/articles/PMC8921387/
23. Jones S, Tillin T, Park C, Williams S, Rapala A, Al Saikhan L, Eastwood SV, Richards M, Hughes AD, Chaturvedi N (2020) Cohort profile update: southall and brent revisited (SABRE) study: a UK population-based comparison of cardiovascular disease and diabetes in people of European, South Asian and African Caribbean heritage. Int J Epidemiol 49(5):1441–1442e. https://doi.org/10.1093/ije/dyaa135
24. Kaissis GA, Makowski MR, Rückert D, Braren RF (2020) Secure, privacy-preserving and federated machine learning in medical imaging. Nature Mach Intell 2(6):305–311. https://doi.org/10.1038/s42256-020-0186-1. https://www.nature.com/articles/s42256-020-0186-1
25. Kang M, Zhu JY, Zhang R, Park J, Shechtman E, Paris S, Park T (2023) Scaling up GANs for text-to-image synthesis. https://doi.org/10.1109/cvpr52729.2023.00976. https://arxiv.org/abs/2303.05511v2
26. Karras T, Laine S, Aila T (2019) A style-based generator architecture for generative adversarial networks. In: Proceedings of the IEEE computer society conference on computer vision and pattern recognition, vol 2019, pp 4396–4405. https://doi.org/10.1109/CVPR.2019.00453
27. Karras T, Laine S, Aila T (2021) A style-based generator architecture for generative adversarial networks. IEEE Trans Pattern Anal Mach Intell 43(12):4217–4228. https://doi.org/10.1109/TPAMI.2020.2970919
28. Kazerouni A, Aghdam EK, Heidari M, Azad R, Fayyaz M, Hacihaliloglu I, Merhof D (2023) Diffusion models in medical imaging: a comprehensive survey. Med Image Anal 88:102846. https://doi.org/10.1016/J.MEDIA.2023.102846
29. Khader F, Müller-Franzes G, Tayebi Arasteh S, Han T, Haarburger C, Schulze-Hagen M, Schad P, Engelhardt S, Baeßler B, Foersch S, Stegmaier J, Kuhl C, Nebelung S, Kather JN, Truhn D (2023) Denoising diffusion probabilistic models for 3D medical image generation. Sci Rep 13(1):1–12. https://doi.org/10.1038/s41598-023-34341-2. https://www.nature.com/articles/s41598-023-34341-2
30. Kingma DP, Welling M (2014) Auto-encoding variational bayes. CoRR abs/1312.6
31. LaMontagne PJ, Benzinger TLS, Morris JC, Keefe S, Hornbeck R, Xiong C, Grant E, Hassenstab J, Moulder K, Vlassenko AG, Raichle ME, Cruchaga C, Marcus D (2019) OASIS-3: longitudinal neuroimaging, clinical, and cognitive dataset for normal aging and alzheimer disease. medRxiv p 2019.12.13.19014902. https://doi.org/10.1101/2019.12.13.19014902. http://medrxiv.org/content/early/2019/12/15/2019.12.13.19014902.abstract
32. Larsen ABL, Sønderby SK, Larochelle H, Winther O (2016) Autoencoding beyond pixels using a learned similarity metric. In: Balcan MF, Weinberger KQ (eds) Proceedings of the 33rd international conference on machine learning. Proceedings of machine learning research, New York, vol 48, pp 1558–1566. http://proceedings.mlr.press/v48/larsen16.html
33. Ma J, He Y, Li F, Han L, You C, Wang B (2024) Segment anything in medical images. Nat Commun 15(1):1–9. https://doi.org/10.1038/s41467-024-44824-z. https://www.nature.com/articles/s41467-024-44824-z

34. Menze BH, Jakab A, Bauer S, Kalpathy-Cramer J, Farahani K, Kirby J, Burren Y, Porz N, Slotboom J, Wiest R, Lanczi L, Gerstner E, Weber MA, Arbel T, Avants BB, Ayache N, Buendia P, Collins DL, Cordier N, Corso JJ, Criminisi A, Das T, Delingette H, Demiralp Ç, Durst CR, Dojat M, Doyle S, Festa J, Forbes F, Geremia E, Glocker B, Golland P, Guo X, Hamamci A, Iftekharuddin KM, Jena R, John NM, Konukoglu E, Lashkari D, Mariz JA, Meier R, Pereira S, Precup D, Price SJ, Raviv TR, Reza SMS, Ryan M, Sarikaya D, Schwartz L, Shin HC, Shotton J, Silva CA, Sousa N, Subbanna NK, Szekely G, Taylor TJ, Thomas OM, Tustison NJ, Unal G, Vasseur F, Wintermark M, Ye DH, Zhao L, Zhao B, Zikic D, Prastawa M, Reyes M, Van Leemput K (2015) The multimodal brain tumor image segmentation benchmark (BRATS). IEEE Trans Med Imag 34(10):1993–2024. https://doi.org/10.1109/TMI.2014.2377694. https://pubmed.ncbi.nlm.nih.gov/25494501. https://www.ncbi.nlm.nih.gov/pmc/articles/PMC4833122/
35. Osuala R, Skorupko G, Lazrak N, Garrucho L, García E, Joshi S, Jouide S, Rutherford M, Prior F, Kushibar K, Diaz O, Lekadir K (2022) Medigan: a Python library of pretrained generative models for medical image synthesis. J Med Imag 10(06), 061403. https://doi.org/10.1117/1.JMI.10.6.061403. http://arxiv.org/abs/2209.14472http://dx.doi.org/10.1117/1.JMI.10.6.061403
36. Park T, Liu MY, Wang TC, Zhu JY (2019) Semantic image synthesis with spatially-adaptive normalization. In: Proceedings of the IEEE conference on computer vision and pattern recognition
37. Pinaya WHL, Tudosiu PD, Dafflon J, Da Costa PF, Fernandez V, Nachev P, Ourselin S, Cardoso MJ (2022) Brain imaging generation with latent diffusion models. In: Mukhopadhyay A, Oksuz I, Engelhardt S, Zhu D, Yuan Y (eds) Deep generative models. Springer, Cham, pp 117–126
38. Ramesh A, Dhariwal P, Nichol A, Chu C, Chen M (2022) Hierarchical text-conditional image generation with CLIP latents. https://arxiv.org/abs/2204.06125v1
39. Rombach R, Blattmann A, Lorenz D, Esser P, Ommer B (2022) High-resolution image synthesis with latent diffusion models. In: 2022 IEEE/CVF Conference on Computer Vision and Pattern Recognition (CVPR), 2022-June, pp 10674–10685. https://doi.org/10.1109/CVPR52688.2022.01042
40. Ronneberger O, Fischer P, Brox T (2015) U-net: convolutional networks for biomedical image segmentation. In: Lecture notes in computer science (including subseries lecture notes in artificial intelligence and lecture notes in bioinformatics), vol. 9351, pp. 234–241. https://doi.org/10.1007/978-3-319-24574-4_28/COVER. https://link.springer.com/chapter/10.1007/978-3-319-24574-4_28
41. Rusak F, Santa Cruz R, Bourgeat P, Fookes C, Fripp J, Bradley A, Salvado O (2020) 3d brain MRI gan-based synthesis conditioned on partial volume maps. In: Simulation and synthesis in medical imaging. Springer Science and Business Media Deutschland GmbH. Lecture Notes in Computer Science, vol 12417, pp 11–20. Springer, Berlin. https://doi.org/10.1007/978-3-030-59520-3_2/FIGURES/5. https://link.springer.com/chapter/10.1007/978-3-030-59520-3_2
42. Saragih D, Tyrrell P (2023) Using diffusion models to generate synthetic labelled data for medical image segmentation. https://arxiv.org/abs/2310.16794v1
43. Skandarani Y, Painchaud N, Jodoin PM, Lalande A (2020) On the effectiveness of GAN generated cardiac MRIs for segmentation. https://arxiv.org/abs/2005.09026v2
44. Song J, Meng C, Ermon S (2020) Denoising diffusion implicit models. In: ICLR 2021 - 9th international conference on learning representations. https://arxiv.org/abs/2010.02502v4
45. Stojanovski D, Hermida U, Lamata P, Beqiri A, Gomez A (2023) Echo from noise: synthetic ultrasound image generation using diffusion models for real image segmentation. Lecture notes in computer science (including subseries lecture notes in artificial intelligence and lecture notes in bioinformatics). Lecture Notes in Computer Science, vol 14337, pp 34–43. https://doi.org/10.1007/978-3-031-44521-7_4/FIGURES/5. https://link.springer.com/chapter/10.1007/978-3-031-44521-7_4
46. Usman Akbar M, Larsson M, Blystad I, Eklund A (2024) Brain tumor segmentation using synthetic MR images - a comparison of GANs and diffusion models. Sci Data 11(1):1–17. https://doi.org/10.1038/s41597-024-03073-x. https://www.nature.com/articles/s41597-024-03073-x

47. Vaswani A, Shazeer N, Parmar N, Uszkoreit J, Jones L, Gomez AN, Kaiser Ł, Polosukhin I (2017) Attention is all you need. In: Advances in neural information processing systems, pp. 5999–6009. https://arxiv.org/abs/1706.03762v7
48. Zhang Z, Deng H, Li X (2023) Unsupervised liver tumor segmentation with pseudo anomaly synthesis. In: Wolterink JM, Svoboda D, Zhao C, Fernandez V (eds) Simulation and synthesis in medical imaging. SASHIMI 2023. Lecture Notes in Computer Science, vol 14288. Springer, Cham. https://doi.org/10.1007/978-3-031-44689-4_9

Chapter 2
Diffusion Models for Histopathological Image Generation

Aman Shrivastava and P. Thomas Fletcher

Abstract Diffusion models have revolutionized artificial intelligence with their ability to generate unprecedentedly realistic imagery. This chapter explores the application of diffusion models for generating histopathological images, and their potential to address issues with limited high-quality and annotated pathology datasets. It highlights how diffusion models, with their iterative denoising process, create realistic and diverse synthetic images that can be conditioned on a semantic mask of nuclei locations. These models improve the diversity of the data set, support robust training for diagnostic algorithms, and mitigate the need for extensive annotated medical data. By examining foundational principles and recent advances, this chapter demonstrates the potential of diffusion models to improve diagnostic accuracy, assist pathologists, and transform the field of histopathology. Additionally, the chapter introduces a first-of-its-kind nuclei-aware semantic tissue generation framework (NASDM) which can synthesize realistic tissue samples given a semantic instance mask of up to six different nuclei types, enabling pixel-perfect nuclei localization in generated samples.

2.1 Introduction

The advent of deep learning has revolutionized numerous fields, and histopathology is no exception. Histopathology is dependent on biopsies stained with hematoxylin and eosin (H&E) for microscopic inspection to identify visual evidence of diseases. Hematoxylin exhibits a deep blue-purple color, and acidic structures such as DNA in cell nuclei are stained by it. Alternatively, eosin is red-pink, and nonspecific proteins in the cytoplasm and the stromal matrix are stained by it. Highlighted tissue characteristics are then examined by pathologists to diagnose diseases, including different cancers. Therefore, the correct diagnosis depends on the pathologist's training and prior exposure to a wide variety of disease subtypes [23]. One of

A. Shrivastava (✉) · P. T. Fletcher
University of Virginia, Charlottesville, VA, USA
e-mail: as3ek@virginia.edu; ptf8v@virginia.edu

L. Zhang et al. (eds.), *Generative Machine Learning Models in Medical Image Computing*, https://doi.org/10.1007/978-3-031-80965-1_2

the primary challenges is the scarcity of certain disease subtypes, which makes visual identification difficult and dependent on the pathologist's exposure to a wide variety of disease presentations. This has spurred interest in the development of computational methods to aid and enhance diagnostic accuracy.

In recent years, generative models, particularly diffusion models, have emerged as powerful tools in the realm of image generation. These models have shown remarkable success in generating realistic images across various domains. In the context of histopathology, diffusion models offer a promising avenue to address some of the inherent challenges. Histopathological images with specific characteristics, such as visual patterns that identify rare cancer subtypes, can be generated by generative models [5]. As such, generative models can be sampled to emphasize each disease subtype equally and more balanced datasets can be generated, thus preventing dataset biases from being amplified by the models [8]. The pedagogy, trustworthiness, generalization, and coverage of disease diagnosis in the field of histology can be improved by generative models by aiding both deep learning models and human pathologists. Privacy concerns surrounding medical data sharing can also be addressed by synthetic datasets. Further value is added to the proposition by conditional generation of annotated data, since tremendous time, labor, and training costs are involved in labeling medical images. Extraordinary success in the conditional and unconditional generation of real-world images has been achieved recently by denoising diffusion probabilistic models (DDPMs) [4, 10]. Diffusion models operate by iteratively refining a noisy image until a high-fidelity, realistic image is produced. This process, known as denoising, is particularly suited for the complexities of histopathological image generation, where fine details and subtle variations are critical.

This chapter delves into the application of diffusion models for histopathological image generation. The chapter begins by exploring the foundational principles of diffusion models and their relevance to medical imaging. In addition, through a combination of theoretical insights and practical examples, this chapter aims to provide a comprehensive understanding of the transformative impact of diffusion models in histopathological image generation. The chapter demonstrates how the recently discovered capabilities of DDPMs can be leveraged to design a first-of-its-kind nuclei-aware semantic diffusion model (NASDM) [19] that can generate realistic tissue patches given a semantic mask comprising multiple nuclei types. NASDM is trained on the Lizard dataset [7] consisting of colon histology images and achieves state-of-the-art generation capabilities, validated through extensive ablative, qualitative and quantitative analyzes to establish the proficiency of the framework on the histopathology generation task.

2.2 Denoising Diffusion Probabilistic Models (DDPMs)

Denoising diffusion probabilistic models (DDPMs) [10] represent a fairly recent and significant advance in generative modeling, harnessing a sequential denoising process inspired by principles of non-equilibrium thermodynamics to synthesize high-fidelity data. A DDPM comprises of a forward diffusion process that iteratively perturbs data with Gaussian noise, transforming it into a tractable noise distribution through a Markov chain of latent variables. The reverse diffusion process, which is the key innovation of DDPMs, involves training a neural network to approximate the reverse transitions, effectively learning to denoise the perturbed data step-by-step. This reverse process is modeled as a series of Gaussian transitions conditioned on the current state, with the neural network effectively denoising the perturbed samples. This method ensures stable training dynamics, mitigating issues commonly encountered in Generative Adversarial Networks (GANs) [6], and achieves state-of-the-art performance in various generative tasks, including high-resolution image synthesis, audio generation, and more. Consequently, DDPMs have established themselves as a robust and versatile framework for high-dimensional data generation with remarkable fidelity and diversity. The following subsections describe the formulations of the forward and the reverse diffusion process in detail.

2.2.1 Forward Diffusion Process

DDPMs are formulated from the variational perspective where the forward diffusion systematically transforms data into a noise distribution through a series of incremental additions of Gaussian noise. Formally, this process yields a Markov Chain of latent variables $\{x_t\}_{t=0}^{T}$, which are of the same dimensionality as the original data, where x_0 is the original data sample, and x_T converges to an isotropic Gaussian distribution. The data is sampled from $q(x_0)$, which represents the real data distribution. At each time step t, Gaussian noise is added to the data controlled by a predefined variance schedule controlled by parameters $\{\beta\}_{t=1}^{T}$. Specifically, each step of the forward diffusion is defined as,

$$q(x_t \mid x_{t-1}) = \mathcal{N}(x_t; \sqrt{1-\beta_t}x_{t-1}, \beta_t \mathbf{I}), \tag{2.1}$$

$$q(x_{1:T} \mid x_0) = \prod_{t=1}^{T} q(x_t \mid x_{t-1}), \tag{2.2}$$

where $\{\beta\}_{t=1}^{T} \in [0, 1)$ is the variance schedule across diffusion steps, $\mathbf{I}$ is the identity matrix and $\mathcal{N}(x; \mu, \sigma)$ represents a normal distribution with mean μ and covariance σ. Note that a key property of Gaussian distributions is that the composition of multiple Gaussian perturbations remains Gaussian. This means if we add Gaussian noise to a Gaussian-distributed variable, the resulting distribution is still Gaussian. This property allows us to combine the noise addition steps over multiple time steps into a single Gaussian distribution. Given the forward process transitions, we can derive the marginal distribution of x_t conditioned on the original data x_0 by recursively applying the transition probabilities. Due to the linear nature of the noise addition and the properties of Gaussian distributions, the marginal distribution $q(x_t \mid x_0)$ can be expressed as a Gaussian distribution,

$$q(x_t \mid x_0) = \mathcal{N}(x_t; \sqrt{\bar{\alpha}_t} x_0, (1 - \bar{\alpha}_t)\mathbf{I}), \tag{2.3}$$

where $\alpha_t = (1 - \beta_t)$ and $\bar{\alpha}_t = \prod_{s=1}^{t} \alpha_s$. This property is particularly advantageous, as it enables the efficient sampling of noisy data at any intermediate time step without requiring an iterative simulation from x_0 to x_t.

2.2.2 *Reverse Diffusion Process*

The reverse diffusion process in DDPMs is a generative mechanism which inverts the forward diffusion process through a sequence of learned denoising steps. This process is designed to transform samples from the noise distribution back into coherent data samples. Specifically, the reverse process aims to approximate the conditional distributions $p_\theta(x_{t-1}|x_t)$ through a neural network, where each x_{t-1} depends only on x_t. The reverse transitions are modeled as Gaussian distributions as follows,

$$p_\theta(x_{t-1} \mid x_t) = \mathcal{N}(x_{t-1}; \mu_\theta(x_t, t), \Sigma_\theta(x_t, t)), \tag{2.4}$$

$$p_\theta(x_{0:T}) = p(x_T) \prod_{t=1}^{T} p_\theta(x_{t-1} \mid x_t), \tag{2.5}$$

where p_θ is a neural network that represents the learned reverse process with parameters θ. During sampling, the model begins with a noise vector $x_T \sim \mathcal{N}(0, \mathbf{I})$ and iteratively applies the reverse transitions $p_\theta(x_{t-1} \mid x_t)$ using the trained denoising neural network to generate a sequence of latent variables that culminate in the reconstructed data sample x_0. This iterative process effectively denoises the initial noise, step by step, reconstructing the data distribution in reverse order. The success of the reverse diffusion process is contingent on a well-trained denoising network p_θ as it ensures that the final samples are realistic and diverse, closely matching the original data distribution.

2.2.3 *Training the Model*

Optimizing the parameters θ of the denoising neural network involves minimizing a variational lower bound on the negative log-likelihood of the data,

$$\mathbb{E}[-\log p_\theta(x_0)] \leq \mathbb{E}_q\left[-\log \frac{p_\theta(x_{0:T})}{q(x_{1:T} \mid x_0)}\right] \tag{2.6}$$

$$\leq \mathbb{E}_q\left[-\log p\left(x_T\right)-\sum_{t \geq 1} \log \frac{p_\theta\left(x_{t-1} \mid x_t\right)}{q\left(x_t \mid x_{t-1}\right)}\right]=L, \tag{2.7}$$

which decomposes into a series of Kullback-Leibler (KL) divergence terms between the true posterior of the forward process and the learned reverse process, along with a reconstruction term:

$$L=L_T+\sum_{t>1} L_{t-1}+L_0, \tag{2.8}$$

$$L_T=D_{KL}\left(q\left(x_T \mid x_0\right) \| p\left(x_T\right)\right), \tag{2.9}$$

$$L_{t-1}=D_{KL}\left(q\left(x_{t-1} \mid x_t, x_0\right) \| p_\theta\left(x_{t-1} \mid x_t\right)\right), \tag{2.10}$$

$$L_0=-\log p_\theta\left(x_0 \mid x_1\right). \tag{2.11}$$

Except for L_0, each term of the decomposition in Eq. 2.8 is a KL-divergence between two Gaussian distributions and hence has a closed-form solution. The KL-divergence terms ensure that the neural network accurately captures the denoising process by aligning the learned distributions $p_\theta(x_{t-1}|x_t)$ with the true posteriors $q(x_{t-1}|x_t, x_0)$. Notice that L_T does not depend on the parameters θ and can be ignored safely during optimization. Upon simplification via Bayes theorem, the posteriors $q(x_{t-1}|x_t, x_0)$ can be represented in terms of parameters β_t and $\bar{\alpha}_t$ as follows,

$$q\left(x_{t-1} \mid x_t, x_0\right)=\mathcal{N}\left(x_{t-1} ; \tilde{\mu}\left(x_t, x_0\right), \tilde{\beta}_t \mathbf{I}\right), \tag{2.12}$$

where,

$$\tilde{\mu}_t\left(x_t, x_0\right)=\frac{\sqrt{\bar{\alpha}_{t-1}} \beta_t}{1-\bar{\alpha}_t} x_0+\frac{\sqrt{\alpha_t}\left(1-\bar{\alpha}_{t-1}\right)}{1-\bar{\alpha}_t} x_t, \tag{2.13}$$

$$\tilde{\beta}_t=\frac{1-\bar{\alpha}_{t-1}}{1-\bar{\alpha}_t} \beta_t. \tag{2.14}$$

For $p_\theta(x_{t-1} \mid x_t) = \mathcal{N}(x_{t-1}; \mu_\theta(x_t, t), \Sigma_\theta(x_t, t))$, the original DDPM work [10] suggests setting $\Sigma_\theta(x_t, t) = \sigma_t^2\mathbf{I}$ to untrained time-dependent constants. They find that both extremes of $\sigma_t^2 = \beta_t$ and $\sigma_t^2 = \tilde{\beta}_t = \frac{1-\bar{\alpha}_{t-1}}{1-\bar{\alpha}_t}\beta_t$ performed similarly. Now with $p_\theta(x_{t-1} \mid x_t) = \mathcal{N}(x_{t-1}; \mu_\theta(x_t, t), \sigma_t^2\mathbf{I})$, the loss terms can be calculated in a Rao-Blackwellized fashion with closed-form expressions as follows,

$$L_{t-1}=\mathbb{E}_q\left[\frac{1}{2 \sigma_t^2}\left\|\tilde{\mu}_t\left(x_t, x_0\right)-\mu_\theta\left(x_t, t\right)\right\|^2\right]+C, \tag{2.15}$$

where C includes the constant terms independent of θ. There are multiple other ways to parameterize $\mu_\theta(x_t, t)$. For instance, the network could also predict the noise ϵ added to x_0, and this noise could be used to predict x_0 via

$$x_0 = \frac{1}{\sqrt{\alpha_t}} \left(x_t - \frac{\beta_t}{\sqrt{1-\bar{\alpha}_t}} \epsilon \right). \tag{2.16}$$

Ho et al. [10] found that predicting ϵ works best with the following simplified loss function,

$$L_{t-1} = \mathbb{E}_{x_0,\epsilon} \left[\frac{\beta_t^2}{2\sigma_t^2 \alpha_t (1-\bar{\alpha}_t)} \left\| \epsilon - \epsilon_\theta \left(\sqrt{\bar{\alpha}_t} x_0 + \sqrt{1-\bar{\alpha}_t} \epsilon, t \right) \right\|^2 \right]. \tag{2.17}$$

The network is trained using stochastic gradient descent, where each training step involves adding noise to a data sample and then predicting the noise to minimize the objective function. The amount of noise added can be determined by uniformly sampling t for each image in each minibatch. Overall, the reverse process mean function approximator, μ_θ, can be used to predict $\tilde{\mu}_t$, or, it can be reparameterized to instead predict ϵ. Ho et al. [10] report that the ϵ-prediction parameterization not only resembles Langevin dynamics but also simplifies the diffusion model's variational bound to an objective akin to denoising score matching [20]. Therefore, efficient training can be achieved by optimizing random terms of L using stochastic gradient descent.

2.2.4 Generating Samples

Sampling from a diffusion model involves simulating the reverse denoising process to systematically transform noise into data through a sequence of learned probabilistic steps. This process begins with an initial sample drawn from a standard Gaussian distribution which serves as the prior. Specifically, the process starts by initializing a noise vector $x_T \sim \mathcal{N}(0, \mathbf{I})$, where T represents the total number of diffusion steps. The idea of the reverse diffusion process is to iteratively apply the reverse transition model to progressively denoise the sample. At each time step t, from T down to 1, the model computes x_{t-1} using the following Gaussian distribution:

$$x_{t-1} \sim p_\theta(x_{t-1} \mid x_t) = \mathcal{N}(x_{t-1}; \mu_\theta(x_t, t), \Sigma_\theta(x_t, t)). \tag{2.18}$$

Here, $\mu_\theta(x_t, t)$ and $\Sigma_\theta(x_t, t)$ are the mean and variance predicted by a neural network parameterized by θ. As described above, typically, the neural network predicts the mean, while the variance can either be fixed or predicted by the network as well. Alternatively, when using the ϵ-based parameterization involves predicting the noise added at each step, instead of predicting the mean directly. This approach can be formalized as:

$$\mu_\theta (x_t, t) = \frac{1}{\sqrt{\alpha_t}} \left(x_t - \frac{\beta_t}{\sqrt{1 - \bar{\alpha}_t}} \epsilon_\theta (x_t, t) \right). \tag{2.19}$$

The iterative denoising process involves repeating the sampling step for each time step, gradually refining x_t until x_0 is obtained. This stepwise process effectively removes the noise added during the forward diffusion, reconstructing a sample from the data distribution. By the end of the iterations, the final output, x_0, represents a sample from the learned data distribution. Due to the stochastic nature of each reverse transition, each run of this process can generate a unique data sample.

In summary, the diffusion model uses the learned reverse transitions to convert initial noise into high-quality data samples, effectively reversing the forward diffusion process. This ensures that the generated samples are consistent with the original data distribution, showcasing the model's ability to produce realistic and diverse outputs.

2.2.5 Conditional Sampling from Diffusion Models Using Guidance

Diffusion models can be used to generate samples conditioned on desired information such as class labels, text descriptions, or other attributes. This is achieved by incorporating a mechanism known as guidance in the sampling process. Guidance-based sampling in diffusion models is a technique designed to enhance the fidelity and controllability of the generated samples by incorporating additional information or constraints into the sampling process. This approach modifies the reverse diffusion process to include guidance from an auxiliary model or a predefined condition, which can steer the generative model towards more desirable outputs. One common implementation of guidance-based sampling involves using a classifier to guide the diffusion model, where the gradients from the classifier are combined with the reverse diffusion steps to bias the sample generation towards specific classes or features. Another approach, known as classifier-free guidance, directly conditions the diffusion model on the desired attributes, enabling the generation of samples that adhere to specified conditions without requiring an explicit classifier. By integrating these guidance mechanisms, diffusion models can produce higher quality, more targeted samples, thereby expanding their applicability in tasks requiring controlled generation such as conditional image synthesis, text-to-image generation, and other domains where adherence to specific criteria is crucial. Following sections describe both these mechanisms in further detail.

2.2.5.1 Classifier Guidance

Classifier guidance [4] is a mechanism used in diffusion probabilistic models to perform conditional generation by incorporating gradients from a pretrained classifier into the sampling process. This method involves using a separate classifier to guide the diffusion model towards generating samples that satisfy specific conditions, such as class labels. The primary objective of classifier guidance is to bias the reverse diffusion process such that the generated samples adhere to a desired condition. This is achieved by using the gradient of an independently trained classifier's output with respect to the input data, effectively steering the generation towards higher probability regions of the conditioned distribution.

Training For classifier guidance, the training phase of the diffusion model remains unchanged. The model is trained to learn the reverse denoising processes without any conditioning. The forward process progressively adds noise to the data, while the reverse process learns to denoise, reconstructing the original data distribution as described above. Critically, a separate classifier $p_\phi(y \mid x_t)$, with parameters ϕ, is trained to predict the condition y (e.g., a class label) given a noisy sample x_t from the diffusion process. Note that this classifier needs to be trained on noisy data generated by the forward diffusion process at various time steps t in order to provide meaningful guidance.

Sampling During the sampling phase, classifier guidance modifies the standard reverse diffusion process to incorporate guidance signal from the classifier using its gradients. Specifically, the sampling process begins with initializing an initial noise vector $x_T \sim \mathcal{N}(0, \mathbf{I})$. Then for each time step t from T down to 1, the reverse transition is adjusted from the one highlighted in Eq. 2.18 using the gradient of the classifier's log-probability with respect to x_t, resulting in

$$x_{t-1} \sim p_{\theta\phi}(x_{t-1} \mid x_t, y), \tag{2.20}$$

where,

$$p_{\theta\phi}(x_{t-1} \mid x_t, y) = \mathcal{N}(x_{t-1}; \mu_\theta(x_t, t) + \alpha \nabla_{x_t} \log p_\phi(y \mid x_t), \Sigma_\theta(x_t, t)). \tag{2.21}$$

Here, α is a scaling factor that determines the strength of the guidance, $\mu_\theta(x_t, t)$ and $\Sigma_\theta(x_t, t)$ are the mean and variance predicted by the diffusion model, and $\nabla_{x_t} \log p_\phi(y|x_t)$ is the gradient provided by the classifier.

Overall, the classifier p_ϕ predicts the probability of the condition y given the current noisy sample x_t. Hence, the gradient $\nabla_{x_t} \log p_\phi(y|x_t)$ indicates the direction in which the sample x_t should be adjusted to increase the probability of the desired condition y. This computed gradient is scaled by a hyper-parameter α and added to the predicted mean $\mu_\theta(x_t, t)$ of the reverse transition. This adjustment effectively biases the sample generation process towards samples that the classifier deems more likely to belong to the desired condition y.

Conclusion Classifier guidance enables the generation of high-quality conditional samples without needing to retrain the entire diffusion model with the conditions. However, there are some considerations. The scaling factor α must be carefully tuned. If α is too high, the guidance may overly distort the samples, leading to poor quality. If too low, the guidance may be insufficient to influence the sampling effectively. Additionally, the effectiveness of this method depends on the robustness of the classifier. The classifier must accurately predict conditions from noisy data at various time steps. Finally, computing the gradients for each time step adds computational overhead, making the sampling process more resource-intensive.

2.2.5.2 Classifier-Free Guidance

Classifier-free guidance [9] is a technique used to generate conditional samples without relying on an explicit classifier to provide gradients. Instead, the model itself is trained to handle both conditional and unconditional sampling, allowing for a more integrated and flexible approach to conditional generation. This method involves training the model with and without conditioning, allowing it to take advantage of both types of information during sampling.

Training For classifier-free guidance, during the training phase, the diffusion model is trained on both conditioned and unconditioned data. Specifically, the model learns to predict the reverse diffusion steps for samples with and without a given condition. This dual training approach involves augmenting the dataset with conditions (e.g., class labels or other attributes) and also training on the same data without these conditions to allow the model to generalize effectively. Formally, this involves training the model with two formulations both $p_\theta(x_{t-1} \mid x_t, y)$ and $p_\theta(x_{t-1} \mid x_t)$ where y is the condition. The model is trained to minimize the loss for both conditioned and unconditioned predictions, thereby learning to handle both scenarios. Practically, this is done by randomly dropping the condition during training for a certain percentage (e.g., $\sim 10\%$) of optimization iterations.

Sampling During sampling, classifier-free guidance combines the predictions from the conditional and unconditional models to guide the generation process. The key idea is to leverage the unconditioned model to adjust the conditioned generation, ensuring that the samples adhere to the desired attributes while maintaining high quality. After starting with an initial noise vector $x_T \sim \mathcal{N}(0, \mathbf{I})$, for each time step t from T down to 1, compute the reverse transition for both the conditioned and unconditioned models,

$$x_{t-1}^{(cond)} \sim p_\theta(x_{t-1} \mid x_t, y), \tag{2.22}$$

$$x_{t-1}^{(uncond)} \sim p_\theta(x_{t-1} \mid x_t). \tag{2.23}$$

These transitions are then combined using a guidance scale factor w to control the influence of the condition as,

$$x_{t-1} \sim x_{t-1}^{(cond)} + w\left(x_{t-1}^{(cond)} - x_{t-1}^{(uncond)}\right), \tag{2.24}$$

where w adjusts the strength of the guidance, effectively interpolating between the conditioned and unconditioned predictions.

Conclusion The combination of the conditioned and unconditioned predictions allows the model to generate samples that adhere to the desired conditions while leveraging the unconditioned model's ability to produce high-quality samples. By adjusting the guidance scale w, the generation process can be fine-tuned to balance adherence to the condition with overall sample quality. Classifier-free guidance offers several advantages over classifier-based methods. By integrating the condition directly into the model, it eliminates the need for a separate classifier, simplifying the overall architecture and reducing the potential for mismatches between the classifier and the diffusion model. Additionally, this method provides more flexibility in handling various types of conditions, including those that may be difficult to encode with a classifier. However, careful tuning of the guidance scale w is essential to achieve the desired balance between conditional fidelity and sample quality. If w is too high, the generated samples may become distorted; if too low, the samples may not adequately reflect the desired conditions.

2.3 DDPMs For Histopathological Image Generation

This section will demonstrate the use of DDPMs for conditional histopathological image generation. Histopathological images require intricate details and accurate representation of tissue structures. Traditional methods for generating synthetic images often fall short in capturing the complex textures and patterns characteristic of histopathological samples. The step-by-step denoising in a DDPM allows it to generate highly realistic synthetic histopathological images from pure noise. When trained on large datasets, DDPMs generate new images that are virtually indistinguishable from real samples. The conditional sampling capabilities of DDPMs allow for the generation of images with specific attributes, such as a nuclei semantic mask. In this section, a conditional DDPM is described that leverages the detailed spatial information encoded in a nuclei segmentation mask, which outlines the positions and shapes of cell nuclei within a tissue sample. By inputting this mask as a condition, a diffusion model can learn to synthesize the surrounding histological context, filling in the cytoplasm, extracellular matrix, and other tissue components with realistic textures and colors that align with the given nuclei arrangement. This method is particularly useful for augmenting datasets in computational pathology, as it allows for the generation of diverse and anatomically accurate histological images tailored to specific cellular configurations. These synthetic images can enhance the training of machine learning algorithms for tasks such as disease classification, anomaly detection, and biomarker discovery, ultimately improving the robustness and accuracy of automated diagnostic tools.

This section demonstrates a framework for generating tissue patches conditioned on semantic layouts of nuclei. Given a nuclei segmentation mask, the model aims to generate realistic synthetic patches. For this demonstration, (1) the first-of-its-kind Nuclei-Aware Semantic Diffusion Model (NASDM) [19] is described that can generate realistic tissue patches given a semantic mask comprising multiple nuclei types, (2) it is trained on the Lizard dataset [7] consisting of colon histology images, achieving state-of-the-art generation capabilities, and (3) extensive ablative, qualitative, and quantitative analyses are provided to establish the proficiency of the framework on this semantics driven tissue generation task.

2.3.1 Data Description

The Lizard dataset [7] is used to demonstrate the NASDM method. This dataset comprises histology image regions of colon tissue from six different data sources at 20× objective magnification. Full segmentation annotation for different types of nuclei—namely, epithelial cells, connective tissue cells, lymphocytes, plasma cells, neutrophils, and eosinophils accompanies the images. A generative model trained on this dataset can be employed to effectively synthesize colonic tumor micro-environments. The dataset includes 238 image regions, with an average size of 1055 × 934 pixels. Due to substantial visual variations across images, a representative test set is constructed by randomly sampling a 7.5% area from each image and its corresponding mask to be held out for testing. The test and train image regions are further divided into smaller image patches of 128 × 128 pixels at two different objective magnifications: (1) at 20×, the images are directly split into 128 × 128 pixel patches, whereas (2) at 10×, 256 × 256 patches are generated and resized to 128 × 128 for training. To utilize the data exhaustively, patching is performed with a 50% overlap in neighboring patches. Consequently, at (1) 20×, a total of 54,735 patches are extracted for training, with 4991 patches held out, while at (2) 10× magnification, 12,409 training patches are generated, and 655 patches are held out.

2.3.2 Stain Normalization

A common issue in training models with H&E stained histopathology slides is the visual bias introduced by variations in the staining protocol and the raw materials of chemicals, leading to different colors across slides prepared at different labs [1]. To address this, several stain-normalization methods have been proposed to normalize all tissue samples to mimic the stain distribution of a given target slide. The earliest approaches to stain normalization mainly involved basic style transfer techniques. One such method, histogram specification, aimed to match the histogram statistics of the source image with those of the target image [3]. This technique is effective only when the source and target images have similar color distributions. Enforcing this normalization can introduce artifacts that compromise the structural integrity of the source image. Reinhard [18] further demonstrated that color transfer using histogram specification could be conducted in the decorrelated CIELAB color space, which approximates the human visual system. For H&E stained histology images, the appropriate color space should accurately represent the presence or absence of each stain in each pixel. Researchers developed advanced stain normalization methods that surpass the performance of the histogram specification technique by utilizing stain separation. These methods begin by converting an RGB image into Optical Density (OD), using the formula $OD = \log \frac{I_0}{I}$, where I_0 represents the maximum possible illumination intensity of the image and I is the RGB image. In the OD space, color deconvolution (CD) becomes more straightforward because the stains exhibit a linear relationship with the OD values. The CD process is typically represented as $OD = VS$, where V is the matrix of stain vectors and S is the stain density map. The stain density map preserves the cell structures of the source image, while the stain vectors are adjusted to match the stain colors of the target image. One such method, the structure-preserving color normalization scheme introduced by Vahadane et al. [21] is used for its effectiveness and simplicity in this demonstration, to transform all slides to match the stain distribution of an empirically chosen slide from the training dataset.

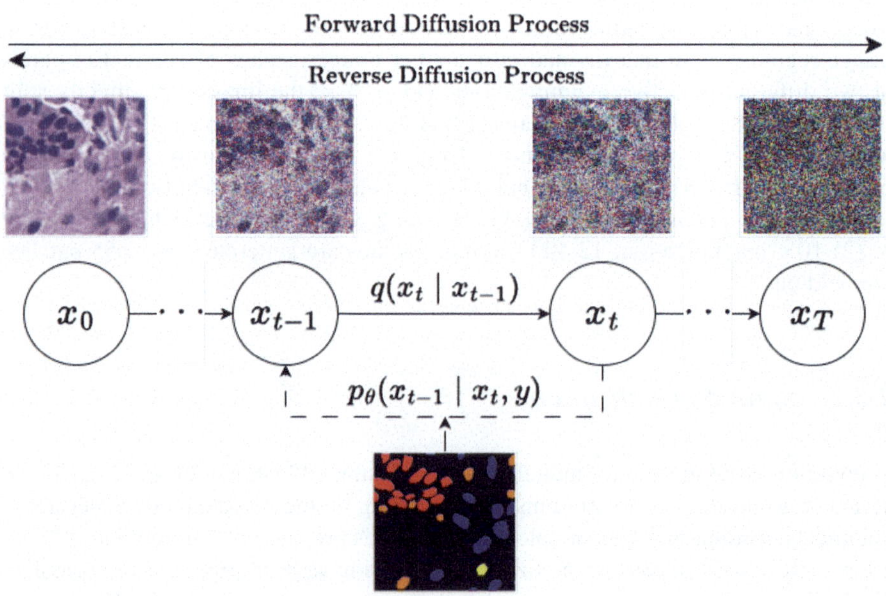

Fig. 2.1 Graphical model of the described conditional diffusion model

2.3.3 Nuclei-Aware Semantic Diffusion Model

The formulation of NASDM derives from conditional diffusion models. A conditional diffusion model aims to maximize the likelihood $p_\theta(x_0 \mid y)$, where data x_0 are sampled from the conditional data distribution, $x_0 \sim q(x_0 \mid y)$, and y represents the conditioning signal. As discussed above, a diffusion model consists of two intrinsic processes. The forward diffusion process that systematically destroys the information in a given sample and the reverse diffusion process which incrementally adds information by denoising a corrupted sample. When formulating a conditional diffusion model, the forward diffusion process can ignore the conditioning signal and Gaussian noise can be incrementally added to corrupt the data sample x_0 using the same description in Sect. 2.2.1. However, the denoising process is designed to incorporate the conditioning signal and is defined as a Markov chain with learned Gaussian transitions starting from pure noise, $p(x_T) \sim \mathcal{N}(0, \mathbf{I})$ and is parameterized as a neural network with parameters θ as

$$p_\theta(x_{0:T} \mid y) = p(x_T) \prod_{t=1}^{T} p_\theta(x_{t-1} \mid x_t, y). \tag{2.25}$$

Hence, for each denoising step from t to $t-1$,

$$p_\theta(x_{t-1} \mid x_t, y) = \mathcal{N}(x_{t-1}; \mu_\theta(x_t, y, t), \Sigma_\theta(x_t, y, t)). \tag{2.26}$$

It has been shown that the combination of q and p here is a form of a variational auto-encoder [12], and hence the variational lower bound (VLB) can be described as a sum of independent terms, $L_{vlb} := L_0 + \ldots + L_{T-1} + L_T$, where each term corresponds to a noising step as described earlier in Eq. 2.8. As described in previous sections, the time step t is randomly sampled during training, and the expectation $E_{t,x_0,y,\epsilon}$ is used to estimate the loss L_{vlb} and optimize the parameters θ. The denoising neural network, as discussed, can be parameterized in various ways. In NASDM, a noise prediction-based formulation results in superior image quality. Consequently, the NASDM denoising model is trained to predict the noise added to the input image given the semantic layout y and the time step t using the loss described below:

$$L_{\text{simple}} = E_{t,x,\epsilon}\left[\|\epsilon - \epsilon_\theta(x_t, y, t)\|_2\right]. \tag{2.27}$$

It is important to note that the given simplified loss function does not provide a training signal for $\Sigma_\theta(x_t, y, t)$. To address this, following the improved DDPMs strategy [16], a network is trained to predict an interpolation coefficient v for each dimension. This coefficient is then converted into variances,

$$\Sigma_\theta(x_t, y, t) = \exp\left(v \log \beta_t + (1 - v) \log \widetilde{\beta}_t\right). \tag{2.28}$$

This is then directly optimized using L_{vlb}, which is the KL divergence between the estimated distribution $p_\theta(x_{t-1} \mid x_t, y)$ and the diffusion posterior $q(x_{t-1} \mid x_t, x_0)$, formulated as,

$$L_{vlb} = D_{KL}(p_\theta(x_{t-1} \mid x_t, y) \parallel q(x_{t-1} \mid x_t, x_0)) \tag{2.29}$$

During this optimization, a stop gradient is applied to $\epsilon(x_t, y, t)$, allowing overall L_{vlb} to guide $\Sigma_\theta(x_t, y, t)$, while L_{simple} in Eq. 2.27 primarily guides $\epsilon(x_t, y, t)$. The overall loss is then a weighted sum of these two objectives, as follows:

$$L_{\text{hybrid}} = L_{\text{simple}} + \lambda L_{\text{vlb}}. \tag{2.30}$$

2.3.4 *Conditioning on a Semantic Mask*

NASDM requires our neural network noise predictor $\epsilon_\theta(x_t, y, t)$ to effectively process the information from the nuclei semantic map. For this purpose, we leverage a modified U-Net architecture described in Wang et al. [22], where the time step is injected into the encoder of the denoising network via scaling and shifting features, while the semantic information is injected into the decoder using multi-layer, spatially-adaptive normalization operators.

Encoder The encoder of the network processes the noisy image with stacked semantic diffusion encoder resblocks and attention blocks. These resblocks consists of convolution, SiLU and group normalization. Where SiLU [17] is a non-linearity of the form $f(x) = x \cdot \text{sigmoid}(x)$ which tends to work better than ReLU [15] on deeper models. In order to inject the time step t at different time steps, the resblock involves scaling and shifting the intermediate activation with learnable weight $w(t) \in \mathbb{R}$ and bias $b(t) \in \mathbb{R}$ formulated as, $f_{i+1} = w(t) \cdot f_i + b(t)$ where $f_i, f_{i+1} \in \mathbb{R}$ are the input and output features.

Decoder The semantic label map is injected into the decoder of the denoising network by the semantic diffusion decoder resblock in multi-layer spatially adaptive manner. Different from the resblocks in the encoder, here the spatially-adaptive normalization is used instead of the group normalization. This normalization layer injects the semantic label map into the denoising streams by regulating the feature in a spatially-adaptive, learnable transformation, which is formulated as follows,

$$f^{i+1} = \gamma^i(x) \cdot \text{Norm}\left(f^i\right) + \beta^i(x), \tag{2.31}$$

where f^i and f^{i+1} are the input and output features and $\text{Norm}(\cdot)$ refers to the parameter-free group normalization. $\gamma^i(x)$, $\beta^i(x)$ are the spatially-adaptive weight and bias learned from the semantic layout, respectively.

In the NASDM model, the conditioning signal is constructed using the semantic mask such that each channel of the signal corresponds to a unique nuclei type. In addition, a mask comprising of the edges of all nuclei to further demarcate nuclei instances is also concatenated to the signal.

2.3.5 *Experimental Results*

In this section, the specifics of the NASDM implementation and training process are described first. Subsequently, an ablative study over the objective magnification and the scale of classifier-guidance is conducted, serving to affirm the robustness of the model. The prowess of our model, specifically designed for generating nuclei-aware semantic histopathology patches, is then illustrated through both qualitative and quantitative evaluations. All subsequent experiments involve the generation of images using the semantic masks belonging to a subset of the dataset that is set aside at two different objective magnifications. The calculation and comparision of metrics such as Fréchet Inception Distance (FID) and Inception Score (IS) between the synthesized and actual images within the isolated group is then carried out.

2.3.5.1 Implementation Details

The NASDM model is implemented using a UNet architecture with conditional resblocks (Sect. 2.3.4) and trained using the objective in Eq. (2.30). Following previous works [16], the trade-off parameter λ is set as 0.001. The AdamW optimizer is used to train the model. Following DDPM [10], the total number of diffusion steps is set to 1000, and linear noising schedule with respect to time step t for the forward process is used. After normal training with a learning rate of $1e-4$, the learning rate is decayed to $2e-5$ to further finetune the model with a drop rate of 0.2 to enhance the classifier-free guidance capability during sampling. The whole framework is implemented using Pytorch and trained on 4 NVIDIA Tesla A100 GPUs with a batch-size of 40 per GPU. Code is available at https://github.com/4m4n5/NASDM.

2.3.5.2 Quantitative Analysis

NASDM is the only model that possesses the capability to synthesize histology images given a semantic mask, which presents a challenge for direct quantitative comparison with other methods. Nevertheless, the standard generative metric, Fréchet Inception Distance (FID), which measures the divergence between the distributions of synthetic and real images within the latent space of the Inception-V3 [13] model. Smaller FID score denotes the model's ability to create images highly similar to the actual data. Consequently, a comparison of FID and IS metrics

Table 2.1 Quantitative assessment: the performance of the NASDM method is demonstrated using Fréchet Inception Distance (FID) and Inception Score (IS) against the metrics reported in existing works. (–) denotes that corresponding information was not reported in original work. *Note that performance reported for best competing method on the colon data is from a custom implementation, performances for both this and NASDM should improve with better tuning

Method	Tissue type	Conditioning	FID($\downarrow$)	IS($\uparrow$)
BigGAN [2]	Bladder	None	158.4	–
AttributeGAN [24]	Bladder	Attributes	53.6	–
ProGAN [11]	Glioma	Morphology	53.8	1.7
Morph-Diffusion [14]	Glioma	Morphology	20.1	2.1
Morph-Diffusion* [14]	Colon	Morphology	18.8	2.2
NASDM (Ours)	Colon	Semantic mask	14.1	2.7

is made against the values cited in original works [14, 24] (refer to Table 2.1), maintaining their respective conditions. It can be observed that the NASDM approach surpasses all previous methods, which encompass both GANs-based techniques and the recently introduced morphology-centered generative diffusion model.

2.3.5.3 Qualitative Analysis

A review of the model-generated patches was conducted by 3 expert pathologists. For this review, a total of 30 patches are utilized, comprising 17 synthetic and 13 real ones. The assessment of the overall medical quality of the patches and their consistency with the associated nuclei masks on a Likert scale is carried out by two experts. A public Google survey, which was employed for the review, can be accessed via the provided link[1] From this survey (Fig. 2.3), it can be inferred that the model-generated patches are deemed more realistic than the patches in our real set. A qualitative discussion is now undertaken regarding our model's ability to generate realistic visual patterns in synthetic histopathology images (refer to Fig. 2.2). Evidence shows that the model can successfully reproduce convincing visual structure for each type of nuclei. In the synthetic images, it is observed that lymphocytes are accurately circular, while neutrophils and eosinophils exhibit a more lobed structure. Additionally, the model's ability to emulate accurate nucleus-to-cytoplasm ratios for each type of nuclei is noted. Epithelial cells, which are less dense, possess a distinct chromatin structure, and are larger compared to other white blood cells, are the most challenging to generate convincingly. However, it is observed that the model can well capture these complexities and accurately replicate chromatin distributions.

[1] https://forms.gle/1dLAdk9XKhp6FWMY6.

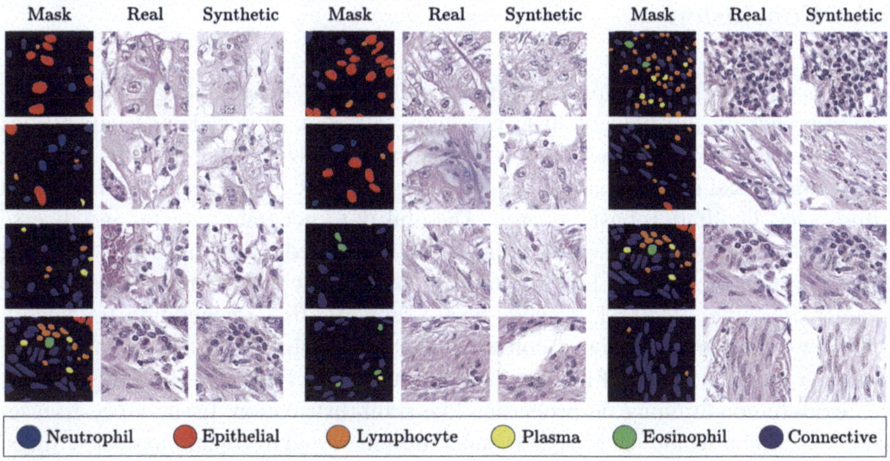

Fig. 2.2 Qualitative results: the generated synthetic images are shown with the semantic masks with each type of nuclei in different environments to demonstrate the proficiency of the model to generate realistic nuclei arrangements. Legend at bottom denotes the mask color for each type of nuclei

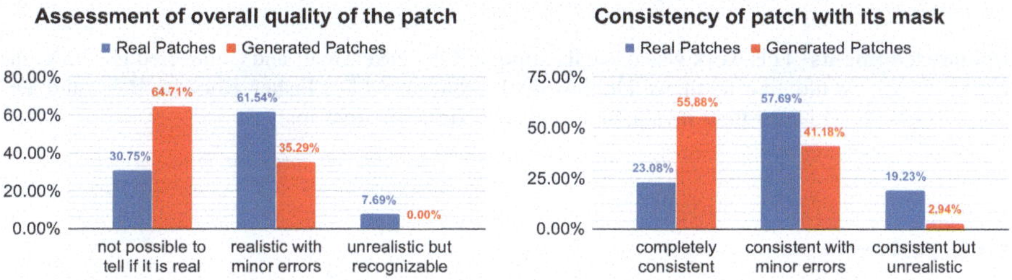

Fig. 2.3 Qualitative review: compiled results from a pathologist review. Experts assess patches for, their overall medical quality (left), as well as, their consistency with the associated mask (right). It can be observed that the patches generated by the model do better on all metrics and majority are imperceptible from real patches

Obj. Mag.	**FID($\downarrow$)**	**IS($\uparrow$)**
10×	38.1	2.3
20×	**20.7**	**2.5**

2.3.5.4 Ablation Over Objective Magnification

As outlined in Sect. 2.3.1, patches are produced at two distinct objective magnifications: 10× and 20×. This section describes the generative capabilities of the models individually trained at these magnification levels. It is discernible from Table on the right that superior generative metrics are yielded by the model trained at an objective magnification of 20×. It should be noted that training is confined to a subset at 20× magnification in order to maintain a consistent volume of training data when compared to the training set at magnification 10×.

2.4 Conclusion

This chapter explored diffusion models which have emerged as a transformative approach in the field of histopathology, offering unprecedented capabilities in controllable image generation. These models provide high-quality synthetic histopathological images that can enhance diagnostic accuracy, support educational efforts, and facilitate robust research. The ability to generate realistic and diverse pathological images addresses the limitations of limited data availability, enabling better training of machine learning models and more comprehensive studies. The chapter presented NASDM, a nuclei-aware semantic tissue generation framework which was demonstrated on a colon dataset and qualitatively and quantitatively establish the proficiency of the framework at this task. Future work in this domain can explore conditioning on properties like stain-distribution, tissue-type, disease-type, etc. which would enable patch generation in varied histopathological settings. As the field progresses, the integration of diffusion models into histopathological workflows holds promise for improving patient outcomes, streamlining pathology processes, and advancing our understanding of various diseases. The continued refinement and adoption of these models will undoubtedly play a crucial role in the future of digital pathology.

Acknowledgments This work was partially supported by NSF Smart and Connected Health grant 2205417. We would like to thank Dr. Shyam Raghavan, M.D., Fisher Rhoads, B.S., and Dr. Lubaina Ehsan, M.D. for their invaluable inputs for our qualitative analysis.

References

1. Bejnordi BE, Timofeeva N, Otte-Höller I, Karssemeijer N, van der Laak JA (2014) Quantitative analysis of stain variability in histology slides and an algorithm for standardization. Med Imag 9041:45–51
2. Brock A, Donahue J, Simonyan K (2018) Large scale gan training for high fidelity natural image synthesis. arXiv preprint 1809.11096
3. Coltuc D, Bolon P, Chassery JM (2006) Exact histogram specification. IEEE Trans Image Process 15(5):1143–1152
4. Dhariwal P, Nichol A (2021) Diffusion models beat gans on image synthesis. Adv Neural Inf Process Syst 34:8780–8794
5. Fajardo VA, Findlay D, Jaiswal C, Yin X, Houmanfar R, Xie H, Emerson DB, et al (2021) On oversampling imbalanced data with deep conditional generative models. Exp Syst Appl 169:114463
6. Goodfellow I, Pouget-Abadie J, Mirza M, Xu B, Warde-Farley D, Ozair S, Bengio Y, et al (2020) Generative adversarial networks. Commun ACM 63(11):139–144
7. Graham S, Jahanifar M, Azam A, Nimir M, Tsang YW, Dodd K, Rajpoot NM, et al (2021) Lizard: a large-scale dataset for colonic nuclear instance segmentation and classification. In: Proceedings of the IEEE/CVF International Conference on Computer Vision, pp 684–693
8. Hall M, van der Maaten L, Gustafson L, Jones M, Adcock A (2022) A systematic study of bias amplification. arXiv preprint 2201.11706
9. Ho J, Salimans T (2022) Classifier-free diffusion guidance. arXiv preprint 2207.12598

10. Ho J, Jain A, Abbeel P (2020) Denoising diffusion probabilistic models. Adv Neural Inf Process Syst 33:6840–6851
11. Karras T, Aila T, Laine S, Lehtinen J (2017) Progressive growing of gans for improved quality, stability, and variation. arXiv preprint 1710.10196
12. Kingma DP, Welling M (2013) Auto-encoding variational bayes, arXiv preprint 1312.6114
13. Kynkäänniemi T, Karras T, Aittala M, Aila T, Lehtinen J (2022) The role of imagenet classes in fréchet inception distance. arXiv preprint 2203.06026
14. Moghadam PA, Van Dalen S, Martin KC, Lennerz J, Yip S, Farahani H, Bashashati A (2023) A morphology focused diffusion probabilistic model for synthesis of histopathology images. In: Proceedings of the IEEE/CVF winter conference on applications of computer vision, pp 2000–2009
15. Nair V, Hinton GE (2010) Rectified linear units improve restricted Boltzmann machines. In: Proceedings of the 27th international conference on machine learning (ICML-10), pp 807–814
16. Nichol AQ, Dhariwal P (2021) Improved denoising diffusion probabilistic models. In: International conference on machine learning. Proceedings of machine learning research, pp 8162–8171
17. Ramachandran P, Zoph B, Le QV (2017) Searching for activation functions. arXiv preprint 1710.05941
18. Reinhard E, Adhikhmin M, Gooch B, Shirley P (2001) Color transfer between images. IEEE Comput Graph Appl 21(5):34–41
19. Shrivastava A, Fletcher PT (2023) NASDM: nuclei-aware semantic histopathology image generation using diffusion models. In: International conference on medical image computing and computer-assisted intervention. Springer, Cham, pp 786–796
20. Song Y, Sohl-Dickstein J, Kingma DP, Kumar A, Ermon S, Poole B (2020) Score-based generative modeling through stochastic differential equations. arXiv preprint 2011.13456
21. Vahadane A, Peng T, Sethi A, Albarqouni S, Wang L, Baust M, Navab N, et al (2016) Structure-preserving color normalization and sparse stain separation for histological images. IEEE Trans Med Imag 35(8):1962–1971
22. Wang W, Bao J, Zhou W, Chen D, Chen D, Yuan L, Li H (2022) Semantic image synthesis via diffusion models. arXiv preprint 2207.00050
23. Xie L, Qi J, Pan L, Wali S (2020) Integrating deep convolutional neural networks with marker-controlled watershed for overlapping nuclei segmentation in histopathology images. Neurocomputing 376:166–179
24. Ye J, Xue Y, Liu P, Zaino R, Cheng KC, Huang X (2021) A multi-attribute controllable generative model for histopathology image synthesis. In: Medical image computing and computer assisted intervention–MICCAI 2021: 24th international conference, Strasbourg, September 27–October 1, 2021, Proceedings, Part VIII 24. Springer, Berlin, pp 613–623

Chapter 3
Generative AI Techniques for Ultrasound Image Reconstruction

Zixia Zhou, Wei Guo, Yi Guo, and Yuanyuan Wang

Abstract In recent years, ultrasound imaging equipment has developed in diverse ways to meet the needs of various clinical applications. However, the in-herent characteristics of ultrasound imaging, including phenomena like diffraction, attenuation, interference, and refraction, as well as issues like speckle, artifacts, and noise, adversely affect spatial resolution. This signifi-cantly impacts the accuracy of clinical diagnosis and poses an obstacle to its widespread application. To improve the quality of ultrasound imaging, traditional methods have focused mainly on hardware enhancements and reconstruction method optimization. However, hardware improvements increase manufacturing difficulty and cost, while reconstruction algorithm optimization often comes at the expense of temporal resolution. Therefore, finding more exquisite methods to break through the spatio-temporal resolution limits of ultrasound imaging, promoting the preci-sion, intelligence, miniaturization, and cost-effectiveness of medical ultra-sound equipment, and ensuring accurate diagnosis are foundational keys to advancing precision intelligent ultrasound healthcare. In this chapter, we introduced advanced deep learning techniques applied to ultrasound image reconstruction and explored the challenges and potential future trends in this evolving field.

Z. Zhou (✉)
Department of Radiation Oncology, Stanford University, Stanford, CA, USA
e-mail: zixia@stanford.edu

W. Guo
Vinno Research Institute, Suzhou City, China

Y. Guo · Y. Wang
Department of Electronic Engineering, Fudan University, Shanghai, China
e-mail: yywang@fudan.edu.cn

L. Zhang et al. (eds.), *Generative Machine Learning Models in Medical Image Computing*, https://doi.org/10.1007/978-3-031-80965-1_3

3.1 Introduction

Ultrasound imaging has been utilized in the medical field for nearly seventy years and is widely adopted for clinical diagnosis [1]. Compared to other medical imaging modalities such as MRI and CT, ultrasound imaging offers several advantages: it is non-invasive, radiation-free, real-time, and cost-effective. These features make it a important tool in clinical diagnosis and disease detection. However, ultrasound imaging has long been plagued by issues related to low image quality. Specifically, it faces challenges such as poor signal noise ratio, blurred lesion boundaries, and posterior echo interference [2]. These issues significantly impact the accuracy of clinical applications, including diagnosis and prognosis, based on ultrasound images. To achieve reliable diagnostic results, higher imaging quality is required from ultrasound devices. Recent years have seen a diversification in ultrasound imaging equipment to cater to different clinical applications, such as ultrafast imaging, 3D/4D imaging, and portable imaging devices [3–6]. However, these devices often sacrifice imaging quality to meet specific application requirements, significantly affecting their clinical usability. Therefore, research into high-quality ultrasound imaging is crucial for enhancing the diagnostic capabilities of medical ultrasound devices. Traditional methods to improve imaging quality generally fall into hardware improvements and reconstruction method optimizations. Hardware improvements typically involve replacing affordable or compact components with expensive or larger ones, increasing manufacturing difficulty and cost while reducing portability. On the other hand, beamformer and postprocessing optimizations often come at the expense of temporal resolution and may not adequately address the diverse problems for low imaging quality in ultrasound systems. With the advance of AI technology [7–9], regression-based deep learning techniques have been proposed to tackle various factors leading to low-quality imaging in ultrasound systems, potentially offering cost-effective, robust, and highly generalizable high-quality ultrasound imaging solutions.

3.2 Ultrasound Imaging System and Imaging Quality Trade-Offs

Medical ultrasound devices emit ultrasound pulses through transducers and receive echo signals reflected from tissue boundaries [10]. The strength of these echo signals is proportional to the difference in acoustic impedance between two media. If adjacent tissues have identical acoustic impedance, no echo signal is generated at their boundary. Conversely, if the tissues have similar impedance, a low-intensity echo signal is produced, while a significant difference in impedance (e.g., between soft tissue and bone) results in a very strong echo signal. In clinical, ultrasound devices utilize this characteristic to create images or videos of the inside of the body. Generally, these devices consist of several key components that are highly correlated with imaging quality as shown in Fig. 3.1.

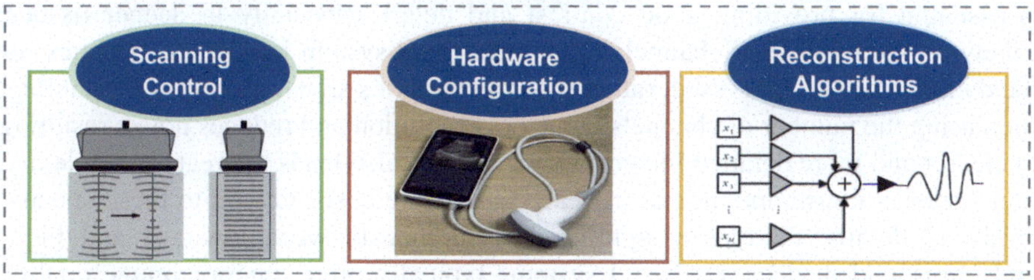

Fig. 3.1 Key components that are highly correlated with ultrasound imaging quality

3.2.1 Ultrasound Scanning Control

The frequency, pulse length, and mode of emitted ultrasound waves are critical for determining imaging resolution and penetration depth. High-frequency waves offer better resolution but limited depth, while low-frequency waves penetrate deeper with reduced resolution [11]. The shape and duration of the pulse affect axial resolution and signal-to-noise ratio (SNR); shorter pulses improve resolution but may decrease SNR, requiring optimized pulse parameters for balanced imaging performance. Additionally, the choice of transmission mode affects imaging resolution [12]. The commonly used focused line-scan emission mode provides high-quality imaging during static scans but requires multiple signal transmissions and receptions, significantly reducing temporal resolution and making it unsuitable for clinical applications requiring high frame rates (e.g., elastography and echocardiography). Thus, research has suggested using plane wave emissions for ultrafast imaging. While plane wave modes significantly increase frame rates, they suffer from poor imaging quality. Coherent plane wave compounding (CPWC), an algorithm that integrates information from multiple angles, addresses this challenge by enhancing overall imaging quality at the cost of reducing frame rate. Other emission modes include wide beam/weak focus and multi-line transmission techniques, which aim to balance between frame rate and image quality, but each comes with its own trade-offs and specific application contexts.

3.2.2 Ultrasound Hardware Configuration

The materials, process and design of the transducer significantly influence the efficiency and sensitivity of ultrasound wave emission and reception. Piezoelectric materials, for instance, are commonly used due to their effectiveness in converting electrical signals to mechanical waves and vice versa [13]. The design includes considerations for transducer shape and array configuration, impacting imaging capabilities [14]. The sensitivity of the transducer impacts the overall SNR of the imaging system. Highly sensitive transducers can detect weaker echoes, which is essential for providing good contrast and detail, especially in deeper tissues. Likewise, the number of channels in an ultrasound system impacts the richness of the data that can be processed, rather than the system's signal processing capability. Increasing the number of channels enhances resolution and reduces noise, resulting in clearer and more detailed images. However, this also leads to greater complexity, higher power consumption, and increased hardware costs. Owing to these specific hardware details, there is a significant difference between low-cost and high-end ultrasound devices. High-end systems typically offer superior image quality, more advanced features, and greater flexibility in clinical applications. Conversely, portable ultrasound devices, as a new emerging technology, have advantages such as low cost, ease of use, and quick imaging, making them promising for rural, community, and remote medical care [15]. However, these devices often compromise on image resolution and depth penetration compared to their high-end counterparts.

3.2.3 Reconstruction Algorithms

The backend algorithms used in signal processing, such as beamforming, filtering, image enhancement, and speckle suppression, play a significant role in enhancing image clarity and contrast. Among these, beamforming algorithms are in the core position, as they remap and focus the signals received from transducers to produce the fundamental image, thereby directly influencing the eventual ultrasound imaging quality [16]. The traditional yet most widely used delay-and-sum (DAS) beamformer is relatively simple and computationally efficient. However, the quality of its beamforming results is often suboptimal, with limited spatial resolution and higher side-lobe artifacts. Advanced beamforming algorithms, including adaptive and coherence beamforming, improve the focusing and steering of ultrasound beams. These algorithms contribute to better spatial resolution and reduced side-lobe artifacts [17, 18] but also require higher computational burdens for implementation.

3.2.4 Combined Impact and Other Factors

The interplay between transmission setup, hardware configuration, and reconstruction algorithms determines the overall performance of the ultrasound imaging system. Synchronizing these aspects through techniques like harmonic imaging can enhance image quality by improving contrast and reducing noise. Additionally, the ultrasound imaging quality may also be affected by operator-dependent and environmental factors. The skill and experience of the operator in positioning the transducer, adjusting settings, and interpreting images greatly affect the quality of the ultrasound images. The interaction with the patient, including their body habitus, the degree of respiratory and cardiac motion, and the ability to maintain a proper acoustic window during scanning, all influences image quality. Environmental factors such as the presence of acoustic windows can also affect imaging quality. Structures like bone or air-filled organs can block or scatter ultrasound waves, reducing image quality for structures behind these barriers. Tissue characteristics, including variations in density and composition, can affect the propagation and reflection of ultrasound waves, impacting image quality.

In conclusion, understanding and addressing the combined impact of these factors, along with considering other influential aspects, is crucial for achieving the best possible imaging performance in clinical practice.

3.3 Integrating Deep Learning for Enhanced Ultrasound Reconstruction

Given that deep learning has demonstrated its applicability across various fields in recent years, it has also emerged as a powerful tool for enhancing ultrasound image reconstruction and improving diagnostic accuracy with minimal trade-offs. Various deep learning-based methods have been proposed, focusing on different modules of the ultrasound system. These techniques aim to address the limitations of ultrasound imaging, offering solutions that enhance image quality while retaining the inherent benefits of ultrasound technology, such as real-time imaging, portability, and cost-effectiveness. In this section, we will explore existing works that utilize deep learning techniques to address the trade-offs in ultrasound imaging.

3.3.1 Quality Enhancement via Ultrasound Scanning Control

Before the advent of deep learning algorithms, ultrasound transmit control focused on meeting the specific requirements of different medical applications, developing different wave scan modes to cater to diverse diagnostic needs. However, conventional methods still suffer from trade-offs. Deep learning techniques have revolutionized this trend, allowing for significant enhancements in imaging quality without compromising the inherent benefits of ultrasound technology. By leveraging prior information, deep learning models can map quality enhancement rules while maintaining specific ultrasound wave emission settings. Traditional focused line-scan mode is the most commonly used scanning mode but requires hundreds of transmissions and receptions of sound beams, resulting in a frame rate typically less than 50 frames per second (fps). To address this limitation, ultrafast ultrasound imaging technology has emerged. Prada et al. [19] introduced plane wave ultrasound imaging to improve temporal resolution, achieving full-field imaging with a single pulse transmission by utilizing all array elements to transmit and receive simulta-

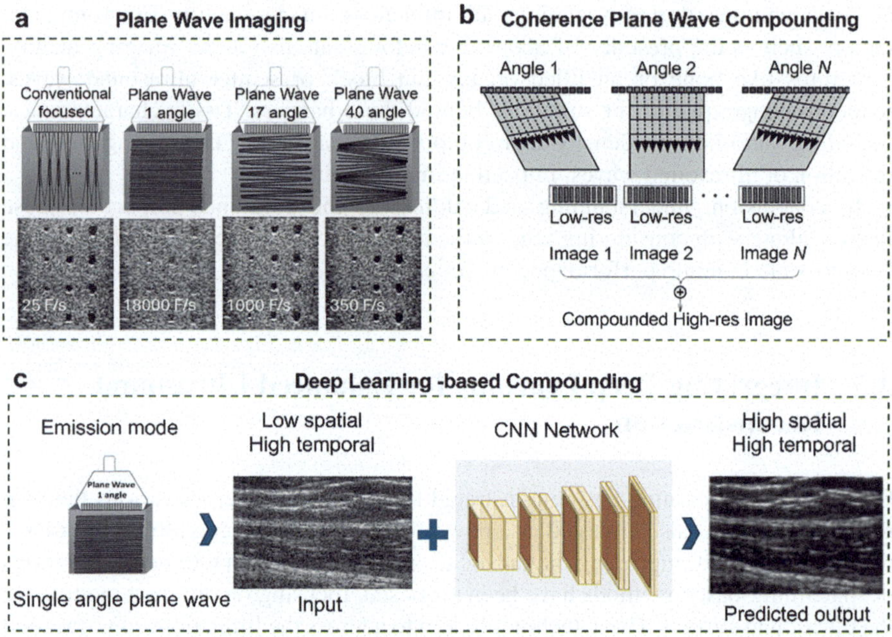

Fig. 3.2 Quality enhancement via ultrasound emission end. (**a**) Plane wave imaging: Comparison between conventional focused line scan mode, single-angle plane wave mode, and compounded plane wave mode. (**b**) Workflow of the conventional multi-angle compounding method for plane wave imaging. (**c**) An example network for deep learning-based compounding

neously. This approach can raise frame rates up to 5000 fps but suffers from high side-lobe noise, leading to poor image quality.

To enhance plane wave imaging quality, Montaldo et al. [20] proposed the CPWC method, which sequentially transmits ultrasound signals at multiple angles and integrates the received multi-frame echo signals to obtain a high-quality composite image as shown in Fig. 3.2b. Figure 3.2c compares the results of plane wave compounding with traditional focused imaging. While this method significantly improves image quality, it reduces temporal resolution, making it unsuitable for applications requiring extremely high frame rates. Deep learning methods have been proposed to overcome the limitations of plane wave imaging while maintaining high frame rates as exampled in Fig. 3.2d. For instance, Zhou et al. [21] proposed a multichannel multiscale convolutional neural network (MMCNN) to reconstruct high-quality images from single plane-wave ultrasound images. The multiscale network architecture captures both local and global features, significantly improving spatial and temporal resolution, preserving speckle information through wavelet postprocessing. In [22], Qi et al. proposed a Deep Neural Network (DNN) to convert RF channel data of plane-wave imaging to those of focused ultrasound scanning, maintaining high imaging quality and frame rate. Another approach, proposed by Senouf et al. [23] uses an convolutional neural network (CNN) to improve cardiac ultrasound MLA image quality, achieving single-line acquisition-like decorrelation while maintaining multi-line acquisition's high frame rate. Chen et al. [24] introduced ApodNet for high frame rate synthetic transmit aperture (STA) ultrasound imaging, providing optimized binarized apodizations to guide plane wave transmissions.

In summary, by considering the aspect of scanning control, deep learning-based techniques can achieve high frame-rate imaging without compromising spatial resolution.

3.3.2 Quality Enhancement for Hardware Complement

In the realm of ultrasound equipment, hardware configuration significantly impacts imaging quality, especially when it comes to cost-effective and portable solutions. Portable ultrasound devices offer several unique advantages, including being user-friendly, rapid, cost-effective, and lightweight. These attributes make portable ultrasound devices an excellent choice in specific scenarios compared to large-scale ultrasound equipment. For instance, in community healthcare, portable ultrasound devices can serve as valuable tools for pre-check, sub-check and early disease screening. In developing countries or rural areas where high-end ultrasound equipment is prohibitively expensive, affordable portable devices present a viable alternative. In telemedicine, these devices facilitate convenient home health management, while in emergency rescue and intensive care situations, they enable quick preliminary diagnoses of critical patients. Despite their extended applications, portable ultrasound devices are limited by their compact size and specs, resulting in lower imaging resolution and higher noise artifacts compared to high-end equipment, as illustrated in Fig. 3.3a. This weakness in imaging quality significantly diminishes the diagnostic reliability of portable devices, emphasizing the need to enhance imaging quality in clinical settings.

Deep learning methods have emerged as a powerful solution to this challenge, offering the potential to improve ultrasound imaging quality without compromising portability or increasing costs. Specifically, Zhou et al. [25] proposed a two-stage generative adversarial network (GAN) together with transfer learning to enhance the image quality of hand-held ultrasound devices, improving tissue structure and detail while minimizing artifacts and deformation impacts. With a similar goal, Dong et al. [26] introduced a feature-guided denoising convolutional neural network for portable ultrasound images improvement, utilizing a hierarchical denoising framework with a feature masking layer and an explainable feature extraction algorithm to remove noise while preserving critical features. Wang et al. [27] also proposed a sparse skip connection U-Net, combining encoder-decoder and U-Net models with a novel loss function to enhance portable ultrasound image quality by preserving more details and improving spatial resolution. Further, researchers have extended these advancements from static images to video, as video can provide more comprehensive information about lesion details under dynamic physiological

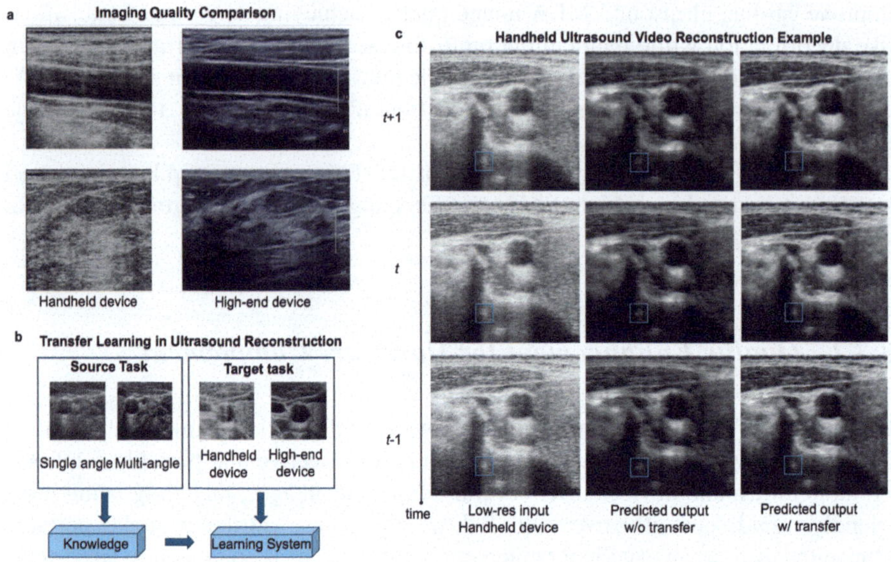

Fig. 3.3 Quality enhancement for hardware complement. (**a**) Comparison between ultrasound images generated handheld device and high-end device. (**b**) Overview of the transfer learning concept in Zhou et al. [25]. (**c**) An example of handheld ultrasound video reconstruction predicted by Zhou et al. [25]

processes. To achieve this goal, Zhou et al. [28] proposed a multi-pathway GAN to reconstruct high-quality video from handheld ultrasound devices, effectively addressing the challenges of low resolution and high noise. This approach combines low-rank representation with GAN-based reconstruction and incorporates adjacent neighborhood information to improve the continuity of the reconstructed video. A brief workflow and an example of the generated ultrasound video is shown in Fig 3.3b, c. With a more targeted objective, Mamistvalov et al. [29] focused on reducing the dependency on high-cost hardware by using deep learning to reconstruct images from sub-Nyquist channel data, thereby lowering overall system costs. Similarly, Xiao et al. [30] addressed the challenge of maintaining image quality after reducing the number of channels in plane-wave ultrasound. By leveraging deep learning, this method reconstructs high-quality images with fewer channels, thereby reducing computational load and data storage requirements, making it a cost-effective solution for high-quality imaging.

Briefly, low-cost imaging methods through deep learning are crucial for expanding access to high-quality ultrasound imaging in resource-limited settings.

3.3.3 Quality Enhancement with Low-Complexity Beamforming

In ultrasound systems, the beamforming module plays a crucial role in determining imaging quality. Currently, the most widely used beamforming method is the non-adaptive DAS approach, known for its low complexity and high robustness. However, DAS often comes along with high sidelobe, leading to low imaging resolution and poor contrast. In recent years, several adaptive beamforming methods have been proposed to enhance ultrasound imaging quality, such as the Coherence Factor (CF) method and the Minimum Variance (MV) method. The CF method suppresses sidelobes and clutter based on the relative proportion of noise in the array signals, but its performance is unstable and can easily oversuppress speckle and cause signal distortion. The MV method improves imaging resolution by minimizing the desired output energy of the beamformer, yet still requires better noise suppression. The Eigen-Space Minimum Variance (ESBMV) method further enhances MV contrast by projecting the weights of the MV method into the eigen-space. Despite these advancements, the high complexity of adaptive beamforming methods makes them difficult to implement on cart, underscoring the need for a low-complexity method that achieves high imaging quality. To address this, Vignon et al. [31] proposed an imaging method that uses only a subset of the transmit or receive array elements to simplify computational complexity. However, this reduction in complexity comes at the cost of imaging resolution. Asl et al. [32] suggested optimizing the computation of the spatial covariance matrix using Toeplitz matrices to reduce the runtime of the MV method. Nonetheless, since the eigen-decomposition of the covariance matrix is the most time-consuming part of the ESBMV method, this approach offers limited improvement in computational complexity.

To overcome these complexity challenges in use, deep learning regression networks have proven to be a promising solution for reducing the time required for beamforming by learning its rules. Deep learning methods generally achieve higher computational efficiency, for instance, Wiacek et al. [33] develop CohereNet, a deep learning model that estimates spatial coherence functions for ultrasound beamforming, achieving enhanced image quality and computational efficiency compared to traditional CPU and GPU implementations. Similarly, Nair et al. [34] present a deep learning approach that simultaneously generates ultrasound images and segmentation maps from raw channel data, enhancing image quality and segmentation accuracy without traditional beamforming. In [35], Luijten et al. demonstrate that deep neural networks can efficiently perform fast high-quality adaptive ultrasound beamforming, maintaining image quality with reduced data-rates and undersampled array design. Further, Khan et al. [36] explore deep learning methods for adaptive and compressive beamforming in medical ultrasound, achieving high-resolution images with low computational burden and robust performance under varying data conditions. Building on these advancements, Zhou et al. [37] introduce a multiconstrained hybrid GAN for ultrasound adaptive beamforming, achieving high-quality imaging by fusing RF-based and image-based features, enhancing spatial resolution and contrast while reducing computational complexity. Additionally, Huang et al. [38] addresses defocusing and distortion in flexible array transducers with deep learning techniques, enhancing lateral resolution and contrast in ultrasound images by learning proper time delays from RF data.

In conclusion, current deep learning-based methods demonstrate significant potential to revolutionize ultrasound beamforming, providing high-resolution, high-contrast imaging with reduced complexity and less processing time.

3.3.4 Ultrasound Domain Transfer for Higher Adaptability

Variations in ultrasound image collection and reconstruction settings can lead to discrepancies in data distribution, which hinders the effective application of pre-trained networks. Thus, research on multi-source or multi-configuration domain adaptation is essential to ensure broader applicability of these models. Generative AI models have been applied to transform within different ultrasound domains, addressing issues of dataset bias and enhancing the adaptability of diagnostic algorithms.

To address these issues, several studies have been conducted, yielding promising results. Huang et al. [39] introduced a stability-enhanced CycleGAN for normalizing ultrasound images across medical centers, reducing database bias and improving deep learning analysis by preserving details and ensuring training stability. Building on this, Huang et al. [40] also proposed M2O-DiffGAN (see Fig. 3.4), a domain transformation model addressing domain shift in ultrasound images, achieving high-fidelity image synthesis and improved generalizability across multiple clinical datasets using a cycle-consistent adversarial learning architecture. To further enhance image quality, Liu et al. [41] proposed aself-supervised CycleGAN for ultrasound image super-resolution. This approach addresses low spatial resolution without paired training data, ensures perceptual consistency, and demonstrates superior performance on benchmark datasets. Similarly, Zhou et al. [42] developed an ultrasound-transfer GAN to perform domain transfer from the plane wave domain to the more frequently used line-scan domain, significantly extending potential applications and improving frame rates. Tierney et al. [43] proposed a domain adaptation scheme using cycle-consistent GANs, leveraging simulated and unlabeled in vivo data to improve image quality consistently. For specific clinical applications, Wildeboer et al. [44] introduced synthetic shear-wave elastography (sSWE) using deep learning to generate SWE images from conventional B-mode ultrasound, achieving accurate elasticity estimates and demonstrating potential for broader clinical applications.

In summary, generative AI models offer great potential in enhancing the adaptability of ultrasound imaging algorithms across different domains.

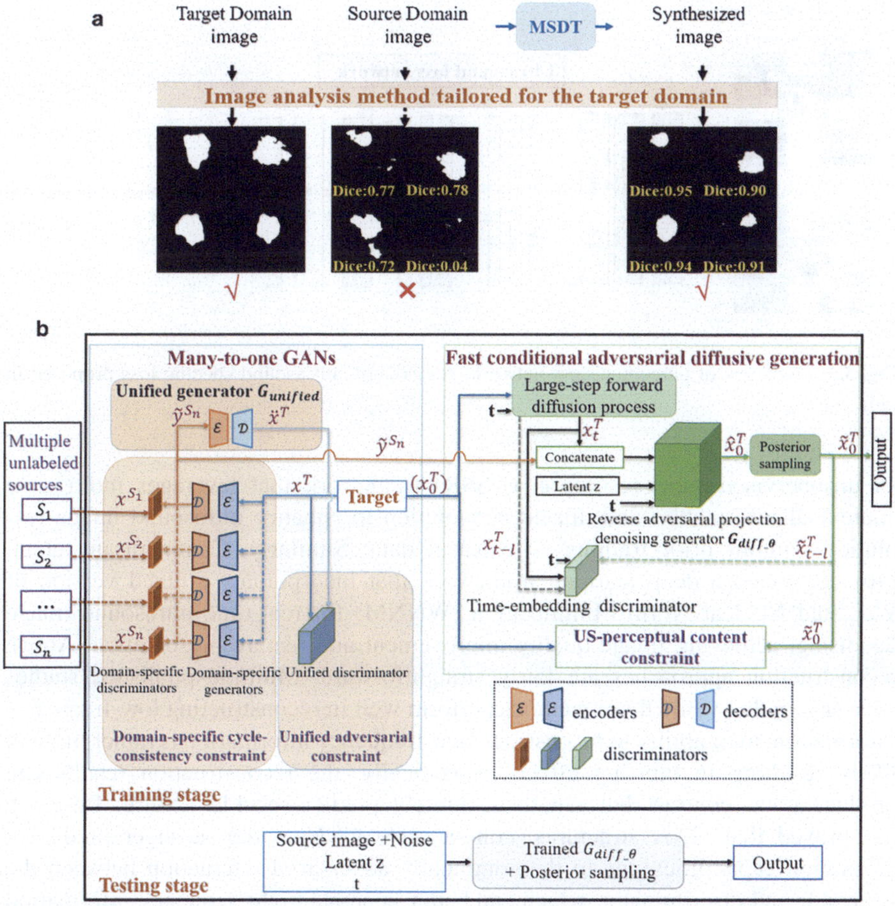

Fig. 3.4 Ultrasound domain transfer for higher adaptability. (**a**) Performance degradation of image analysis methods tailored for the target domain is caused by domain shifts; however, high performance is achieved by the synthesized images after the domain transfer method. (**b**) Overview of the M2O-DiffGAN proposed by Huang et al. [40]

3.4 Technical Summary and Analysis

Technically, deep learning-based ultrasound imaging methods can be categorized into three main classes: image-to-image, RF-to-image generation, and fusion-style techniques.

The image-to-image approach typically operates in a post-processing manner, learning an end-to-end mapping between low-quality and high-quality images or across different ultrasound imaging domains. This kind of method commonly employs U-Net based CNN networks. For instance, Lu and Liu [45] introduced

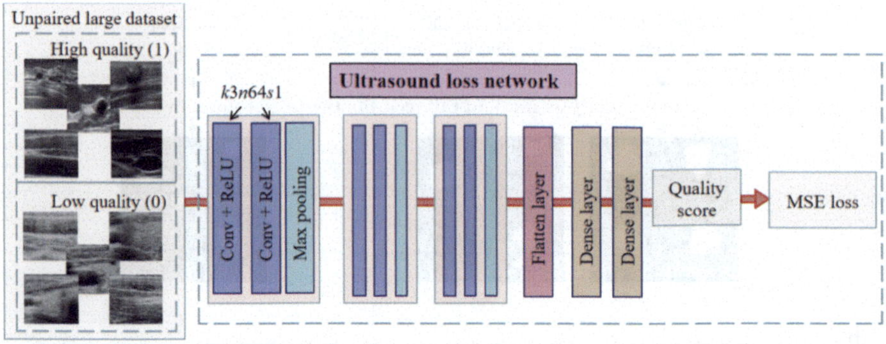

Fig. 3.5 Overview of perceptual loss network. An example ultrasound specific loss proposed in [28]

an unsupervised super-resolution (USSR) framework that leverages multi-scale contextual information and dilated convolution to enhance ultrasound image resolution without prior training or external data. Similarly, Cammarasana et al. [46] developed a deep learning framework that incorporates a tuned version of Weighted Nuclear Norm Minimization (WNNM) for real-time ultrasound image denoising, achieving image quality improvement and feature preservation. Above reconstruction approaches are fairly straightforward. Multiple published studies have shown that while these methods perform well in reconstructing low-frequency information, their ability to reconstruct high-frequency information is rather limited, likely resulting in blurring effects. Specifically, the reconstruction results can produce good contrast but fail to accurately predict speckle texture. Research has proved that GAN structures, compared to CNNs, offer stronger predictive generation capabilities due to the continually adversarial interaction between the generator and discriminator, which can better generate high-frequency information and thus become a promising improvement direction. For example, Khor et al. [47] proposed a wavelet-based generative adversarial network (WGAN-DUS) that incorporates wavelet residual channel attention blocks and a wavelet-based discriminator, significantly enhancing de-speckling performance while preserving fine image details. Some research efforts focus on enhancing ultrasound reconstruction performance by introducing more powerful regression-based loss functions. For instance, in [28], Zhou et al. proposed an ultrasound perceptual loss function, which better extracts ultrasound-specific features. As illustrated in Fig. 3.5, the ultrasound-specific perceptual loss is obtained using an a pretrained classification CNN model. This pretrained model was forced to differentiate between low-end and high-end device images using a large, unpaired ultrasound dataset.

The RF-to-Image approach, on the other hand, inputs raw or initially time-delay-corrected RF signals and utilizes networks to learn the mapping relationships from RF to beamformed images. Some studies have employed multilayer perceptron (MLP) to sequentially process each channel or depth [48], while others have used generative AI models to predict multi-channel or global images [49, 50]. Compared to the image-to-image approach, RF-to-Image methods that sequentially process each channel typically require less network memory but can be time-consuming due to the iterative generation for different channels/depths. Additionally, the lack of spatial texture information from neighboring regions may limit the results. Conversely, global image generation does not require iteration and is relatively straightforward but demands more network memory resources and longer training time. Multi-channel/depth generation is a compromise between these two approaches.

Furthermore, some studies have employed RF-to-RF conversion, such as predicting more channels of RF signals from fewer channels, followed by traditional beamforming based on multi-channel RF. Another type of study involves predicting the weight matrix of adaptive beamforming algorithms from raw RF signals, replacing the most time-consuming algorithmic part with mapping. For instance, in [37] (see Fig. 3.6), a hybrid generator processes the raw RF signal using two distinct learning modules: an intrinsic learning module that determines the 3D adaptive weights, and a perceptual learning module that generates 2D adaptive beamformed images. These outputs are then combined through a fusion module to produce high-quality beamformed ultrasound images. This fusion-style method considers multimodal features in both the image and signal domains, offering higher interpretability compared to purely black-box deep learning methods.

3.5 Clinical Usability and Reliability

To fully realize the potential of deep learning in clinical practice, integrating it with specific clinical scenarios is crucial. Recent studies have increasingly targeted specialized applications of deep learning in ultrasound reconstruction, underscoring the importance of clinical usability. For example, Bar-Shira et al. [51] used a deep neural network for super-resolution ultrasound localization microscopy in breast cancer detection, achieving rapid microvasculature imaging without prior knowledge of the point spread function. Another study by Blanken et al. [52] presented a one-dimensional dilated CNN for super-resolution imaging with direct deconvolution of RF signals, significantly improving detection-localization in dense microbubble environments. Yan et al. [53] integrated microbubble image features into a Kalman tracking framework with sparsity-based deconvolution, enhancing the accuracy of microbubble localization in deep tissue imaging. Sloun et al. [54] introduced Deep-ULM, a deep learning-based enhancement of ultrasound localization microscopy, enabling real-time analysis of high-density contrast-enhanced ultrasound data, making it suitable for clinical applications.

Transitioning from promising research to practical clinical tools requires rigorous validation. This involves extensive testing across diverse patient populations and clinical settings to ensure robustness and generalizability. While these studies have shown the potential of deep learning in specific imaging applications, a general-

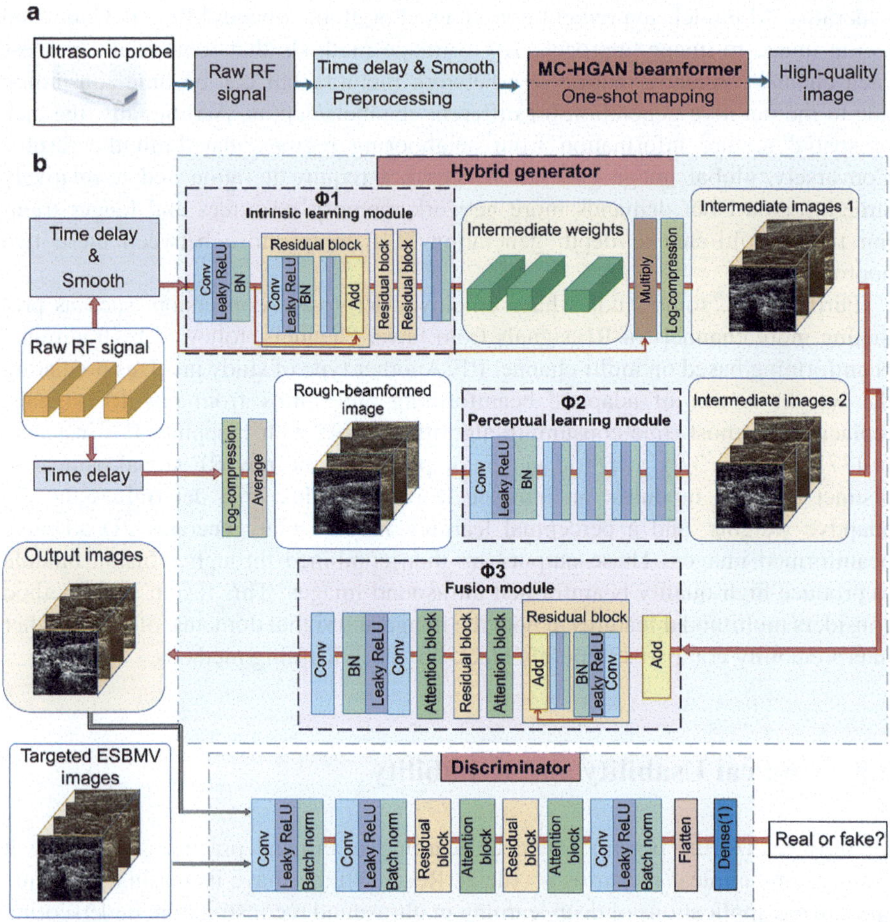

Fig. 3.6 An example method of reconstruction between raw RF data and an intermediate refined RF data. (**a**) A brief workflow of the MC-HGAN beamformer [37]. (**b**) Detailed network structure of MC-HGAN beamformer

specific-general transformation approach is necessary. This involves validating the potential efficacy and generalizability of technologies, applying them to specialized scenarios, and confirming their reliability across diverse scenarios. Currently, there is a lack of comprehensive clinical multi-scenario systematic evaluation studies for ultrasound reconstruction. Advanced models like GANs and diffusion models have expanded the applications of generative AI in natural image generation. However, the medical field demands a higher standard of precision and detail due to its close link to human health. Reliability analysis of medical generative AI is crucial, especially in reconstructing speckle patterns in ultrasound imaging. Speckles provide essential information but can also introduce noise and artifacts, posing a unique challenge. Accurately reconstructing speckles without compromising image quality is essential for trustworthy ultrasound reconstruction. Moreover, usability studies should address integrating these technologies into existing clinical workflows, emphasizing user-friendliness for sonographers and technicians.

3.6 Limitations and Future Directions

Despite the advancements from deep learning for ultrasound reconstruction, several challenges remain that need to be solved to fully realize its potential.

3.6.1 Explainability and Effectiveness of Deep Learning Models

The explainability and effectiveness of deep learning models in ultrasound reconstruction remain significant concerns. Many current models operate as "black boxes," providing little insight into how they arrive at their conclusions. This lack of transparency can hinder clinical adoption, as practitioners need to trust and understand the tools they use. Future research should prioritize developing models with built-in explainability features, such as attention mechanisms or interpretability modules, to provide clearer insights into the decision-making process and enhance clinician confidence in these technologies.

3.6.2 Public Data Collection and Diversity

The effectiveness of deep learning models depends on diverse and comprehensive datasets. Many researchers use proprietary datasets, which leads to resource wastage as models need retraining for different datasets. Establishing a robust, public ultrasound dataset that covers a wide range of conditions and imaging scenarios would streamline research efforts, foster collaboration, and enhance model performance and generalizability.

3.6.3 Comprehensive Clinical Reliability Validation

Ensuring the clinical reliability of reconstructed images across various diseases is paramount. Various pathologies present unique challenges in image reconstruction, and the reliability of deep learning models must be thoroughly validated across a spectrum of conditions. Future research should focus on extensive clinical trials and validation studies to evaluate the performance of these models in reconstructing images of diverse lesions. A comprehensive analysis of the model's ability to handle different types of pathological features is essential to ensure its robustness and reliability in clinical practice.

3.6.4 Unbalance in Training Data

Class imbalance in training datasets can significantly impact the performance of deep learning models. In ultrasound reconstruction, rare conditions or features may be underrepresented, leading to biased models that perform poorly on these cases. Addressing this imbalance through data augmentation, synthetic data generation, or weighted loss functions can improve model training.

Generally, future research should continue to explore avenues that advance ultrasound reconstruction technologies towards greater effectiveness and wider adoption. Key directions include enhancing model explainability, establishing comprehensive public datasets, and conducting thorough clinical reliability validation, all of which are crucial challenges to address. Additionally, incorporating continuous learning concepts will be valuable to research, enabling models to adapt and improve over time with new data. The potential of large models for medical image reconstruction may also be investigated, as their capacity for handling complex patterns and large datasets could significantly enhance diagnostic accuracy and robustness.

References

1. Rumack CM, Levine D (2023) Diagnostic ultrasound. Elsevier, Amsterdam
2. Contreras Ortiz SH, Chiu T, Fox MD (2021) Ultrasound image enhancement: a review. Biomed Signal Process Control 7(5):419–428. https://doi.org/10.1016/j.bspc.2012.02.002
3. Tanter M, Fink M (2014) Ultrafast imaging in biomedical ultrasound. IEEE Trans Ultrason Ferroelectr Freq Control 61(1):102–119. https://doi.org/10.1109/TUFFC.2014.6689779
4. Liebgott H, Molares AR, Jensen JA, Cervenansky F, Jensen JA, Bernard O (2016) Plane-wave imaging challenge in medical ultrasound: 2016 IEEE international ultrasonics symposium. In: Proceedings of 2016 IEEE international ultrasonics symposium. https://doi.org/10.1109/ULTSYM.2016.7728908
5. Fenster A, Parraga G, Bax J (2011) Three-dimensional ultrasound scanning. Interface Focus 1(4):503–519. https://doi.org/10.1098/rsfs.2011.0019
6. Kimura BJ, Amundson SA, Willis CL, Gilpin EA, DeMaria AN (2002) Usefulness of a hand-held ultrasound device for bedside examination of left ventricular function. Am J Cardiol 90(9):1038–1039. https://doi.org/10.1016/s0002-9149(02)02699-1
7. Amisha MP, Pathania M, Rathaur VK (2019) Overview of artificial intelligence in medicine. J Family Med Prim Care 8(7):2328–2331. https://doi.org/10.4103/jfmpc.jfmpc_440_19
8. Ahishakiye E, Bastiaan Van Gijzen M, Tumwiine J, Wario R, Obungoloch J (2021) A survey on deep learning in medical image reconstruction. Intell Med 01(03):118–127. https://doi.org/10.1016/j.imed.2021.03.003

9. Rajpurkar P, Chen E, Banerjee O, Topol EJ (2022) AI in health and medicine. Nat Med 28(1):31–38. https://doi.org/10.1038/s41591-021-01614-0
10. Wells PNT (2006) Ultrasound imaging. Phys. Med. Biol. 51(13):R83. https://doi.org/10.1088/0031-9155/51/13/R06
11. R Lg (1996) Applications of high-frequency ultrasound imaging. IEEE Eng. Med. Biol. 15(6):60–71
12. Abu-Zidan FM, Hefny AF, Corr P (2011) Clinical ultrasound physics. J. Emerg Trauma Shock 4(4):501 (2011). https://doi.org/10.4103/0974-2700.86646
13. Li J, Ma Y, Zhang T, Shung KK, Zhu B (2022) Recent advancements in ultrasound transducer: from material strategies to biomedical applications. BME Front **2022**, 9764501. https://doi.org/10.34133/2022/9764501
14. La TG, Le LH (2022) Flexible and wearable ultrasound device for medical applications: a review on materials, structural designs, and current challenges. Adv Mater Technol 7(3):2100798. https://doi.org/10.1002/admt.202100798
15. Becker DM, Tafoya CA, Becker SL, Kruger GH, Tafoya MJ, Becker TK (2016) The use of portable ultrasound devices in low- and middle-income countries: a systematic review of the literature. Tropical Med. Int. Health 21(3):294–311. https://doi.org/10.1111/tmi.12657
16. Matrone G, Savoia AS, Caliano G, Magenes G (2015) The delay multiply and sum beamforming algorithm in ultrasound B-mode medical imaging. IEEE Trans Med Imag 34(4):940–949. https://doi.org/10.1109/TMI.2014.2371235
17. Zeng X, Wang Y, Yu J, Guo Y (2013) Beam-domain eigenspace-based minimum variance beamformer for medical ultrasound imaging. IEEE Trans Ultrason Ferroelectr Freq Control 60(12):2670–2676. https://doi.org/10.1109/tuffc.2013.2866
18. Sasso M, Cohen-Bacrie C (2005) Medical ultrasound imaging using the fully adaptive beamformer. In: Proceedings. (ICASSP'05). IEEE international conference on acoustics, speech, and signal processing. https://doi.org/10.1109/icassp.2005.1415448
19. Prada C, Wu F, Fink M (1991) The iterative time reversal mirror: a solution to self-focusing in the pulse echo mode. J. Acoust Soc Am 90(2):1119–1129. https://doi.org/10.1121/1.402301
20. Montaldo G, Tanter M, Bercoff J, Benech N, Fink M (2009) Coherent plane-wave compounding for very high frame rate ultrasonography and transient elastography. IEEE Trans Ultrason Ferroelectr Freq Control 56(3):489–506. https://doi.org/10.1109/tuffc.2009.1067
21. Zhou Z, Wang Y, Yu J, Guo Y, Guo W, Qi Y (2018) High spatial-temporal resolution reconstruction of plane-wave ultrasound images with a multichannel multiscale convolutional neural network. IEEE Trans Ultrason Ferroelectr Freq Control 65(11):1983–1996. https://doi.org/10.1109/tuffc.2018.2865504
22. Lu JY, Lee PY, Huang CC (2022) Improving image quality for single-angle plane wave ultrasound imaging with convolutional neural network beamformer. IEEE Trans Ultrason Ferroelectr Freq Control 69(4):1326–1336. https://doi.org/10.1109/tuffc.2022.3152689
23. Senouf O, et al (2018) High frame-rate cardiac ultrasound imaging with deep learning. In: Frangi AF, Schnabel JA, Davatzikos C, Alberola-López C, Fichtinger G (eds), Medical image computing and computer assisted intervention – MICCAI 2018. Springer, Cham, pp. 126–134. https://doi.org/10.1007/978-3-030-00928-1_15
24. Chen Y, Liu J, Luo X, Luo J (2021) ApodNet: learning for high frame rate synthetic transmit aperture ultrasound imaging. IEEE Trans Med Imag 40(11):3190–3204. https://doi.org/10.1109/tmi.2021.3084821
25. Zhou Z, Wang Y, Guo Y, Qi Y, Yu J (2020) Image quality improvement of hand-held ultrasound devices with a two-stage generative adversarial network. IEEE Trans Biomed Eng 67(1):298–311. https://doi.org/10.1109/TBME.2019.2912986
26. Dong G, Ma Y, Basu A (2021) Feature-guided CNN for denoising images from portable ultrasound devices. IEEE Access 9:28272–28281. https://doi.org/10.1109/ACCESS.2021.3059003
27. Wang R, et al (2019) High-resolution image reconstruction for portable ultrasound imaging devices. EURASIP J Adv Signal Process 2019(1):56. https://doi.org/10.1186/s13634-019-0649-x

28. Zhou Z, Guo Y, Wang Y (2021) Handheld ultrasound video high-quality reconstruction using a low-rank representation multipathway generative adversarial network. IEEE Trans Neural Netw Learn Syst 32(2), 575–588. https://doi.org/10.1109/TNNLS.2020.3025380
29. Mamistvalov A, Amar A, Kessler N, Eldar YC (2022) Deep-learning based adaptive ultrasound imaging from sub-nyquist channel data. IEEE Trans Ultrason Ferroelectr Freq Control 69(5):1638–1648. https://doi.org/10.1109/TUFFC.2022.3160859
30. Xiao D, Pitman WMK, Yiu BYS, Chee AJY, Yu ACH (2022) Minimizing image quality loss after channel count reduction for plane wave ultrasound via deep learning inference. IEEE Trans Ultrason Ferroelectr Freq Control 69(10):2849–2861. https://doi.org/10.1109/tuffc.2022.3192854
31. Vignon F, Burcher MR (2008) Capon beamforming in medical ultrasound imaging with focused beams. IEEE Trans Ultrason Ferroelectr Freq Control 55(3):619–628. https://doi.org/10.1109/tuffc.2008.686
32. Asl BM, Mahloojifar A (2012) A low-complexity adaptive beamformer for ultrasound imaging using structured covariance matrix. IEEE Trans Ultrason Ferroelectr Freq Control 59(4):660–667. https://doi.org/10.1109/tuffc.2012.2244
33. Wiacek A, González E, Bell MAL (2020) CohereNet: a deep learning architecture for ultrasound spatial correlation estimation and coherence-based beamforming. IEEE Trans Ultrason Ferroelectr Freq Control 67(12):2574–2583. https://doi.org/10.1109/TUFFC.2020.2982848
34. Nair AA, Washington KN, Tran TD, Reiter A, Lediju Bell MA (2020) Deep learning to obtain simultaneous image and segmentation outputs from a single input of raw ultrasound channel data. IEEE Trans Ultrason Ferroelectr Freq Control 67(12):2493–2509. https://doi.org/10.1109/TUFFC.2020.2993779
35. Luijten B, et al (2020) Adaptive ultrasound beamforming using deep learning. IEEE Trans Med Imag 39(12):3967–3978. https://doi.org/10.1109/TMI.2020.3008537
36. Khan S, Huh J, Ye JC (2020) Adaptive and compressive beamforming using deep learning for medical ultrasound. IEEE Trans Ultrason Ferroelectr Freq Control 67(8):1558–1572. https://doi.org/10.1109/TUFFC.2020.2977202
37. Zhou Z, Guo Y, Wang Y (2021) Ultrasound deep beamforming using a multiconstrained hybrid generative adversarial network. Med Image Anal 71:102086. https://doi.org/10.1016/j.media.2021.102086
38. Huang X, Lediju Bell MA, Ding K (2021) Deep learning for ultrasound beamforming in flexible array transducer. IEEE Trans Med Imag 40(11):3178–3189. https://doi.org/10.1109/TMI.2021.3087450
39. Huang L, Zhou Z, Guo Y, Wang Y (2022) A stability-enhanced CycleGAN for effective domain transformation of unpaired ultrasound images. Biomed Signal Process Control 77:103831. https://doi.org/10.1016/j.bspc.2022.103831
40. Huang L, et al (2024) Standardization of ultrasound images across various centers: M2O-DiffGAN bridging the gaps among unpaired multi-domain ultrasound images. Med Image Anal 95:103187. https://doi.org/10.1016/j.media.2024.103187
41. Liu H, Liu J, Hou S, Tao T, Han J (2023) Perception consistency ultrasound image super-resolution via self-supervised CycleGAN. Neural Comput Appl 35(17):12331–12341. https://doi.org/10.1007/s00521-020-05687-9
42. Zhou Z, Wang Y, Guo Y, Jiang X, Qi Y (2020) Ultrafast plane wave imaging with line-scan-quality using an ultrasound-transfer generative adversarial network. IEEE J Biomed Health Inf 24(4):943–956. https://doi.org/10.1109/JBHI.2019.2950334
43. Tierney J, Luchies A, Khan C, Byram B, Berger M (2020) Domain adaptation for ultrasound beamforming. In: Martel AL, Abolmaesumi P, Stoyanov D, Mateus D, Zuluaga MA, Zhou SK, Racoceanu D, Joskowicz L (eds) Medical image computing and computer assisted intervention – MICCAI 2020. Springer, Cham, pp. 410–420. https://doi.org/10.1007/978-3-030-59713-9_40
44. Wildeboer RR, et al (2020) Synthetic elastography using b-mode ultrasound through a deep fully convolutional neural network. IEEE Trans Ultrason Ferroelectr Freq Control 67(12):2640–2648. https://doi.org/10.1109/TUFFC.2020.2983099

45. Lu J, Liu W (2018) Unsupervised super-resolution framework for medical ultrasound images using dilated convolutional neural networks. In: 2018 IEEE 3rd international conference on image, vision and computing (ICIVC), pp. 739–744. https://doi.org/10.1109/ICIVC.2018.8492821
46. Cammarasana S, Nicolardi P, Patanè G (2022) Real-time denoising of ultrasound images based on deep learning. Med Biol Eng Comput 60(8):2229–2244. https://doi.org/10.1007/s11517-022-02573-5
47. Khor HG, Ning G, Zhang X, Liao H (2022) Ultrasound speckle reduction using wavelet-based generative adversarial network. IEEE J Biomed Health Inf 26(7):3080–3091. https://doi.org/10.1109/jbhi.2022.3144628
48. Perdios D, Besson AGJ, Arditi M, Thiran JP (Eds) (2017) A deep learning approach to ultrasound image recovery. In: 2017 IEEE International Ultrasonics Symposium (IUS). https://doi.org/10.1109/ULTSYM.2017.8092746
49. Yoon YH, Khan S, Huh J, Ye JC (2019) Efficient b-mode ultrasound image reconstruction from sub-sampled RF data using deep learning. IEEE Trans Med Imag 38(2):325–336. https://doi.org/10.1109/tmi.2018.2864821
50. Khan S, Huh J, Ye JC (2022) Switchable and tunable deep beamformer using adaptive instance normalization for medical ultrasound. IEEE Trans Med Imag 41(2):266–278. https://doi.org/10.1109/TMI.2021.3110730
51. Bar-Shira O, et al (2021) Learned super resolution ultrasound for improved breast lesion characterization. In: Medical image computing and computer assisted intervention – MICCAI 2021. Springer, Cham, pp. 109–118. https://doi.org/10.1007/978-3-030-87234-2_11
52. Blanken N, Wolterink JM, Delingette H, Brune C, Versluis M, Lajoinie G (2022) Super-resolved microbubble localization in single-channel ultrasound RF signals using deep learning. IEEE Trans Med Imag 41(9):2532–2542. https://doi.org/10.1109/tmi.2022.3166443
53. Yan J, Zhang T, Broughton-Venner J, Huang P, Tang MX (2022) Super-resolution ultrasound through sparsity-based deconvolution and multi-feature tracking. IEEE Trans Med Imag 41(8):1938–1947. https://doi.org/10.1109/TMI.2022.3152396
54. van Sloun RJG, Solomon O, Bruce M, Khaing ZZ, Eldar YC, Mischi M (2019) Deep learning for super-resolution vascular ultrasound imaging. In: 2019 IEEE international conference on acoustics, speech, and signal processing, ICASSP 2019 - proceedings, pp. 1055–1059. https://doi.org/10.1109/ICASSP.2019.8683813

Chapter 4
Conditional Image Synthesis Using Generative Diffusion Models: Application to Pathological Prostate MR Image Generation

Shaheer U. Saeed and Yipeng Hu

Abstract In this work, we propose an image synthesis mechanism based on diffusion, which models the reversal of the sequential addition of noise to an image. We further develop conditioning mechanisms for this approach, such that image synthesis can be conditioned on information relevant to the clinical tasks-of-interest. We demonstrate the conditional synthesis capabilities of such models via an example application of multi-sequence prostate MR image synthesis, conditioned on text, to control lesion presence and sequence, and on images, to generate paired MR sequences e.g., generating diffusion-weighted MR from T2-weighted MR, which are two challenging tasks in pathological image synthesis. We validate our method using 2D image slices from real suspected prostate cancer patients. The realism of the synthetic images was validated through a blind evaluation by an expert radiologist, specialising in urological MR with 4 years of experience. The radiologist was able to distinguish between real and fake images with an accuracy of 59.4%, only slightly above the random chance of 50%. For the first time, we also evaluate the realism of the generated pathology by blind expert identification of the presence of suspected lesions. We find that the clinician performs similarly for both real and synthesised images, with a 2.9 percentage point difference in lesion identification accuracy between real and synthesised images, demonstrating the potentials for radiological training. Additionally, we demonstrated that a machine learning model trained for lesion identification exhibited improved performance (76.2% vs 70.4%, a statistically significant increase) when augmented with synthesised data compared to training solely on real images, highlighting the utility of synthesised images in enhancing model performance.

S. U. Saeed · Y. Hu (✉)
University College London, London, UK
e-mail: shaheer.saeed.17@ucl.ac.uk; yipeng.hu@ucl.ac.uk

L. Zhang et al. (eds.), *Generative Machine Learning Models in Medical Image Computing*, https://doi.org/10.1007/978-3-031-80965-1_4

4.1 Introduction

4.1.1 Image Synthesis in Medical Imaging

Image synthesis plays a pivotal role in medical imaging for a variety of applications [13]. For training machine learning models, image synthesis is used to augment exisiting real training data, to ensure robustness and generalisability of the models to varied appearances of anatomical and pathological regions-of-interest [2, 8]. This is especially beneficial for training, or adapting existing models, when training data for the application-of-interest is scarce. Under these data-constrained scenarios it can alleviate issues with generalisability by training models with a large breadth of samples, of the kinds that may be encountered at inference [2, 8]. In such applications, synthetic training data, in conjunction with real data, often leads to improved task performance for automated tasks like organ segmentation [2, 8]. In addition to machine learning model training, image synthesis has also been proposed for radiological simulations, to enhance training experiences or pre-procedure planning [7].

4.1.2 Necessity of Conditional Image Synthesis

While these applications benefit from realistic synthetic data, it is important to ensure that synthesised images have features of-interest that are relevant to the clinical application [13, 32]. Conditioning image synthesis on such features-of-interest, known as conditional image synthesis, ensures that the information relevant to the clinical context is adequately captured in the synthetic data [13, 32].

4.1.3 Types of Conditional Image Synthesis

Various approaches have been adopted for conditional image synthesis, to capture features-of-interest in synthesised images. Examples of these sythesis techniques are outlined below.

4.1.3.1 Physics-Based Simulations

Physics-based simulators, often inspired by the underlying physics of the imaging process, have continually been proposed for medical image synthesis since before the advent of deep learning [3, 23, 29]. Models of features-of-interest either artificially constructed, or derived from pre-operative images, are used to capture clinically-relevant information. The synthesis then involves the simulation of the imaging process for these modelled structures. An example of this type of simulation-based synthesis is generating intra-operative ultrasound data from larger and higher-resolution pre-operative images such as computed tomography (CT) images [3, 29]. These types of simulation methods are strongly conditioned on the modelled features-of-interest, where models are derived from higher-resolution pre-operative data. While useful for generating intra-operative data, utility of these methods for generating pre-operative data is limited, as model construction for features-of-interest is often infeasible without pre-operative images.

4.1.3.2 Generative Adversarial Networks (GAN)

Machine learning approaches for medical image synthesis have largely focused on using GANs, or conditional GANs (cGANs). The adversarial setup of cGANs is based on two functions: (1) the generator to generate an image, given a specific condition; and (2) the discriminator to distinguish between real and generated images. The training is conducted by first training the discriminator using real samples and synthetic samples created by the generator, such that it can discriminate between the two, with higher scores for real samples. The generator is then trained by maximising the discriminator score, such that it aims to produce more realistic samples. This adversarial training leads to the generator being able to produce more realistic samples as training progresses.

Such cGANs have extensively been used for both pre- and intra-operative image synthesis, without relying on patient anatomy being available for synthesis [13, 31, 32]. They have also been utilised to condition the synthesis on features-of-interest e.g., blood vessels [4, 5, 9, 12, 35] and tumours [16, 19], where complete model of the features are not a pre-requisite. Another common use-case is for learning inter-modality correspondence e.g. for generating CT from MR or vice versa [2, 21, 33, 34].

Despite realistic synthesis, GANs often suffer from problems such as under-represented features of interest [13], poor performance on class-imbalanced data-sets [13], especially for under-represented classes, and other common problems encountered during training, e.g. unstable training, mode collapse and diminishing gradients [28], which prevent them from being widely usable [17]. Preliminary experiments for our application of prostate cancer synthesis on magnetic resonance images (see Fig. 4.2) were consistent with these identified limitations, with unconvincing results including broken anatomical or in-painted anatomical structures, lacking details (see Fig. 4.2). These results show lack of generative modelling ability or ineffective conditioning, for challenging applications such as prostate cancer image synthesis, with often subtle and sometimes radiologically undetermined pathology.

4.1.3.3 Diffusion Probabilistic Models (DPM)

Recent work on DPMs has demonstrated their generative capabilities on a variety of image synthesis tasks [11, 20, 25, 27]. These models are based on the idea of 'diffusion' in computer vision, which refers to the sequential addition of Gaussian noise to an image, for a fixed number of steps. DPMs then learn to reconstruct the original (un-noised) image at the first step by reversing the noise addition processes. The data for learning such a reversion is derived from the forward noise addition process itself. The reverse diffusion process, of synthesising an image from random noise, is then used at inference to generate new synthetic images.

Compared to cGANs, DPMs have shown improved image synthesis capabilities for a wide array of problems while incorporating both image-based and text-based conditioning [11, 20, 24, 25, 27]. Their use in medical image synthesis remains limited, with studies mostly focusing on either unconditional synthesis or conditioning only on text-based variables.

4.1.4 Conditional Image Synthesis for Prostate Cancer

In this chapter we investigate an example application of synthesising abdominal magnetic resonance (MR) images showing pathological regions-of-interest such as tumours or lesions within the prostate gland. The generation of pathological images can potentially aid the training of radiologists and clinicians, and the development of machine learning models, which are often hindered by the low sample availability to diversity ratio in disease conditions such as prostate cancer.

4.1.4.1 Challenging Synthesis of Pathological Images

In such applications, where pathologies are diverse, under-represented in the data, and difficult to manually localise, conditioning directly on local pathology may be under-specific. Instead, conditioning on other image sequences, e.g., multi-parametric MR for the prostate, where subtle features or different appearances of such pathology may be captured, is beneficial or even inevitably required. This conditional synthesis for pathological prostate MR images, based on other sequences, is further supported by modern uro-radiological guidelines such as PiRADS. For example, peripheral zone lesions are primarily graded on DW images, while transition zone cancers are predominantly determined on T2 images but their risk may be upgraded with positive findings on DW images. The ability to model the conditional distribution of these paired image data and to synthesise diffusion images, given other complementary sequences are essential for the, above-discussed, machine learning data augmentation and clinical training applications.

To this end, we investigate the example application of conditional prostate MR image synthesis. Since models of anatomy or pathology are not available to us prior to imaging, physics-based simulators prove infeasible to implement. GANs, while able to generate synthetic images, suffer from broken or in-painted anatomical structures, lacking details, as discussed in Sect. 4.1.3.2. This motivates the use of conditional DPMs for the synthesis of pathological prostate MR images.

4.1.4.2 Using DPM for Conditional Image Synthesis of Prostate MR Images

We present a DPM approach for synthesis of prostate MR images, conditioned not only on text to control variables such as the presence of cancer and sequence of MR acquisition, i.e. T2-weighted (T2W), apparent diffusion contrast (ADC), or diffusion-weighted (DW), but on images to facilitate generation of corresponding image pairs by generating DW images conditioned on T2W images. Our text- and image-based conditional synthesis for DPMs, presents flexible conditional synthesis, compared to the previous unconditional generation, only text-based conditioning, or image modification e.g., in-painting or super-resolution.

We evaluate our conditional DPM approach for our application of prostate cancer MR image synthesis by: (1) presenting images to a clinician to identify synthesised images, to test the efficacy of the image synthesis, to demonstrate the realism of the synthesised images; (2) presenting corresponding T2-weighted and diffusion-weighted, generated and real, images to a clinician for a cancer detection task, to test the realism of the generated lesions; and (3) testing the segmentation accuracy for a neural network-based multi-parametric MR lesion identification task with real data versus with a dataset augmented using synthesised images. The image synthesis is thus evaluated for both the clinical training and machine learning model development applications.

4.1.5 Summary of Contributions

The contributions of this chapter are summarised:

1. We present a conditional DPM for synthesis of prostate MR images with challenging pathology.
2. We propose conditioning the synthesis on text-based inputs to control presence of lesions and MR sequence.
3. We propose conditional image synthesis to generate DW images from corresponding T2W images as a means of generating corresponding multi-sequence images.
4. We conduct an evaluation to demonstrate the effectiveness of the synthesised images not only for clinical training use cases but also for machine learning model training for a task carried out with the MR images i.e. lesion identification.

4.2 Methods

A DPM relies on diffusion—the sequential addition of Gaussian noise to an image. The synthesis is learnt as a reverse diffusion process—sequentially removing noise from an image until the image is completely de-noised. The forward and reverse diffusion processes are described in the sections below along with conditioning mechanisms to enable conditional synthesis. An overview of the entire framework is presented in Fig. 4.1.

4.2.1 *Forward Diffusion Process*

Assume that a forward diffusion adds noise in sequential steps, to a given input image $\mathbf{x}_0 \sim q(x|y)$ sampled from a data distribution of real samples $q(x)$, the distribution to be modelled. The conditioning variable y is used to condition the data. At each step t, for $t \in \{1, T\}$, the added Gaussian noise follows a Markov

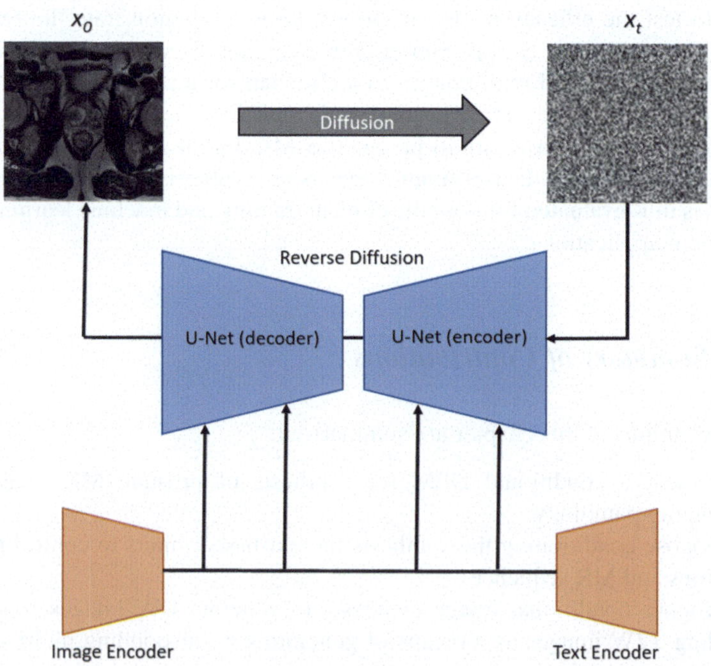

Fig. 4.1 An overview of the diffusion process. The text and image encoders provide a mechanism to condition image synthesis on either text prompts or other images, respectively. In our application, text prompts control aspects such as presence of pathology and MR image sequence, and image conditioning controls paired MR sequence generation i.e., generating one sequence conditioned on another

chain with T steps, with variance β_t, and only depends on the sample from the previous step and the variable used for conditioning. The distribution can then be written as $q(\mathbf{x}_t|\mathbf{x}_{t-1}, y)$, with $\mathbf{x}_t$ as a latent variable.

The forward diffusion process is thus formulated as:

$$q(\mathbf{x}_t|\mathbf{x}_{t-1}, y) = \mathcal{N}(\mathbf{x}_t; \boldsymbol{\mu}_t = \sqrt{1-\beta_t}\mathbf{x}_{t-1}, \boldsymbol{\sigma}_t = \beta_t \mathbf{I}) \tag{4.1}$$

In a closed form, going from sample $\mathbf{x}_0$ to the sample $\mathbf{x}_T$ can be denoted as:

$$q(\mathbf{x}_{1:T}|\mathbf{x}_0, y) = \prod_{t=1}^{T} q(\mathbf{x}_t|\mathbf{x}_{t-1}, y) \tag{4.2}$$

This formulation, however, requires t time-steps of applying q to get sample $\mathbf{x}_t$.

We can re-parameterise to allow computation of $\mathbf{x}_t$ without requiring computation of all samples at previous steps. As detailed in previous works [11, 20, 25], it can be shown that by defining $\alpha_t = 1 - \beta_t$, $\bar{\alpha}_t = \prod_{s=0}^{t} \alpha_s$, a sample $\mathbf{x}_t$ may be sampled as follows:

$$\mathbf{x}_t \sim q(\mathbf{x}_t|\mathbf{x}_{t-1}, y) = \mathcal{N}(\mathbf{x}_t; \sqrt{\bar{\alpha}_t}\mathbf{x}_0, (1-\bar{\alpha}_t)\mathbf{I} \tag{4.3}$$

A cosine schedule is adopted for β [20], increasing from 10^{-4} to 0.02 over T steps, where the cosine schedule may formally be defined as:

$$f(t) = \cos \frac{t/T + s}{1+s} \cdot \frac{\pi}{2} \tag{4.4}$$

where s is configured as $s = 0.008$, empirically [20].

4.2.2 Additional Inputs for Conditioning

An encoder τ_γ, with weights γ, may be used for any conditioning variables y. The conditioning variables could take any form that can be used to condition the image synthesis. In our work, we use text to condition the image synthesis on factors such as presence of pathology and on images to condition synthesis of a particular MR image sequence on another MR sequence. The encoder maps to an intermediate representation $\tau_\gamma(y) \in \mathbb{R}^{M \times d_\tau}$, which is then mapped to the intermediate layers of the diffusion-reversing network (as outlined in the next section). For sample $\mathbf{x}_t$, conditioned on y (e.g., consisting of the image and text conditioning) this gives us $\mathbf{x}_t \sim q(\mathbf{x}_t|\mathbf{x}_{t-1}, \tau_\gamma(y))$. For notational brevity, however, we use y in-place of $\tau_\gamma(y)$, in the remaining analysis. The specific text- and image-conditioning are discussed further in Sects. 4.3.1.1 and 4.3.1.2.

4.2.3 Reverse Diffusion Process

The distribution approaches an isotropic Gaussian with a sufficiently large T [11]. The data distribution $q(x)$ can, therefore, be modelled by reversing the noise adding process from unit Gaussian distribution $\mathcal{N}(0, \mathbf{I})$ samples. However, the reverse $q(\mathbf{x}_{t-1}|\mathbf{x}_t, y)$ is not known and cannot be statistically estimated since any statistical estimates would involve knowing the data distribution [11].

Approximations of $q(\mathbf{x}_{t-1}|\mathbf{x}_t, y)$, however, can be learnt, using a parameterised function $\epsilon_\theta(\mathbf{x}_t, t, y)$. This can be interpreted as a sequence of de-noising auto-encoders with additional conditioning on the time-step t.

In practice, it is easier to parameterise a Gaussian and then remove the predicted Gaussian noise manually. Thus for sample $\mathbf{x}_{t-1}$ we have:

$$p_\theta(\mathbf{x}_{t-1}|\mathbf{x}_t, t, y) = \mathcal{N}(\mathbf{x}_{t-1}; \mu_\theta(\mathbf{x}_t, t), \sigma_\theta(\mathbf{x}_t, t)) \tag{4.5}$$

Then applying the reverse process for all time-steps:

$$p_\theta(\mathbf{x}_{0:T}, 0 : T, y) = p_\theta(\mathbf{x}_T, T, y) \prod_{t-1}^{T} p_\theta(\mathbf{x}_{t-1}|\mathbf{x}_t, t, y) \tag{4.6}$$

We summarise the entire de-noising process as a de-noising function $\epsilon_\theta(\mathbf{x}_t, t, y)$ which is trained to predict a de-noised version of its input i.e. $\mathbf{x}_0$ from $\mathbf{x}_t$.

To incorporate the encoder τ used to pre-process the conditioning variable we may re-write this de-noising function as $\epsilon_\theta(\mathbf{x}_t, t, \tau_\gamma(y))$.

Note that in actuality the de-noising is a two-step process: (1) predicting the noise in a noised image; (2) subtracting the noise from the noised image. This two-step process ensures stable optimisation as explored in previous works [20]. As shown in previous works [11, 20, 25], the objective for the first step can be simplified to:

$$\mathcal{L} = \mathbb{E}_{x,\epsilon\sim\mathcal{N}(0,1),t,y}\left[||\epsilon - \epsilon_\theta(\mathbf{x}_t, t, y)||_1^1\right] \tag{4.7}$$

This objective can be used to train a neural network to predict noise in a noised image, which can then be subtracted from the image to obtain a de-noised version. Nonetheless, for notational simplicity in further analyses, we summarise the two-step de-noising process as a de-noising function $\mathbf{x}_0 = \epsilon_\theta(\mathbf{x}_t, t, \tau_\gamma(y))$, which predicts the de-noised image from a noised version $\mathbf{x}_t$.

4.2.4 Sampling from the Trained Diffusion Model

Synthesising images from the diffusion model consists of first sampling noise $\mathbf{x}_T \sim \mathcal{N}(0, \mathbf{I})$ and then computing the de-noised sample using our reverse de-noising function $\mathbf{x}_0 = \epsilon_\theta(\mathbf{x}_t, t, \tau_\gamma(y))$. However, it is practically more efficient to add back a portion of the noise using a noise schedule and then de-noise the sample again using the de-noising function, repeating until the noise schedule exhausts. In more concrete terms this means that after the first de-noising of the sample, we add back noise until step $t - 1$, and then use the de-noising function to again de-noise the sample. Then add back noise until step $t - 2$ and again use the de-noising function to de-noise the sample. This is repeated until $t - t$.

4.3 Experiments

4.3.1 Model Implementation and Training

We closely follow the implementation used in [25]. Hyper-parameters are summarised in Table 4.2.

4.3.1.1 Text Conditioning

For text conditioning, a transformer architecture is used as the encoder τ_γ, i.e., the BERT tokeniser together with the provided encoder for encoding text prompts [25]. BERT was chosen due to the vast prior research into BERT-based text encoding for diffusion models. For constructing text prompts, we used the presence of cancer together with MR sequence. Prompts were randomly generated from a list of 8 phrases with the MR sequence or lesion presence being inserted into each of the phrases as appropriate. Example phrases are presented in Table 4.1. Variability in these text prompts may promote learning higher-level concepts such as 'prostate', 'lesion' etc. This BERT-based text prompt encoding allows us to avoid training a binary variable encoder, which may be difficult since auto-encoders have not demonstrated to be suitable to map to dimensions higher than the input as they mostly rely on bottlenecks with lower dimensions compared to the input for encoding.

Table 4.1 Examples of text prompts used

Text prompts
'A T2 image of a prostate with a lesion'
'Prostate DW image with a lesion'
'ADC image of a prostate with no lesion'
'Image of ADC prostate without lesion'

Table 4.2 Hyperparameters used for training the diffusion model which are set empirically based on experiments from [25]

Hyperparameter	Value
Diffusion steps (train)	1000
Number of parameters	396M
Channels	192
Depth	2
Channel multiplier	1, 1, 2, 2 , 4, 4
Batch size	7
Embedding dimension	512
Convergence criterion	Minimum-delta (1e-6)

4.3.1.2 Image Conditioning

For image conditioning, we use a latent representation from a trained auto-encoder as the encoder τ_γ. This is implemented as a convolutional neural network with 3 down-sampling and 3 up-sampling layers, with a 128-dimensional latent representation, which acts as our image encoding. The image encoding is used for cross-sequence translation i.e., T2W to DW.

4.3.1.3 The De-Noising Function

The de-noising function adopts a U-net architecture as in [25] with other hyper-parameters summarised in Table 4.2. The encodings for both text conditioning and image conditioning are mapped to the intermediate layers of the U-net as in [25]. As in [25], we also use compressed representations from a 'perceptual compression model' as inputs to the U-net, for computational efficiency (for further details refer to [25]).

For obtaining a sample, we iterate diffusion reversal 50 times by first generating x_T randomly, obtaining an estimate for x_0 using the reverse diffusion network and then adding back 49/50-th of the noise back. Then we repeat reverse diffusion and add back 48/50th of the noise. We run this for 50 steps until we add back 0/50-th of the noise and obtain our final sample.

4.3.2 Datasets

We used two datasets for training, a large open dataset to train the model and a smaller in-house dataset to fine-tune the model for the paired sequence translation. These datasets are described below. Even though these datasets consist of 3D images, we train all models on individual slices i.e., on slice-level 2D data, for computational/ development efficiency and for use of robust training strategies and hyper-parameter values from previous work, which may not generalise to 3D samples.

4.3.2.1 Open-Source Prostate MR Data

The PICAI dataset [26] had 1285 samples of 3D prostate MR images with both T2W and ADC available. From these, 190 were removed after a semi-manual process, due to porr quality and unclear conformity to radiological reporting standards. 10 central slices from all remaining volumes were used to form our data for training at the 2D slice-level, as these slices contain the majority of the prostate volume. 200 such patient cases were held out from training, to be used for evaluation (details in Sect. 4.3.3).

This dataset was used to generate ADC and T2W images used in Sect. 4.3.3.

4.3.2.2 Closed-Source Multi-Sequence Prostate MR Data

Multi-parametric 3D MR images were acquired from 850 patients undergoing prostate biopsy and therapy as part of trials at University College London Hospitals [1, 6, 10, 18, 22, 30]. The dataset consisted of paired T2W and DW sequences for each patient. Cancerous lesions were delineated manually by a radiologist and used to generate slice-level binary labels of lesion presence. Similar to the open dataset, 10 central slices were used for training the model on the 2D slice-level, due to the majority of the prostate volume existing within these slices. For the purpose of slice-level cancer presence, we deemed all slices with lesions visible with PIRADS ≥ 3 as containing a lesion. Similar to the open dataset, 200 patient cases were held out from training, for evaluation (details in Sect. 4.3.3).

This data was used to train the model for paired synthesis i.e., paired T2W and DW images, as described in Sect. 4.3.3. The model trained on the open-source data was fine-tuned for this dataset, rather than training from scratch.

4.3.3 Usability Study

4.3.3.1 Expert Identification of Synthesised ADC and T2W Images

The aim of this experiment is to demonstrate the realism of the synthesised images. This is done by a clinician, with 4 years experience reading prostate MR images, conducting a comparison of synthesised versus real images, without any prior knowledge of the model, images, labels and synthesis. For this experiment we used 32 2D T2W and 32 2D DW slices from the held-out set (not necessarily from the same patient). These slices had an equal ratio of real to synthetic samples, as well as positive to negative ratio for lesion presence, however, the clinician remained blind to these ratios. The clinician was asked to identify synthesised images from a mixture of real and synthetic images, regardless of lesion presence.

4.3.3.2 Expert Identification of Lesions on ADC and T2W Images

The aim of this experiment is to demonstrate the realism of lesions on synthesised images. With the same data as the above synthesised identification task, we asked the clinician to identify 2D slices that contain a suspected cancerous lesion with PIRADS ≥ 3, regardless of the images being real or synthetic.

4.3.3.3 Expert Identification of Lesions on Paired T2W-DW Images

The aim of this experiment is to demonstrate the realism of lesions on paired data, synthesised using conditional synthesis with DW images generated based on synthetic T2W. We used 32 paired T2W-DW slices, with equal ratio of real to synthetic samples, as well as positive to negative ratio for lesion presence, blind to the clinician. The clinician was asked to identify images with a suspected lesion, PIRADS ≥ 3, regardless of images being real or synthesised.

4.3.3.4 Machine Learning-Automated Lesion Detection

The aim of this experiment is to determine whether the use of synthetic data while training machine learning models aids generalisability and improves model performance. For this experiment we use an automated task of slice-level binary classification of lesion presence.

The machine learning model trained for this task is an AlexNet (4 convolutional and 4 fully connected layers). We note that based on this architecture, performance reported in Table 4.3 is consistent with those reported in similar applications, e.g. [15], therefore justifies the choice of the widely established baseline, which is also competitive in a wide variety of other tasks [14].

We trained two models for comparison, one with only real data and the other with real data augmented by synthetic samples.

For the real case, we used the closed-source dataset with train, validation and holdout sets, with 510, 170 and 170 patients, respectively, resulting in a total of 5100, 1700 and 1700 2D slices in respective sets.

For the dataset augmented with synthetic samples, we added 1600 synthesised 2D images with lesions and 1600 without to the dataset. These were added to the train and validation sets, resulting in a total of 7500, 2500 slices in each of the sets, respectively.

For comparison, the holdout set remains the same with 1700 real samples, with this set being used to report performance for both models to compare the difference between training with and without augmented synthesised images.

4.4 Results

Results for the described experiments are summarised in Table 4.3 and Fig. 4.2. Our stable diffusion model took approximately 8 days to train on a single Nvidia Tesla V100 GPU, with an average of 10 seconds for sample synthesis on the same GPU.

4.4.1 *Expert Identification of Synthesised Images*

As summarised in Table 4.3, an expert clinician was only able to identify synthesised images from a mixture of real and synthetic samples with an average accuracy of 0.594, averaged over all ADC and T2W images, where random chance is 0.500.

Table 4.3 Results for both expert clinician and machine learning model experiments, with details described in Sect. 4.3.3. 'N_{set}' indicates the set size in terms of images

Task	Data	Accuracy
Clinician—synthesised identification $N_{\text{train}} = 8950$ $N_{\text{usability study}} = 32$ T2W, 32 ADC	ADC (overall)	0.563
	ADC (w/ cancer)	0.625
	ADC (w/o cancer)	0.500
	T2W (overall)	0.625
	T2W (w/ cancer)	0.688
	T2W (w/o cancer)	0.563
Clinician—lesion identification $N_{\text{train}} = 8950$ $N_{\text{usability study}} = 32$ T2W, 32 ADC	ADC (overall)	0.688
	ADC (real)	0.625
	ADC (synthesised)	0.750
	T2W (overall)	0.594
	T2W (real)	0.625
	T2W (synthesised)	0.563
Clinician—lesion identification $N_{\text{train}} = 6500$ $N_{\text{usability study}} = 32$ T2W-DW	T2W-DW paired (overall)	0.563
	T2W-DW paired (real)	0.563
	T2W-DW paired (synthesised)	0.563
ML model—lesion identification	Trained with real	0.704 ± 0.035
	Trained with real + synthesised	0.762 ± 0.042

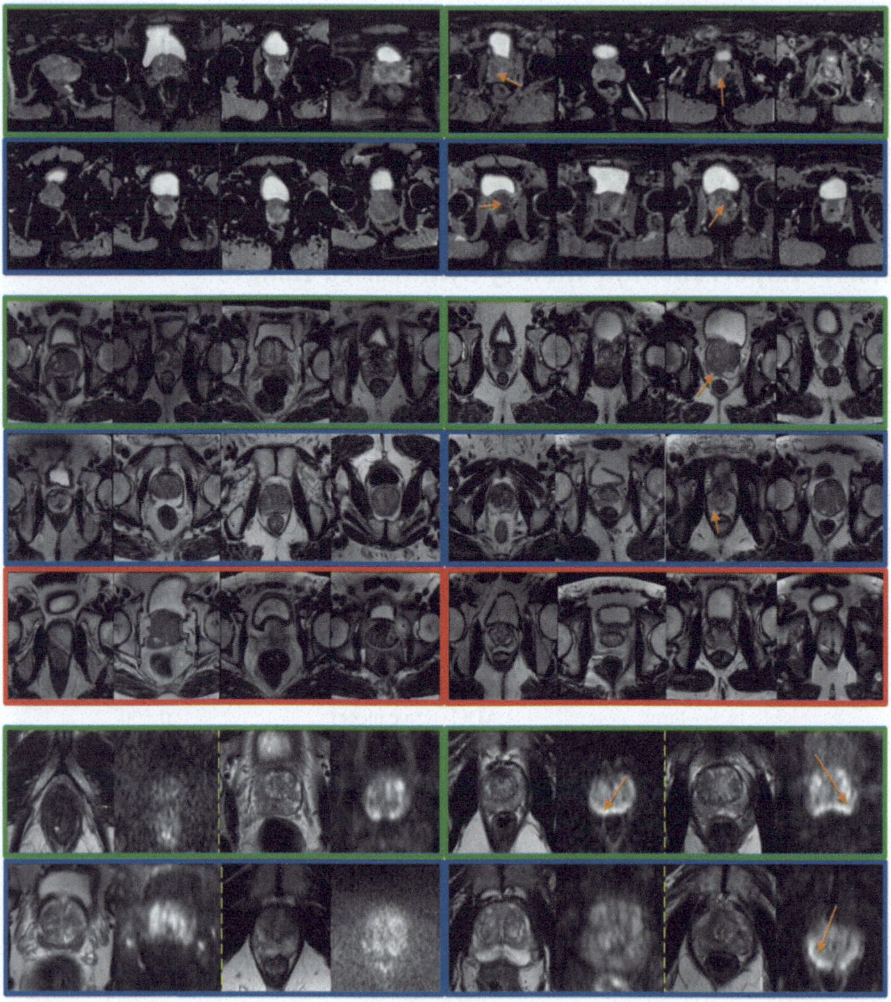

Fig. 4.2 Examples of generated and real images, with keys as follows. Blue: synthesised using DPM, Green: real, Red: synthesised using cGAN. Left: no cancer, Right: cancer (arrows indicating suspected lesions, w.r.t. PIRADS $\geq$3). Top block: ADC, middle block: T2W, Bottom block: paired T2W-DW (left-right)

4.4.2 Expert Identification of Lesions on Real Versus Synthesised Images

From Table 4.3, comparing the lesion identification accuracy, averaged over ADC, T2W and paired T2W-DWI, between real versus synthetic images, we observe similar values of 60.4% for real images versus 62.5% for synthetic images.

This means only a small difference of 2.1 percentage points between the lesion identification performance of the expert for real versus synthesised images.

4.4.3 Machine Learning-Automated Lesion Identification

Summarised in Table 4.3, we observe an improvement of 5.8 percentage points, with statistical significance (p-value=0.004), for the lesion identification task for the model trained with real data augmented with synthetic data, compared to a model trained only with real data.

4.5 Discussion

Based on the presented results, we observed: (1) only marginal improvement over random chance in the expert identification of synthesised versus real images, and (2) similar accuracy in the lesion identification between real and synthetic data. This leads us to conclude that the proposed diffusion-based image synthesis is able to effectively generate realistic synthetic samples that may enable a variety of applications including training tools for radiological or clinical trainees. Due to the paired synthesis or sequence translation, challenging radiological tasks such as DW reading following positive findings from T2W images for a transition-zone prostate lesion, have potential to be simulated using our proposed framework.

Furthermore, performance improvement in lesion identification performance using machine learning models with synthetic data versus those without, suggests a promising approach for data augmentation for clinical tasks.

Our proposed method is currently limited in terms of which areas of prostate can be synthesised since mostly central parts are synthesised by the trained network, partly due to random sampling without explicit positional conditioning. To mitigate this in future work, investigations need to be conducted into further conditioning mechanisms controlling regions of the gland to synthesise e.g., apical, peripheral etc., which are enabled by our flexible text and image-based conditioning. Additionally, investigating conditioning on cancer severity i.e., PIRADS scores would also be an additional mechanism to ensure fine-grained control over the synthetic images. These future directions would indeed be interesting for targeted sample synthesis and could potentially aid both the radiological training and automated machine learning applications discussed.

4.6 Conclusion

In this work we presented a diffusion-based image synthesis method, together with a flexible conditioning mechanism that allows generation of realistic synthetic prostate MR images, with lesion presence, MR sequence and data pairing may be controlled. Experimental findings demonstrate the utility of the presented approach for two applications of radiological training simulation as well as for data augmentation of machine learning models, to improve their task performance.

Attribution Statement

Parts of text, figures and tables in this work are borrowed or adapted from our previous paper:

Saeed, S.U., Syer, T., Yan, W., Yang, Q., Emberton, M., Punwani, S., Clarkson, M.J., Barratt, D. and Hu, Y., 2024. Bi-parametric prostate MR image synthesis using pathology and sequence-conditioned stable diffusion. Medical Imaging with Deep Learning (MIDL), in Proceedings of Machine Learning Research (PMLR), vol. 227, pp. 814–828. URL: https://proceedings.mlr.press/v227/saeed24a.html

Acknowledgments This work was supported by the EPSRC [EP/T029404/1], Wellcome/EPSRC Centre for Interventional and Surgical Sciences [203145Z/16/Z], and the International Alliance for Cancer Early Detection, an alliance between Cancer Research UK [C28070/A30912; C73666/A31378], Canary Center at Stanford University, the University of Cambridge, OHSU Knight Cancer Institute, University College London and the University of Manchester.

References

1. Bosaily AES, Parker C, Brown L, Gabe R, Hindley R, Kaplan R, Emberton M, Ahmed H, Group P, et al (2015) Promis—prostate mr imaging study: a paired validating cohort study evaluating the role of multi-parametric MRI in men with clinical suspicion of prostate cancer. Contemp Clin Trials 42:26–40
2. Chartsias A, Joyce T, Dharmakumar R, Tsaftaris SA (2017) Adversarial image synthesis for unpaired multi-modal cardiac data. In: International workshop on simulation and synthesis in medical imaging. Springer, Berlin, pp 3–13
3. Cong W, Yang J, Liu Y, Wang Y (2013) Fast and automatic ultrasound simulation from CT images. Comput Math Methods Medicine 2013:327613
4. Costa P, Galdran A, Meyer MI, Abramoff MD, Niemeijer M, Mendonça AM, Campilho A (2017) Towards adversarial retinal image synthesis. arXiv:170108974
5. Costa P, Galdran A, Meyer MI, Niemeijer M, Abràmoff M, Mendonça AM, Campilho A (2017) End-to-end adversarial retinal image synthesis. IEEE Trans Med Imag 37(3):781–791
6. Dickinson L, Ahmed HU, Kirkham A, Allen C, Freeman A, Barber J, Hindley RG, Leslie T, Ogden C, Persad R, et al (2013) A multi-centre prospective development study evaluating focal therapy using high intensity focused ultrasound for localised prostate cancer: the index study. Contemp Clin Trials 36(1):68–80
7. Frangi AF, Tsaftaris SA, Prince JL (2018) Simulation and synthesis in medical imaging. IEEE Trans Med Imag 37(3):673–679

8. Frid-Adar M, Klang E, Amitai M, Goldberger J, Greenspan H (2018) Synthetic data augmentation using gan for improved liver lesion classification. In: 2018 IEEE 15th international symposium on biomedical imaging (ISBI 2018), IEEE, Piscataway, pp 289–293
9. Guibas JT, Virdi TS, Li PS (2017) Synthetic medical images from dual generative adversarial networks. arXiv:170901872
10. Hamid S, Donaldson IA, Hu Y, Rodell R, Villarini B, Bonmati E, Tranter P, Punwani S, Sidhu HS, Willis S, et al (2019) The smarttarget biopsy trial: a prospective, within-person randomised, blinded trial comparing the accuracy of visual-registration and magnetic resonance imaging/ultrasound image-fusion targeted biopsies for prostate cancer risk stratification. Eur Urol 75(5):733–740
11. Ho J, Jain A, Abbeel P (2020) Denoising diffusion probabilistic models. Adv Neural Inf Process Syst 33:6840–6851
12. Isola P, Zhu JY, Zhou T, Efros AA (2017) Image-to-image translation with conditional adversarial networks. In: Proceedings of the IEEE conference on computer vision and pattern recognition, pp 1125–1134
13. Kazeminia S, Baur C, Kuijper A, van Ginneken B, Navab N, Albarqouni S, Mukhopadhyay A (2020) Gans for medical image analysis. Artif Intell Med 109:101938. https://doi.org/10.1016/j.artmed.2020.101938. https://www.sciencedirect.com/science/article/pii/S0933365719311510
14. Krizhevsky A, Sutskever I, Hinton G (2012) Imagenet classification with deep convolutional neural networks. NeurIPS
15. Kwon D, dos Reis IM, Breto AL, Tschudi Y, Gautney N, Zavala-Romero O, Lopez C, Ford JC, Punnen S, Pollack A, Stoyanova R (2018) Classification of suspicious lesions on prostate multiparametric MRI using machine learning. J Med Imag 5:034502
16. Li Q, Yu Z, Wang Y, Zheng H (2020) Tumorgan: a multi-modal data augmentation framework for brain tumor segmentation. Sensors 20(15):4203
17. Li X, Jiang Y, Rodríguez-Andina JJ, Luo H, Yin S, Kaynak O (2021) When medical images meet generative adversarial network: recent development and research opportunities. Discov Artif Intell 1:5
18. Linch M, Goh G, Hiley C, Shanmugabavan Y, McGranahan N, Rowan A, Wong Y, King H, Furness A, Freeman A, et al (2017) Intratumoural evolutionary landscape of high-risk prostate cancer: the progeny study of genomic and immune parameters. Ann Oncol 28(10):2472–2480
19. Mukherkjee D, Saha P, Kaplun D, Sinitca A, Sarkar R (2022) Brain tumor image generation using an aggregation of gan models with style transfer. Sci Rep 12(1):1–16
20. Nichol AQ, Dhariwal P (2021) Improved denoising diffusion probabilistic models. In: International conference on machine learning. Proceedings of machine learning research, pp 8162–8171
21. Nie D, Trullo R, Lian J, Petitjean C, Ruan S, Wang Q, Shen D (2017) Medical image synthesis with context-aware generative adversarial networks. In: International conference on medical image computing and computer-assisted intervention. Springer, Berlin, pp 417–425
22. Orczyk C, Barratt D, Brew-Graves C, Peng Hu Y, Freeman A, McCartan N, Potyka I, Ramachandran N, Rodell R, Williams NR, et al (2021) Prostate radiofrequency focal ablation (proraft) trial: a prospective development study evaluating a bipolar radiofrequency device to treat prostate cancer. J Urol 205(4):1090–1099
23. Ramalhinho J, Koo B, Montaña-Brown N, Saeed SU, Bonmati E, Gurusamy K, Pereira SP, Davidson B, Hu Y, Clarkson MJ (2022) Deep hashing for global registration of untracked 2d laparoscopic ultrasound to CT. Int J Comput Assist Radiol Surg 17(8):1461–1468
24. Ramesh A, Dhariwal P, Nichol A, Chu C, Chen M (2022) Hierarchical text-conditional image generation with clip latents. arXiv:220406125
25. Rombach R, Blattmann A, Lorenz D, Esser P, Ommer B (2022) High-resolution image synthesis with latent diffusion models. In: Proceedings of the IEEE/CVF conference on computer vision and pattern recognition, pp 10684–10695

26. Saha A, Bosma J, Twilt J, van Ginneken B, Yakar D, Elschot M, Veltman J, Fütterer J, de Rooij M (2023, April) Artificial intelligence and radiologists at prostate cancer detection in mri-the pi-cai challenge. In: International Conference on Medical Imaging with Deep Learning (MIDL) 2023, short paper track. https://openreview.net/forum?id=XfXcA9-0XxR
27. Saharia C, Chan W, Saxena S, Li L, Whang J, Denton E, Ghasemipour SKS, Ayan BK, Mahdavi SS, Lopes RG, et al (2022) Photorealistic text-to-image diffusion models with deep language understanding. arXiv:220511487
28. Saxena D, Cao J (2021) Generative adversarial networks (gans) challenges, solutions, and future directions. ACM Comput Surv 54(3):1–42
29. Shams R, Hartley R, Navab N (2008) Real-time simulation of medical ultrasound from ct images. In: International conference on medical image computing and computer-assisted intervention. Springer, Berlin, pp 734–741
30. Simmons LA, Kanthabalan A, Arya M, Briggs T, Barratt D, Charman SC, Freeman A, Hawkes D, Hu Y, Jameson C, et al (2018) Accuracy of transperineal targeted prostate biopsies, visual estimation and image fusion in men needing repeat biopsy in the picture trial. J Urol 200(6):1227–1234
31. Singh NK, Raza K (2021) Medical image generation using generative adversarial networks: a review. In: Health informatics: a computational perspective in healthcare. Springer, Berlin, pp 77–96
32. Skandarani Y, Jodoin PM, Lalande A (2021) Gans for medical image synthesis: an empirical study. ArXiv abs/2105.05318
33. Wolterink JM, Dinkla AM, Savenije MH, Seevinck PR, van den Berg CA, Išgum I (2017) Deep MR to CT synthesis using unpaired data. In: International workshop on simulation and synthesis in medical imaging. Springer, Berlin, pp 14–23
34. Wolterink JM, Leiner T, Viergever MA, Išgum I (2017) Generative adversarial networks for noise reduction in low-dose CT. IEEE Trans Med Imag 36(12):2536–2545
35. Zhao H, Li H, Cheng L (2017) Synthesizing filamentary structured images with gans. arXiv:170602185

Part II
Detection and Classification

Chapter 5
Analyzing Tumors by Synthesis

Qi Chen, Yuxiang Lai, Xiaoxi Chen, Qixin Hu, Alan Yuille, and Zongwei Zhou

Abstract Computer-aided tumor detection has shown great potential in enhancing the interpretation of over 80 million CT scans performed annually in the United States. However, challenges arise due to the rarity of CT scans with tumors, especially early-stage tumors. Developing AI with real tumor data faces issues of scarcity, annotation difficulty, and low prevalence. Tumor synthesis addresses these challenges by generating numerous tumor examples in medical images, aiding AI training for tumor detection and segmentation. Successful synthesis requires realistic and generalizable synthetic tumors across various organs. This chapter reviews AI development on real and synthetic data and summarizes two key trends in synthetic data for cancer imaging research: modeling-based and learning-based approaches. Modeling-based methods, like Pixel2Cancer, simulate tumor development over time using generic rules, while learning-based methods, like DiffTumor, learn from a few annotated examples in one organ to generate synthetic tumors in others. Reader studies with expert radiologists show that synthetic tumors can be convincingly realistic. We also present case studies in the liver, pancreas, and kidneys reveal that AI trained on synthetic tumors can achieve performance

Q. Chen
University of Chinese Academy of Sciences, Beijing, China
e-mail: chenqi24@ucas.ac.cn

Y. Lai
Emory University, Atlanta, GA, USA
e-mail: ylai76@emory.edu

X. Chen
University of Illinois Urbana-Champaign, Champaign, IL, USA
e-mail: xiaoxic3@illinois.edu

Q. Hu
University of Southern California, Los Angeles, CA, USA
e-mail: qixinhu@usc.edu

A. Yuille · Z. Zhou (✉)
Johns Hopkins University, Baltimore, MD, USA
e-mail: ayuille1@jhu.edu; zzhou82@jh.edu

L. Zhang et al. (eds.), *Generative Machine Learning Models in Medical Image Computing*, https://doi.org/10.1007/978-3-031-80965-1_5

comparable to, or better than, AI only trained on real data. Tumor synthesis holds significant promise for expanding datasets, enhancing AI reliability, improving tumor detection performance, and preserving patient privacy.

5.1 Introduction

Medical image analysis aims to derive detailed information non-invasively about a patient's medical condition, including the disease's origin, precise location, and its relationship with adjacent tissues. Specifically, for symptoms that cannot be directly diagnosed, medical professionals employ various imaging devices to capture detailed images of target organs for disease screening, diagnosis, and treatment. Therefore, medical imaging systems generate vast amounts of medical image data daily. This data may encompass different organs of the body, as well as tissues and pathological regions associated with diseases.

Medical images come from modalities like X-ray, CT, MRI, and PET. This data, referred to as **real data** in this chapter, can be analyzed using post-processing and artificial intelligence (AI) to reveal details not visible to the naked eye, aiding in disease detection such as detecting tumors at their early stage. However, managing real-world data for AI-driven diagnostics is challenging. **Synthetic data** offers a promising alternative, potentially allowing AI to generalize better to real-world scenarios and overcome the difficulties of using real data for training. Generally, synthetic data refer to artificially generated data that mimic the characteristics and structure of real data without being directly derived from actual observations (Fig. 5.1).

5.1.1 Why Synthetic Data?

Synthetic data are vital in AI research due to the challenges of acquiring real data, including time constraints, high costs, patient privacy concerns, and manual effort [24, 31, 32, 122]. They provide significant advantages by saving time and reducing the need for extensive manual annotation. The use of AI-generated content (AIGC) has proven effective across various domains, including medical imaging, where it serves both as a training resource for AI models and as a means of evaluating their performance with realistic yet hard-to-obtain data (see Table 5.1). Synthetic data offer precise control over properties such as shape, texture, and location, which is particularly valuable in medical applications. This control enables the creation of diverse and representative datasets for model training and provides useful examples for medical education and patient communication. Additionally, controllable synthetic tumors facilitate AI debugging and model diagnostics, enhancing the interpretability of AI behavior. Increasing evidence supports that synthetic data can

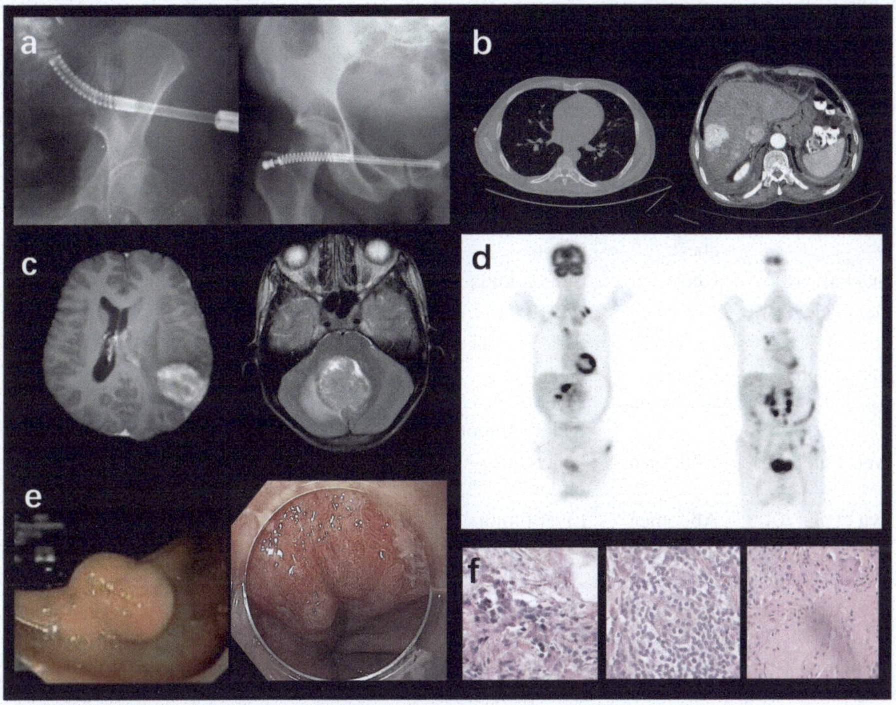

Fig. 5.1 *Can you distinguish synthetic data from real data in different modalities?* (**a**) X-ray image examples [26]. (**b**) CT image examples [33]. (**c**) MR image examples [78]. (**d**) PET image example. (**e**) Endoscopy image example [64]. (**f**) Histopathology image example [4]

improve AI performance, making it a powerful tool for advancing research and improving outcomes in fields like oncology.

5.1.2 Real vs. Synthetic Data

Unlike real data, which are collected from real-world imaging devices and represent true observations, synthetic data are created using algorithms, simulations, or models designed to replicate the properties of real data. We summarize the differences between real data and synthetic data as follows: *First*, real data are collected from actual imaging devices (e.g., X-ray, CT, MRI, PET, ultrasound, histopathology). Synthetic data are generated artificially using computational methods and simulations [43, 59]. *Second*, real data are often limited by practical constraints such as patient privacy, the cost of imaging, and the time required for data collection and annotation [13]. Synthetic data can be produced in large quantities without the ethical and logistical issues associated with real data collection [10]. *Third*, real data require manual annotation by experts, which is time-consuming [77] and prone to

Table 5.1 A summary of existing synthesis methods for medical imaging encompasses various aspects: body part, disease type, imaging modality, dataset utilized, and generative model type. Additionally, we are maintaining a webpage to track the latest publications and corresponding code repositories on data synthesis in medicine more comprehensively

Reference	Body part	Disease	Modality	Dataset	Generative model
Teixeira et al. [97]	Whole body	Anomaly detection	X-ray	Private dataset	GAN
Wu et al. [107]	Chest	Breast cancer	X-ray	DDSM [37]	GAN
Gao et al. [26]	Bone & chest	COVID-19 lesion	X-ray	COVID-19 CXR [101]	GAN
Jin et al. [48]	Chest	Lung nodule	CT	LIDC [3]	GAN
Yao et al. [113]	Chest	COVID-19	CT	LUNA16 [87]	Hand-crafted designs
Jiang et al. [47]	Chest	Covid-19	CT	COVID [112]	GAN
Jin et al. [49]	Abdomen	Liver & Kidney tumors	CT	LiTS [8] & KiTS [38]	GAN
Wei et al. [105]	Abdomen	Pancreatic tumors	CT	Private dataset	GAN
Lyu et al. [70]	Abdomen	Liver tumors	CT	LiTS [8]	GAN
Hu et al. [43]	Abdomen	Liver tumors	CT	LiTS [8]	Hand-crafted designs
Li et al. [63]	Abdomen	Pancreatic tumors	CT	MSD [2]	Hand-crafted designs
Chen et al. [9]	Abdomen	Tumors in liver, pancreas and kidney	CT	MSD [2] & KiTS [38]	Diffusion model
Lai et al. [59]	Abdomen	Tumors in liver, pancreas and kidney	CT	MSD [2] & KiTS [38]	Hand-crafted designs
Yu et al. [117]	Brain	Brain tumors	MRI	BraTS [72]	GAN
Han et al. [34]	Brain	Brain tumors	MRI	BraTS [72]	GAN
Zhao et al. [119]	Abdomen	Liver tumors	MRI	Private dataset	GAN
Mukherkjee et al. [73]	Brain	Brain tumors	MRI	BraTS [72]	GAN
Basaran et al. [6]	Brain	Brain tumors	MRI	WMH [54]	Hand-crafted designs
Wang et al. [103]	Brain	–	PET	Private dataser	GAN
Luo et al. [69]	Brain	–	PET	Private dataset	GAN
Sharan et al. [88]	Mitral valve	Landmark detection	Endo.	surgical simulator [23]	GAN
Yoon et al. [116]	Colon	Polyp detection	Endo.	Private dataset	GAN
Hou et al. [41]	Tissue	Cancer	Histo.	Kumar [55]	GAN
Xue et al. [110]	Tissue	Cancer	Histo.	PCam [100]	GAN
Aversa et al. [4]	Tissue	Cancer	Histo.	Private dataset	Diffusion Model
Du et al. [19]	Skin	Dermatoscopic lesion	Dermo.	ISIC [17]	Diffusion model

GAN stands for Generative Adversarial Network
Endo. refers to Endoscopy, Histo. refers to Histopathology, and Dermo. refers to dermoscopy.

human error [65]. Annotations of synthetic data can be automatically generated as part of the data creation process, ensuring consistency and accuracy [80].

5.2 Detecting Real Tumors in CT Scans

5.2.1 Tumors in Solid Organs

Solid tumors in organs like the liver, kidneys, and brain—such as hepatocellular carcinoma, renal cell carcinoma, and glioma—typically show well-defined margins and growth patterns [85], illustrated in Fig. 5.2. In CT images, early-stage tumors appear as small nodules with slightly blurred edges and homogeneous texture.

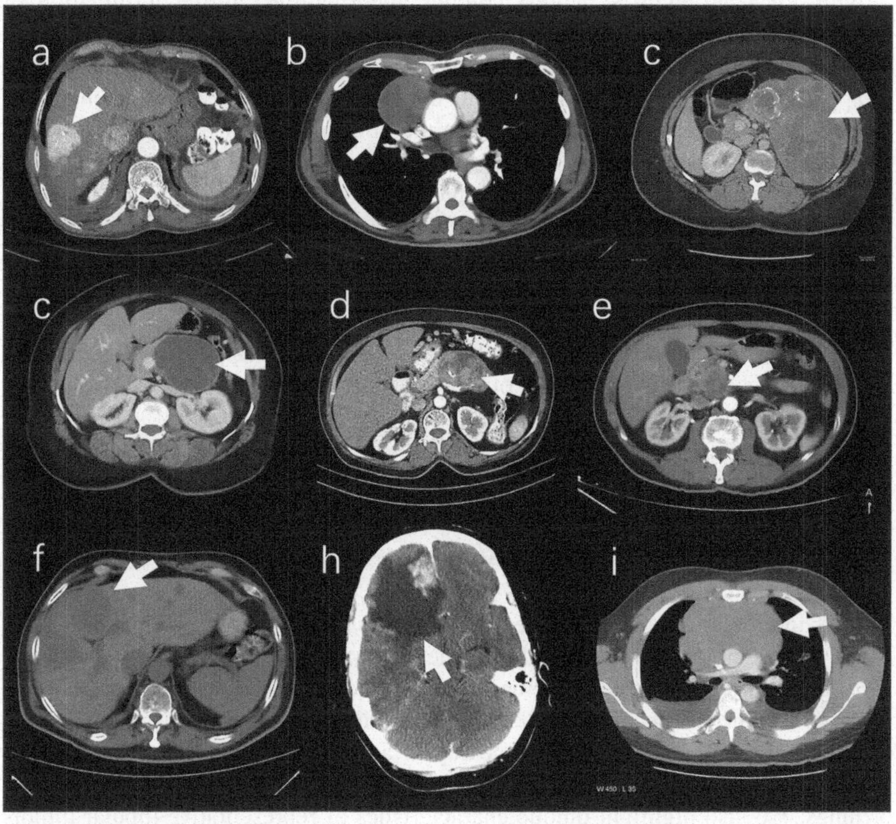

Fig. 5.2 Tumors in solid organs. (**a**) Hepatocellular carcinoma. (**b**) Thymoma. (**c**) Solid pseudopapillary tumor of the pancreas. (**d**) Pancreatic mucinous cystadenoma. (**e**) Pancreatic mucinous cystadenocarcinoma. (**f**) Pancreatic adenocarcinoma. (**g**) Neuroendocrine tumor in liver. (**h**) Meningioma. (**i**) Mediastinal lymphoma

As tumors advance, they grow larger, become irregular in shape, and exhibit significant mass effect and infiltrative growth [20]. Advanced tumors may also show hemorrhage, necrosis, and fibrosis, leading to a heterogeneous appearance [89].

- **Liver tumors:** Hepatocellular carcinoma (HCC) is the most common malignant liver tumor. Early HCC presents as a small, well-differentiated nodule with a good prognosis and low metastatic potential [25]. CT imaging may show mass effect extending beyond the liver, displacement of blood vessels, intrahepatic venous thrombosis, and bile duct obstruction [82]. HCCs often exhibit intense arterial-phase enhancement due to neoangiogenesis and reduced portal triads, and typically appear hypoattenuating on venous phase scans [5].
- **Pancreatic tumors:** Pancreatic ductal adenocarcinoma (PDAC) constitutes the majority of malignant pancreatic tumors and is associated with a very poor prognosis and high morbidity. In the early stages, PDACs typically appear as homogeneous small nodules with blurred edges. Secondary findings associated with advanced PDACs include contour abnormalities, abrupt termination of the biliary or pancreatic duct, pancreatic atrophy upstream from the mass, vascular encasement, etc. [57]. PDACs typically exhibit poor enhancement, appearing hypoattenuating relative to the surrounding pancreatic parenchyma. This hypoenhancement is attributed to the development of a dense fibroblastic stromal component in PDACs [22].
- **Kidney tumors:** Renal cell carcinoma (RCC) is the most common adult renal epithelial cancer, accounting for more than 90% of all renal malignancies [61]. The most prevalent subtype, clear cell RCC, presents as a homogeneously enhancing lesion during the corticomedullary phase and as a hypoattenuating renal lesion surrounded by homogenously enhancing renal parenchyma in the nephrographic phase. Advanced clear cell RCC often appears heterogeneous in imaging due to the presence of hemorrhage, necrosis, and cysts, along with invasion into the renal pelvis, perirenal fat, or renal vessels [104].

5.2.2 Tumors in Tubular Organs

Tumors in tubular organs, illustrated in Fig. 5.3, have distinct growth patterns [74]: exophytic, where the tumor expands into the lumen, and invasive, where it penetrates the organ wall into adjacent structures. For instance, colon cancer progresses from stage 0, confined to the lining, to stage I, invading the submucosa, and stage II, extending through the wall without nearby invasion [21]. Stage III involves spread to lymph nodes, and stage IV features metastasis to distant organs such as the liver or lungs. We also highlight unique characteristics of representative tubular tumors to illustrate their specific behaviors and progression.

- **Esophageal tumors**, though rare, have a poor prognosis if malignant unless detected early and surgically removed [45]. Imaging studies include X-ray

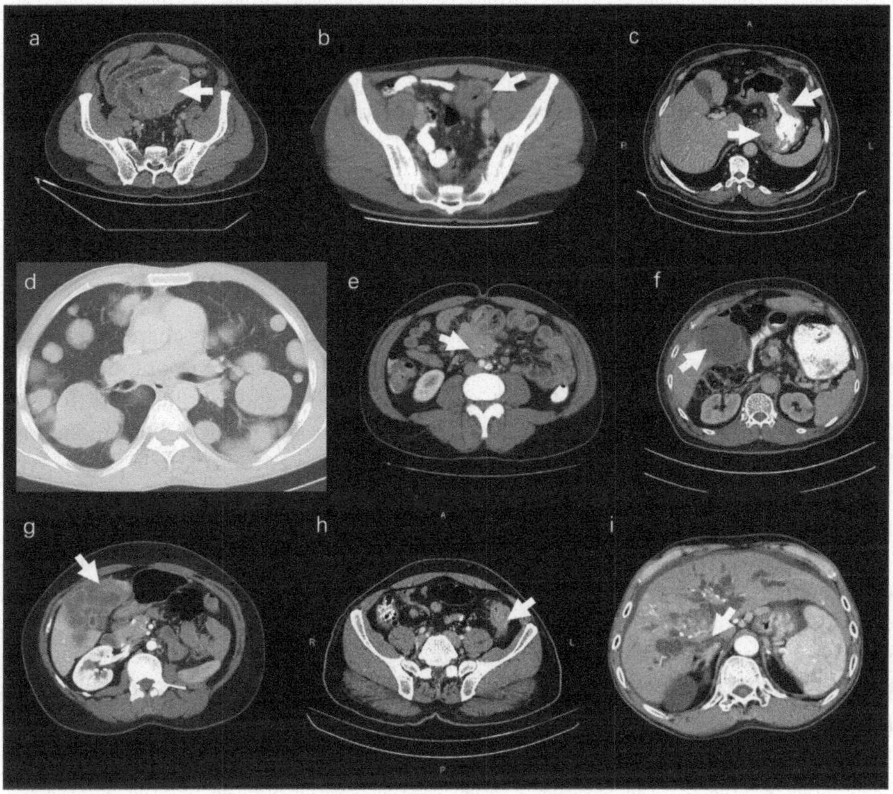

Fig. 5.3 Tumors in tubular organs. (**a**) Gastrointestinal stromal tumor. (**b**) Sigmoid colon cancer. (**c**) Gastric cancer. (**d**) Lung metastases. (**e**) Intestinal carcinoid tumor. (**f**) Gallbladder carcinoma. (**g**) Gallbladder adenocarcinoma. (**h**) Colon cancer. (**i**) Cholangiocarcinoma

esophagography, CT, endoscopic ultrasound, and PET. Malignant strictures often show asymmetric narrowing with abrupt margins and irregular, nodular, or ulcerated surfaces. X-ray esophagography helps evaluate invasion of the muscularis mucosae for early-stage cancers. Key CT features are eccentric or circumferential wall thickening over 5 mm and periesophageal soft tissue and fat stranding [62, 94].

- **Stomach tumors**, primarily adenocarcinoma, are common and often asymptomatic when superficial. Up to 50% of patients may have nonspecific gastrointestinal symptoms like dyspepsia. Endoscopy is the most sensitive method for diagnosis, allowing direct visualization and biopsy. Initial detection is often through radiological methods, with CT imaging using negative contrast to reveal common features such as polypoid masses, wall thickening, or ulceration [18, 62, 93].
- **Colorectal tumors** are a leading gastrointestinal malignancy. Contrast-enhanced CT of the chest, abdomen, and pelvis is used for staging, detecting metastases,

evaluating surgical options, and assessing treatment response. Colorectal cancers typically appear as soft tissue masses that narrow the bowel lumen. Larger tumors often show ulceration, mucinous tumors may appear as low-density masses with low-density lymph nodes, and psammomatous calcifications can be seen in mucinous adenocarcinoma [30, 92].

5.2.3 High Similarity in Early-Stage Tumors

Early-stage tumors ($< 2\,\text{cm}$) frequently exhibit similar imaging characteristics in CT scans, regardless of whether they originate in the liver, pancreas, or kidneys [12]. Should this finding be validated, it could carry profound implications for the application of generative AI in medical imaging. This implies that both modeling-based and learning-based approaches could be developed on a single tumor type with readily available annotated data and subsequently applied to synthesize various tumor types in other organs, for which data/annotation acquisition is more arduous.

A study involving three expert radiologists was conducted to assess their ability to recognize the organ class of early-stage cancers [9]. Three expert radiologists, certified in accordance with the Quality Standards Act, participated in the reader study. Recognition results are presented in Fig. 5.4b. The results were sufficiently compelling that medical professionals, boasting over five years of experience, could potentially mistake the synthetic tumors for genuine ones. The precision and recall scores, which approximate randomness, imply that the similarity in the appearance of early-stage tumors is such that even seasoned radiologists encounter difficulties when attempting to distinguish the organ types of these tumors.

The similarity of early-stage tumors can be evidenced by their Radiomics Feature[1] profiles [9]. From a *qualitative* standpoint, Fig. 5.4a depicts the feature mapping in a two-dimensional space via *t*-SNE. The appearance features of early-stage tumors manifest within a joint feature space, with no discernible segregation among different organ types. From a *quantitative* perspective, we trained a support vector machine (SVM) classifier to identify the organ types of early-stage tumors. To infer a general conclusion, we conducted ten repeated experiments and computed the precision and recall metrics of the SVM classifier for both the training and test sets. The final results indicate that both the precision and recall metrics for the training set are close to 1.0, demonstrating that the SVM is effectively trained and has established a robust decision boundary for the training set. However, the precision scores for the test set approximate random chance, as illustrated in

[1] Utilization of the official radiomics feature repository [99] enables the extraction of appearance features, comprising 3D shape-based features, gray level co-occurrence matrix, gray level run length matrix, gray level size zone matrix, neighboring gray-tone difference matrix, and gray level dependence matrix.

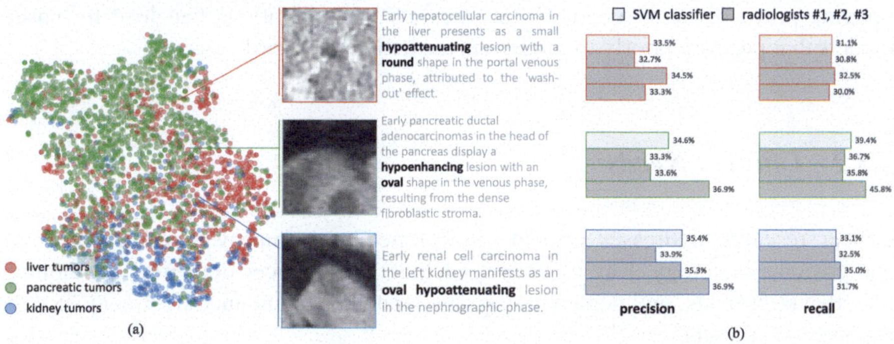

Fig. 5.4 *Feature analysis and reader study.* The left panel features a t-SNE (t-distributed stochastic neighbor embedding) visualization that maps the multidimensional Radiomics features of tumors from the liver, pancreas, and kidneys onto a two-dimensional space. This visualization underscores the substantial overlap in features among early-stage tumors from different organs, which may contribute to the challenges in correctly identifying their organ types. Complementing these findings, this study evaluates the efficacy of a support vector machine (SVM) classifier, which utilizes Radiomics Features [16, 102], in differentiating the organ types for the cropped tumors. The SVM classifier is trained to classify each tumor as originating from either the liver, pancreas, or kidneys—a three-way classification challenge. Parallel to the assessment of the SVM classifier, three expert radiologists conducted a similar evaluation by reviewing the original CT scans containing these tumors. The results displayed on the right panel reveal significant difficulties faced by both the SVM classifier and the radiologists when it comes to accurately pinpointing the origin of early-stage tumors. The precision and recall metrics for both the machine and human methods approximate the performance expected from random selection. (**a**) Feature analysis. (**b**) Reader studies

Fig. 5.4b. This implies that even an effectively trained SVM classifier encounters difficulty in recognizing the organ types of unseen early-stage tumors.

5.3 Technical Barriers and Clinical Needs

5.3.1 Technical Barriers

AI development for real tumors faces key technical barriers: First, **data scarcity**: High-performance models need extensive annotated data, which is limited due to the time and expertise required for medical image and genomic annotation. Rare cancers further exacerbate this issue, leading to poor model performance on less common types [14, 96, 120, 121]. Second, **generalization to different organs**: AI models struggle to generalize across organs due to distinct anatomical structures and imaging modalities. Models trained on one organ, like the lung, perform poorly on others, such as the liver, due to differing tissue compositions and imaging techniques [68, 118]. Third, **generalization to different demographics**: Privacy laws restrict access to diverse datasets, impacting model robustness. Variations in imaging protocols and genetic differences across populations can lead to biased models that perform poorly on underrepresented groups [66].

5.3.2 Clinical Needs

Cancer research addresses critical clinical needs to improve patient outcomes and advance oncology. Key objectives include early cancer detection, developing effective treatments, and personalizing care strategies to enhance treatment success and system efficiency.

Early Detection and Diagnosis Early detection and diagnosis of cancer are crucial for improving patient outcomes, as identifying cancer at an early stage often leads to more effective treatment and better survival rates. There is a critical need for screening methods with high sensitivity (ability to correctly identify those with cancer) and high specificity (ability to correctly identify those without cancer). Improved accuracy reduces false positives and false negatives, which are common issues in current screening practices. Besides, enhanced accuracy can help avoid overdiagnosis, where non-life-threatening cancers are treated unnecessarily, causing undue stress and potential harm to patients.

Health System Efficiency For effective training in tumor detection across multiple organs, AI models traditionally require numerous annotated real tumor examples from each organ [51, 67, 79, 123]. However, these AI models often face difficulties in generalizing their ability to interpret images from different hospitals, a challenge compounded by varying imaging protocols, patient demographics, and scanner manufacturers [75, 111]. While the challenge of domain generalization could be alleviated if the AI is trained on a considerable number of annotated data from various domains [109, 114], it could take up to 25 human years for just annotating tumors in a specific organ [1, 108]. Collecting and annotating a comprehensive dataset that includes tumor examples from several organs (N) and numerous hospitals (M) is a formidable task, denoted by the complexity ($N \times M$). We hypothesize that *tumor synthesis could address this challenge by creating various tumor types across non-tumor images from multiple hospitals, even if only one type of tumor is available and annotated.* This approach can simplify the complexity from $N \times M$ to $1 \times M$.

Personalized Treatment Planning Tumors within the same type of cancer can vary significantly at the genetic and molecular levels. Personalized treatment planning requires comprehensive genomic profiling to identify specific mutations, gene expression patterns, and other molecular characteristics that drive an individual's cancer. This information helps in selecting targeted therapies that are more likely to be effective for that particular tumor profile. Understanding the diversity of cancer cells within a tumor can inform treatment strategies that target multiple pathways and cell populations simultaneously.

5.4 Technology Trend I: Modeling-Based Approaches

Hand-crafted tumor synthesis has been conducted in [42–44, 63]. This approach applies a sequence of hand-crafted morphological image-processing operations, including local selection, texture generation, shape generation, and post-processing, to generate realistic tumors for training AI models. The intrinsic observation about these operations is clinical knowledge. Taking liver tumors as an example, the mean HU intensity of hepatocellular carcinomas (tumors grown from liver cells) was 106 HU (with a range of 36–162 HU) [60]. Milder carcinomas usually lead to smaller, fewer spherical lesions, while multi-focal lesions (which means scattered small tumors) only appear in rare cases. Additionally, larger tumors usually display evident mass effects and are accompanied by capsule appearances that separate the tumor from the liver parenchyma [71]. This medical guidance, together with visual clues, determines the parameters and pipeline of this method.

Cellular Automata are computational models used to simulate complex systems through simple rules and interactions. They employ a grid of cells (pixels), where each cell is initially assigned a state between zero and ten to represent the tumor population. The basic element is the *cell*, which refers to a single *pixel* in the computed tomography (CT) image. Tumor growth and behavior are modeled based on specific rules that simulate processes such as proliferation, invasion, and death. These rules are derived from medical knowledge and are guided by an idealized tumor model that reflects real-world characteristics. The tumor state can then be integrated into the original CT images to generate synthetic tumors in different organs. This tumor synthesis approach allows for sampling tumors at various stages and analyzing tumor-organ interactions. Motivated by this, Lai et al. [59] proposed Pixel2Cancer to simulate tumor growth (Fig. 5.6). Tumors generated by Pixel2Cancer are illustrated in Fig. 5.5.

5.4.1 Property of Pixel2Cancer

(i) **Label-free.** Pixel2Cancer can be applied as a label-free data synthesis approach, eliminating the need for manual per-voxel annotation. Previous learning-based approaches, such as GANs [28] and Diffusion models [40], are

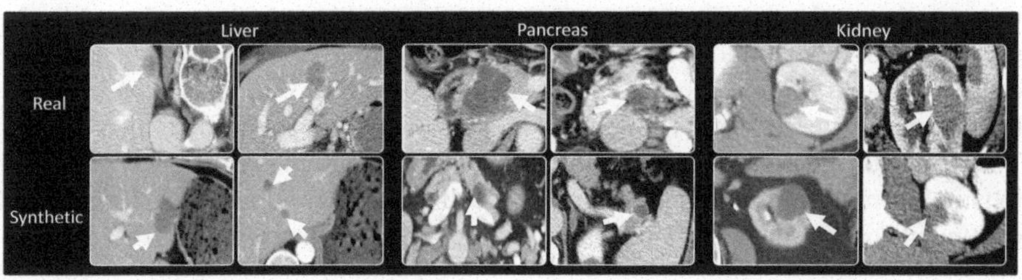

Fig. 5.5 Synthetic liver, pancreatic, and kidney tumors generated by Cellular Automata [59]

designed to learn the representation and distribution of tumors. While these approaches excel in generating natural images, synthesizing tumors in CT scans still requires significant amounts of paired tumor data. Moreover, when generating synthetic tumors, generative models also need masks to indicate the tumor locations and shapes [49], necessitating extensive manual efforts for training and synthesis.

(ii) **Tumor development.** Pixel2Cancer incorporates specific medical knowledge regarding tumor growth and appearance, enabling the simulation of realistic tumors. None of the existing synthetic approaches can adequately simulate tumor development in abdominal CT, and the primary challenges in current synthetic methods are the proliferation and invasion of tumors [36]. These processes in tumor growth are complex and interconnected, highly influenced by the surrounding environment [95, 106]. Consequently, synthetic tumors generated using current methods may conflict with normal organ structures and pose challenges when adapting them to different organs.

(iii) **Early tumor detection and boundary segmentation.** Early detection of small tumors is critical for timely cancer diagnosis. However, real datasets often lack sufficient instances due to the asymptomatic nature of early-stage patients. Pixel2Cancer can generate more small tumors to improve the sensitivity of segmentation models for small tumor detection. Additionally, Pixel2Cancer generates synthetic tumors with precise tumor masks, whereas real data annotations are often inaccurate at the boundaries, leading to *label noise* in boundary segmentation accuracy.

5.4.2 Clinical Perspectives

Tumors and genetic disorders from DNA mutations in single cells undergo complex growth processes [56]. Mutations during cell division lead to uncontrolled proliferation, forming neoplastic lesions that can be benign or malignant [27]. While both types follow similar growth principles, they differ in growth rate and invasiveness. Malignant tumors often grow rapidly, secreting growth factors or inducing surrounding stromal cells to do so, as seen in pancreatic IPMN lesions which grow larger and faster than benign ones [50]. Slow growth rates in renal tumors and hepatocellular carcinoma correlate with lower malignancy [91]. Malignant tumors are invasive, gradually penetrating and destroying surrounding tissues, whereas benign tumors remain confined to their original sites. Even slowly growing malignant tumors can infiltrate neighboring structures. Tumor necrosis, caused by rapid proliferation exceeding vascular supply [39], appears as irregular hypo-attenuating areas in CT images and serves as a poor prognostic indicator [25]. The **death** rule models this necrosis. A hybrid cellular automaton model is proposed to simulate tumor development from single cells to invasive tumors, capturing their continuous progression and interactions within the microenvironment (Fig. 5.6).

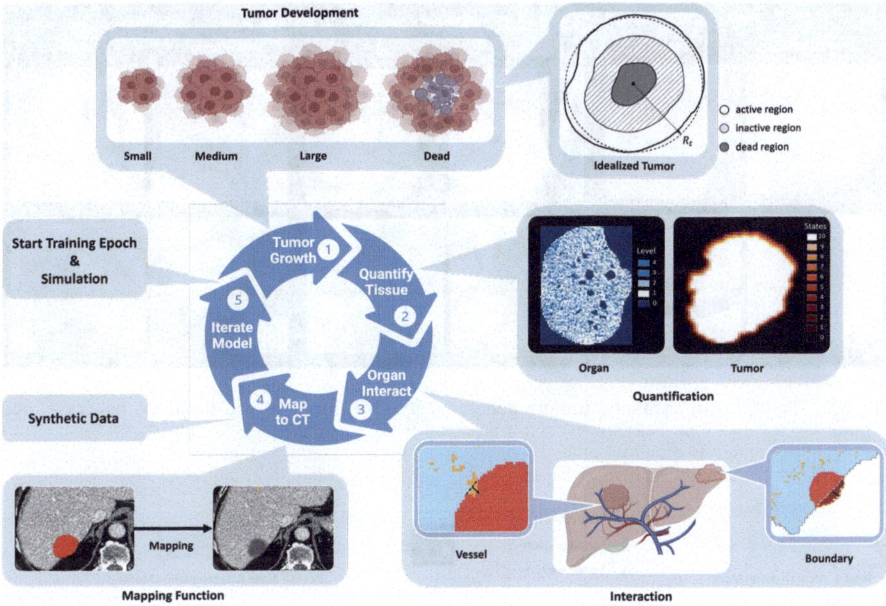

Fig. 5.6 ① Tumor development: The cellular automata simulate tumor growth from a single pixel to various sizes and even tumor death, producing synthetic tumors with diverse sizes, shapes, and textures. An idealized tumor is created to quantify development, with dead cells in the gray region, living quiescent cells in the inactive region, and proliferative cells in the active outer shell. ② Tissue quantification: The organ map in blue transforms CT images into distinct intensity levels affecting tumor development rate, while the red tumor map assigns values representing the tumor cell population. ③ Tumor interaction with boundaries and vessels: The tumor grows and exerts pressure against organ boundaries and deforms as it interacts with vessels. ④ Mapping synthetic tumors to CT images: A mapping function correlates the synthetic tumor with CT values, integrating the tumor's state with the original CT intensity. ⑤ Training segmentation models with synthetic data: Pixel2Cancer generates new synthetic data for each epoch to train the segmentation model

5.5 Technology Trend II: Learning-Based Approaches

Generative Adversarial Networks (GANs) [29] have been extensively explored for generating synthetic tumors. Zhao et al. [119] introduced Tripartite-GAN, which simultaneously achieves contrast-enhanced magnetic resonance imaging synthesis and tumor detection. Mukherkjee et al. [73] proposed AGGrGAN to generate synthetic MRI scans of brain tumors. However, the training process of GANs is often unstable, making it challenging to achieve convergence. Additionally, GANs can suffer from issues such as mode collapse, where the model generates limited diversity in outputs.

Diffusion Models [52, 76] provide more stable and reliable training compared to GANs, as they gradually denoise data, making the optimization process easier to control. Additionally, Diffusion Models are capable of generating high-quality,

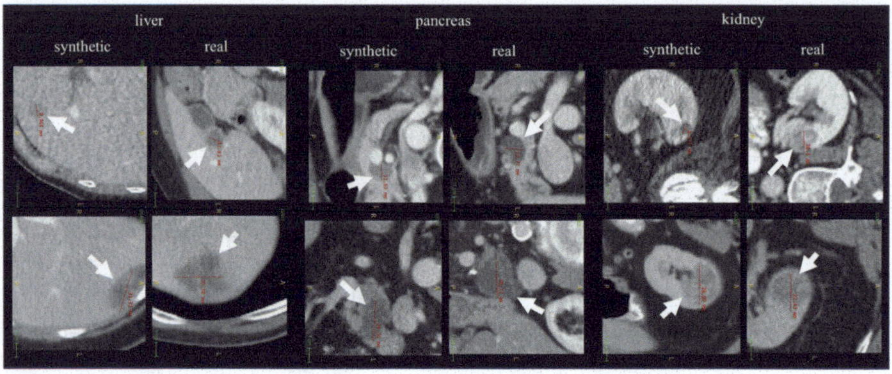

Fig. 5.7 Examples of synthetic tumors generated by DiffTumor [9] on the liver, pancreas, and kidney

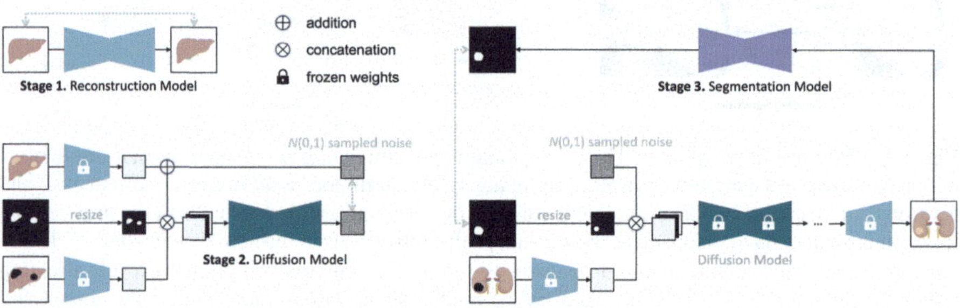

Fig. 5.8 *Overview of DiffTumor framework.* In pursuit of achieving generalizable tumor synthesis, DiffTumor encompasses three stages. ① The first stage is the training of an Autoencoder Model—comprising an encoder and a decoder—to learn comprehensive latent features. The learning objective in this stage entails image reconstruction conducted on 9262 unlabeled three-dimensional CT volumes. Both the trained encoder and decoder are integral to subsequent stages. ② The second stage involves training a Diffusion Model—a specialized generative model—by utilizing latent features and tumor masks as conditions. Once trained, the model is capable of generating the requisite latent features for the reconstruction of CT volumes with tumors, utilizing arbitrary masks. ③ The third stage entails training a Segmentation Model with CT volumes of synthetic tumors, reconstructed by the decoder. Armed with a considerable repository of healthy CT volumes, DiffTumor has the capacity to generate an extensive collection of synthetic tumors, which vary in location, size, shape, texture, and intensity, thus contributing to the enhancement of AI models for tumor detection and segmentation

diverse samples with fewer issues related to mode collapse. DiffTumor [9] is the first to explore tumor synthesis in abdominal organs using Diffusion Models and demonstrates an efficient method for achieving generalizable tumor synthesis. Tumors generated by DiffTumor are illustrated in Fig. 5.7. The network architecture of DiffTumor is shown in Fig. 5.8.

5.5.1 *Property of DiffTumor*

(i) **Reduced annotations for Diffusion Model.** The quality of synthetic data produced by a generative model typically depends heavily on the quantity and diversity of the paired training data used during the training phase [11, 46]. Nevertheless, the relationship between the number of annotated real tumors required for training the Diffusion Model and the performance of the Segmentation Model has not been extensively studied. DiffTumor found that the relationship between the amount of paired training data and the quality of synthetic data is not necessarily linear. Remarkably, it requires only one annotated tumor to train the Diffusion Model and to generate synthetic tumors for the subsequent training of the Segmentation Model. This finding is in contrast to the conventional wisdom in computer vision [81], which often necessitates extensive datasets for training generative models. The results suggest that a smaller number of real tumors may suffice for training the Diffusion Model, particularly for early-stage tumors. Such a discovery could have profound implications for improving efficiency and reducing the costs associated with training generative models in the field of medical imaging.

(ii) **Accelerated tumor synthesis.** The speed at which synthetic tumors are generated is critical for the practical use of synthetic data, particularly for accelerating the training of segmentation models. The synthesis speed of DiffTumor is significantly affected by the choice of timestep (T). An investigation into the influence of timestep on the segmentation performance of the Segmentation Model has been conducted. It is observed that using DDPM [40] with one-step sampling, DiffTumor cannot synthesize realistic textures for both organ and tumor, which negatively affects the training of the Segmentation Model. Conversely, by setting T higher than 1, DiffTumor can produce more realistic textures, leading to an enhanced performance of the segmentation model. Taking into account the balance between performance and synthesis efficiency, DiffTumor selects a timestep of $T = 4$ as the default setting for early tumor synthesis. This selection strikes a balance that allows for the generation of high-quality synthetic data while maintaining an acceptable level of efficiency.

5.5.2 *Clinical Perspectives*

This learning-based approach can be widely applied because of the similar growth dynamics observed in tumors across various types and locations. Tumorigenesis is a complex, multistage process involving cellular and histological transformations, from precancerous lesions to malignant tumors. This progression, driven by genetic mutations and functional changes known as the ‘hallmarks of cancer,’ is consistent across tumor types [12, 35, 58]. Early-stage tumors typically consist of well-to-moderately differentiated cells with mild atypia and invasiveness, showing rare hemorrhage and necrosis. They often appear as homogeneous nodules with slightly indistinct margins and small diameters in CT images [15, 90]. In contrast, advanced tumors exhibit significant infiltration and destruction of surrounding tissues, extending beyond the original site and potentially affecting adjacent structures [5]. As tumors become more malignant, rapid growth leads to ischemia and necrosis due to insufficient vascular supply, resulting in heterogeneous patterns in CT images with features like hemorrhage and fibrosis [84, 115]. These characteristics are consistent across different populations, ages, and genders (Fig. 5.8).

5.6 Tumor Synthesis Benchmark

We evaluate the effectiveness of Pixel2Cancer and DiffTumor by comparing them with supervised models trained on real data and several prominent unsupervised anomaly segmentation methods. Table 5.2 highlights that synthetic data have

Table 5.2 *Comparison with state-of-the-art unsupervised methods.* We compare the initial label-free modeling-based methods with other unsupervised anomaly segmentation baselines, tumor synthesis strategies, and fully-supervised methods. Modeling-based methods significantly outperform all other state-of-the-art unsupervised baseline methods and even surpass the fully-supervised method with detailed *pixel-wise annotation*

Liver tumor segmentation performance					
Tumors	Method	Architecture	Labeled/unlabeled CTs	DSC (%)	NSD (%)
None	PatchCore [83]	Resnet50	0/116	15.9	16.4
None	f-AnoGAN [86]	Customized [7]	0/116	19.0	16.9
None	VAE [53]	Customized [7]	0/116	24.6	23.6
Synt	Yao et al. [113]	U-Net	0/116	32.8	31.3
Real	Fully-supervised	U-Net	101/0	56.7	58.0
Synt	Hand-crafted [43]	U-Net	0/116	59.8	61.3
Synt	Pixel2Cancer [59]	U-Net	0/116	58.9	63.7
Synt	DiffTumor [9]	U-Net	101/116	70.9	71.2
Pancreas tumor segmentation performance					
Tumors	Method	Architecture	Labeled/unlabeled CTs	DSC (%)	NSD (%)
Real	Fully-supervised	U-Net	96/0	57.5	56.5
Synt	Hand-crafted [43]	U-Net	0/104	54.1	52.2
Synt	Pixel2Cancer [59]	U-Net	0/104	60.9	57.1
Synt	DiffTumor [9]	U-Net	96/104	64.8	60.5
Kidney tumor segmentation performance					
Tumors	Method	Architecture	Labeled/unlabeled CTs	DSC (%)	NSD (%)
Real	Fully-supervised	U-Net	96/0	71.3	62.8
Synt	Hand-crafted [43]	U-Net	0/120	63.2	55.4
Synt	Pixel2Cancer [59]	U-Net	0/120	73.2	65.0
Synt	DiffTumor [9]	U-Net	96/120	84.2	76.6

significantly outperformed all these baseline methods, achieving a DSC of 59.77% and NSD of 61.29%. These results highlight the potential of synthetic strategies to avoid per-pixel manual annotation for tumor segmentation.

5.6.1 Case Study: Fake Tumors, Real Results

Synthetic Liver Tumors In synthetic liver tumors, synthetic data have demonstrated significant superiority over real data across all stages, from small to large tumors. The hand-crafted approach proposed by Hu et al. [43] outperforms real data, achieving a 2.3% improvement in DSC and a 3.3% improvement in NSD. Pixel2Cancer has shown superior performance in liver segmentation, with a DSC improvement of 2.2% and an NSD improvement of 5.7%. Additionally, DiffTumor has surpassed the performance of real data by 4.0% in DSC and 4.7% in NSD.

Synthetic Kidney Tumors In kidney tumors, segmentation models have achieved superior performance when using synthetic data as data augmentation. Pixel2Cancer has shown superior performance in kidney segmentation, with a DSC improvement of 2.4% and an NSD improvement of 3.2%. Additionally, DiffTumor has surpassed the performance of real data by 7.0% in DSC and 6.7% in NSD.

Synthetic Pancreatic Tumors Segmentation models also have achieved superior performance in pancreatic tumor segmentation when using synthetic data as data augmentation. Pixel2Cancer has shown superior performance in pancreas segmentation, with a DSC improvement of 3.9% and an NSD improvement of 1.9%. DiffTumor has surpassed the performance of real data by 8.2% in DSC and 9.4% in NSD.

5.6.2 Visual Turing Test

The Turing Test, introduced by Alan Turing in "Computing Machinery and Intelligence" [98], assesses whether a machine can exhibit intelligent behavior indistinguishable from that of a human. We apply the Visual Turing Test to evaluate if synthetic tumors resemble real tumors. For this, we compared CT volumes containing real and synthetic tumors across various organs. Professionals, blinded to the origins of the samples, classified each volume as real or synthetic based on 3D views of continuous slice sequences (see Fig. 5.9).

Modeling-Based Approach (Pixel2Cancer) The outcome metrics, as presented in Table 5.3, unveil the performance evaluations by different radiologists. For the junior radiologist R1 (7 years of experience), metrics such as accuracy, sensitivity, and specificity all register below 40%. Notably, a specificity of 35.5% indicates that 64.5% of synthetic tumors are inaccurately identified as real. The intermediate

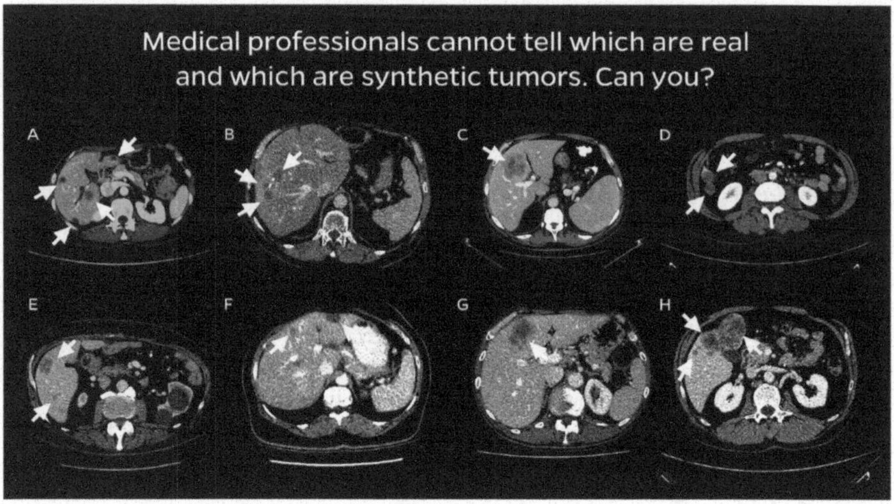

Fig. 5.9 Visual Turing Test. Can you find some examples of synthetic data in the CT images? Answers are in *Johns Hopkins Researchers Create Artificial Tumors to Help AI Detect Early-Stage Cancer*

radiologist R2 (9 years of experience) exhibits comparable metrics around 40%, with 59.2% of synthetic tumors causing confusion. Even the senior radiologist R3 (14 years of experience) misclassifies 44.1% of synthetic tumors as real, underscoring the formidable challenge posed even to seasoned professionals. These results emphasize the efficacy of our modeling-based approach (Pixel2Cancer) in achieving a realistic simulation of tumor development.

Learning-Based Approach (DiffTumor) Two professionals were involved in this test, with 4 and 11 years of experience, respectively. 60 CT volumes were arranged in random order and scrutinized independently by two professionals. The test outcomes are detailed in Table 5.3. Radiologists R1's near-zero specificity scores suggested that synthetic data closely resembled real tumors, resulting in the misclassification of most synthetic tumors as real. Consequently, R1's accuracy scores hovered around 50%. Conversely, R2, with more experience, exhibited higher specificity scores compared to R1, approaching 50%. This implies that nearly 50% of synthetic samples were correctly identified as synthetic, indicating a better discernment between real and synthetic tumors by R2. These findings affirm the effectiveness of DiffTumor in generating visually realistic tumors.

Table 5.3 *Results of reader study.* Pixel2Cancer (top table): The test was conducted with three medical professionals having 7, 9, and 14 years of experience, respectively. Each professional evaluated 50 CT images for each organ, consisting of both real and synthetic tumors. They were tasked with categorizing each CT image as either *real*, *synthetic*, or *unsure*. DiffTumor (bottom table): Visual Turing test over three organs has been conducted with two radiologists (R1 and R2). Both radiologists are provided with 60 three-dimensional CT volumes of each organ, including 30 scans with real tumors and the remaining 30 with synthetic ones. Radiologists are tasked to label each CT volume as *real* or *synthetic*. A lower specificity score indicates a higher number of synthetic tumors being identified as real

Modeling-based Approach: Pixel2Cancer				
Reader	Metric	Liver	Pancreas	Kidneys
R1	Sensitivity (%)	100	95.0	95.5
	Specificity (%)	27.3	22.7	26.7
	Accuracy (%)	60.9	57.1	67.6
R2	Sensitivity (%)	94.7	87.5	90.0
	Specificity (%)	47.8	47.4	56.3
	Accuracy (%)	69.1	65.7	75.0
R3	Sensitivity (%)	100	100	100
	Specificity (%)	45.4	55.6	57.9
	Accuracy (%)	68.4	72.4	75.8
Positives: real tumors (N = 25); negatives: synthetic tumors (N = 25)				
Learning-based Approach: DiffTumor				
Reader	Metric	Liver	Pancreas	Kidneys
R1	Sensitivity (%)	100	97.1	92.9
	Specificity (%)	2.9	0.0	3.1
	Accuracy (%)	45.0	56.7	45.0
R2	Sensitivity (%)	84.6	100	100
	Specificity (%)	47.1	44.0	65.6
	Accuracy (%)	63.3	76.7	81.7

Positives: real tumors (N = 30); negatives: synthetic tumors (N = 30)

5.7 Conclusion

In this chapter, we delved into the concept of synthetic data and its application in medical fields, with a particular focus on cancer research. We defined synthetic data and discussed its critical role in cancer research, such as improving data diversity, protecting patient privacy, and enabling robust research in tumor detection, diagnosis, and treatment. We explored the challenges and opportunities presented in cancer research. Despite these challenges, synthetic data offers significant opportunities, such as enhancing the training of machine learning models, supporting large-scale studies without privacy concerns, and fostering innovation in personalized medicine. Additionally, we highlighted promising approaches and future directions for the use of synthetic data in cancer research, including modeling-based methods and learning-based methods. These methods are opening new avenues for more accurate and comprehensive cancer research, enabling researchers to simulate various scenarios and treatments, and ultimately contributing to better patient outcomes.

Acknowledgments This work was supported by the Lustgarten Foundation for Pancreatic Cancer Research and the Patrick J. McGovern Foundation Award.

References

1. Abi Nader C, Vetil R, Wood LK, Rohe MM, Bône A, Karteszi H, Vullierme MP (2023) Automatic detection of pancreatic lesions and main pancreatic duct dilatation on portal venous CT scans using deep learning. Invest Radiol 58(11):791–798
2. Antonelli M, Reinke A, Bakas S, Farahani K, Kopp-Schneider A, Landman BA, Litjens G, Menze B, Ronneberger O, Summers RM, et al (2022) The medical segmentation decathlon. Nat Commun 13(1):1–13
3. Armato SG III, McLennan G, Bidaut L, McNitt-Gray MF, Meyer CR, Reeves AP, Zhao B, Aberle DR, Henschke CI, Hoffman EA, et al (2011) The lung image database consortium (LIDC) and image database resource initiative (IDRI): a completed reference database of lung nodules on CT scans. Med Phys 38(2):915–931
4. Aversa M, Nobis G, Hägele M, Standvoss K, Chirica M, Murray-Smith R, Alaa AM, Ruff L, Ivanova D, Samek W, et al (2024) Diffinfinite: large mask-image synthesis via parallel random patch diffusion in histopathology. Adv Neural Inf Process Syst 36:78126–78141
5. Ayuso C, Rimola J, Vilana R, Burrel M, Darnell A, García-Criado Á, Bianchi L, Belmonte E, Caparroz C, Barrufet M, et al (2018) Diagnosis and staging of hepatocellular carcinoma (HCC): current guidelines. Eur J Radiol 101:72–81
6. Basaran BD, Zhang W, Qiao M, Kainz B, Matthews PM, Bai W (2023) Lesionmix: a lesion-level data augmentation method for medical image segmentation. In: International conference on medical image computing and computer-assisted intervention. Springer, Berlin, pp. 73–83
7. Baur C, Denner S, Wiestler B, Navab N, Albarqouni S (2021) Autoencoders for unsupervised anomaly segmentation in brain MR images: a comparative study. Med Image Anal 69:101952
8. Bilic P, Christ P, Li HB, Vorontsov E, Ben-Cohen A, Kaissis G, Szeskin A, Jacobs C, Mamani GEH, Chartrand G, et al (2023) The liver tumor segmentation benchmark (LITS). Med Image Anal 84:102680
9. Chen Q, Chen X, Song H, Xiong Z, Yuille A, Wei C, Zhou Z (2024) Towards generalizable tumor synthesis. In: IEEE/CVF conference on computer vision and pattern recognition (2024). https://github.com/MrGiovanni/DiffTumor
10. Chiruvella V, Guddati AK, et al (2021) Ethical issues in patient data ownership. Interact J Med Res 10(2):e22269
11. Chlap P, Min H, Vandenberg N, Dowling J, Holloway L, Haworth A (2021) A review of medical image data augmentation techniques for deep learning applications. J Med Imag Rad Oncol 65(5):545–563
12. Choi JY, Lee JM, Sirlin CB (2014) CT and MR imaging diagnosis and staging of hepatocellular carcinoma: part I. Development, growth, and spread: key pathologic and imaging aspects. Radiology 272(3):635–654
13. Chou YC, Li B, Fan DP, Yuille A, Zhou Z (2024) Acquiring weak annotations for tumor localization in temporal and volumetric data. Mach Intell Res 21:1–13 (2024). https://github.com/johnson111788/Drag-Drop
14. Chou YC, Zhou Z, Yuille A (2024) Embracing massive medical data. arXiv:2407.04687. https://github.com/MrGiovanni/OnlineLearning

15. Chu LC, Goggins MG, Fishman EK (2017) Diagnosis and detection of pancreatic cancer. Cancer J 23(6):333–342
16. Chu LC, Park S, Kawamoto S, Fouladi DF, Shayesteh S, Zinreich ES, Graves JS, Horton KM, Hruban RH, Yuille AL, et al (2019) Utility of CT radiomics features in differentiation of pancreatic ductal adenocarcinoma from normal pancreatic tissue. Am J Roentgenol 213(2):349–357
17. Codella NC, Gutman D, Celebi ME, Helba B, Marchetti MA, Dusza SW, Kalloo A, Liopyris K, Mishra N, Kittler H, et al (2018) Skin lesion analysis toward melanoma detection: a challenge at the 2017 international symposium on biomedical imaging (ISBI), hosted by the international skin imaging collaboration (ISIC). In: 2018 IEEE 15th international symposium on biomedical imaging (ISBI 2018). IEEE, Piscataway, pp. 168–172
18. Davis GB, Blanchard DK, Hatch GF III, Wertheimer-Hatch L, Hatch KF, Foster RS Jr., Skandalakis JE (2000) Tumors of the stomach. World J Surg 24(4):412–420
19. Du S, Wang X, Lu Y, Zhou Y, Zhang S, Yuille A, Li K, Zhou Z (2023) Boosting dermatoscopic lesion segmentation via diffusion models with visual and textual prompts. arXiv:2310.02906
20. Dunnick NR (2016) Renal cell carcinoma: staging and surveillance. Abdomin Radiol 41:1079–1085
21. Edge SB, Compton CC (2010) The American joint committee on cancer: the 7th edition of the AJCC cancer staging manual and the future of TNM. Ann Surg Oncol 17(6):1471–1474
22. Elbanna KY, Jang HJ, Kim TK (2020) Imaging diagnosis and staging of pancreatic ductal adenocarcinoma: a comprehensive review. Insights Imag 11(1):1–13
23. Engelhardt S, Sauerzapf S, Preim B, Karck M, Wolf I, De Simone R (2019) Flexible and comprehensive patient-specific mitral valve silicone models with chordae tendineae made from 3d-printable molds. Int J Comput Assist Radiol Surg 14:1177–1186
24. Feng R, Zhou Z, Gotway MB, Liang J (2020) Parts2whole: self-supervised contrastive learning via reconstruction. In: Domain adaptation and representation transfer, and distributed and collaborative learning. Springer, Berlin, pp 85–95
25. Fowler KJ, Burgoyne A, Fraum TJ, Hosseini M, Ichikawa S, Kim S, Kitao A, Lee JM, Paradis V, Taouli B, et al (2021) Pathologic, molecular, and prognostic radiologic features of hepatocellular carcinoma. Radiographics 41(6):1611–1631
26. Gao C, Killeen BD, Hu Y, Grupp RB, Taylor RH, Armand M, Unberath M (2023) Synthetic data accelerates the development of generalizable learning-based algorithms for x-ray image analysis. Nat Mach Intell 5(3):294–308
27. Golias C, Charalabopoulos A, Charalabopoulos K (2004) Cell proliferation and cell cycle control: a mini review. Int J Clin Pract 58(12):1134–1141
28. Goodfellow I, Pouget-Abadie J, Mirza M, Xu B, Warde-Farley D, Ozair S, Courville A, Bengio Y (2014) Generative adversarial nets. Adv Neural Inf Process Syst 27:2672–2680
29. Goodfellow I, Pouget-Abadie J, Mirza M, Xu B, Warde-Farley D, Ozair S, Courville A, Bengio Y (2020) Generative adversarial networks. Commun ACM 63(11):139–144
30. Griswold D, Corbett TH (1975) A colon tumor model for anticancer agent evaluation. Cancer 36(S6):2441–2444
31. Haghighi F, Hosseinzadeh Taher MR, Zhou Z, Gotway MB, Liang J (2020) Learning semantics-enriched representation via self-discovery, self-classification, and self-restoration. In: International conference on medical image computing and computer-assisted intervention. Springer, Berlin, pp. 137–147. https://github.com/fhaghighi/SemanticGenesis
32. Haghighi F, Taher MRH, Zhou Z, Gotway MB, Liang J (2021) Transferable visual words: exploiting the semantics of anatomical patterns for self-supervised learning. IEEE Trans Med Imag 40(10):2857–2868. https://doi.org/10.1109/TMI.2021.3060634
33. Hamamci IE, Er S, Simsar E, Tezcan A, Simsek AG, Almas F, Esirgun SN, Reynaud H, Pati S, Bluethgen C, et al (2024) Generatect: text-guided 3d chest ct generation. In: Proceedings of the European conference on computer vision (ECCV)
34. Han C, Rundo L, Araki R, Furukawa Y, Mauri G, Nakayama H, Hayashi H (2019) Infinite brain MR images: PGGAN-based data augmentation for tumor detection. In: Neural approaches to dynamics of signal exchanges. Springer, Berlin, pp. 291–303

35. Hanahan D, Weinberg RA (2000) The hallmarks of cancer. Cell 100(1):57–70
36. Harpold HL, Alvord EC Jr, Swanson KR (2007) The evolution of mathematical modeling of glioma proliferation and invasion. J Neuropathol Exp Neurol 66(1):1–9
37. Heath M, Bowyer K, Kopans D, Kegelmeyer P Jr, Moore R, Chang K, Munishkumaran S (1998) Current status of the digital database for screening mammography. In: Digital mammography: Nijmegen. Springer, Berlin, pp. 457–460
38. Heller N, Isensee F, Maier-Hein KH, Hou X, Xie C, Li F, Nan Y, Mu G, Lin Z, Han M, et al (2021) The state of the art in kidney and kidney tumor segmentation in contrast-enhanced ct imaging: results of the kits19 challenge. Med Image Anal 67:101821
39. Hiraoka N, Ino Y, Sekine S, Tsuda H, Shimada K, Kosuge T, Zavada J, Yoshida M, Yamada K, Koyama T, et al (2010) Tumour necrosis is a postoperative prognostic marker for pancreatic cancer patients with a high interobserver reproducibility in histological evaluation. British J Cancer 103(7):1057–1065
40. Ho J, Jain A, Abbeel P (2020) Denoising diffusion probabilistic models. Adv Neural Inf Process Syst 33:6840–6851
41. Hou L, Agarwal A, Samaras D, Kurc TM, Gupta RR, Saltz JH (2019) Robust histopathology image analysis: to label or to synthesize? In: Proceedings of the IEEE/CVF conference on computer vision and pattern recognition, pp. 8533–8542
42. Hu Q, Xiao J, Chen Y, Sun S, Chen JN, Yuille A, Zhou Z (2022) Synthetic tumors make AI segment tumors better. In: NeurIPS workshop on medical imaging meets NeurIPS. https://github.com/MrGiovanni/SyntheticTumors
43. Hu Q, Chen Y, Xiao J, Sun S, Chen J, Yuille AL, Zhou Z (2023) Label-free liver tumor segmentation. In: IEEE/CVF conference on computer vision and pattern recognition, pp. 7422–7432. https://github.com/MrGiovanni/SyntheticTumors
44. Hu Q, Yuille A, Zhou Z (2023) Synthetic data as validation. arXiv:2310.16052. https://github.com/MrGiovanni/SyntheticValidation
45. Iyer R, Dubrow R (2004) Imaging of esophageal cancer. Cancer Imag 4(2):125
46. Jaipuria N, Zhang X, Bhasin R, Arafa M, Chakravarty P, Shrivastava S, Manglani S, Murali VN (2020) Deflating dataset bias using synthetic data augmentation. In: Proceedings of the IEEE/CVF conference on computer vision and pattern recognition workshops, pp. 772–773
47. Jiang Y, Chen H, Loew M, Ko H (2020) Covid-19 CT image synthesis with a conditional generative adversarial network. IEEE J Biomed Health Inf 25(2):441–452
48. Jin D, Xu Z, Tang Y, Harrison AP, Mollura DJ (2018) CT-realistic lung nodule simulation from 3d conditional generative adversarial networks for robust lung segmentation. In: Medical image computing and computer assisted intervention. Springer, Berlin, pp. 732–740
49. Jin Q, Cui H, Sun C, Meng Z, Su R (2021) Free-form tumor synthesis in computed tomography images via richer generative adversarial network. Knowl Based Syst 218:106753
50. Kang MJ, Jang JY, Kim SJ, Lee KB, Ryu JK, Kim YT, Yoon YB, Kim SW (2011) Cyst growth rate predicts malignancy in patients with branch duct intraductal papillary mucinous neoplasms. Clin Gastroenterol Hepatol 9(1):87–93
51. Kang M, Li B, Zhu Z, Lu Y, Fishman EK, Yuille A, Zhou Z (2023) Label-assemble: leveraging multiple datasets with partial labels. In: IEEE international symposium on biomedical imaging. IEEE, Piscataway, pp. 1–5. https://github.com/MrGiovanni/LabelAssemble
52. Khader F, Müller-Franzes G, Tayebi Arasteh S, Han T, Haarburger C, Schulze-Hagen M, Schad P, Engelhardt S, Baeßler B, Foersch S, et al (2023) Denoising diffusion probabilistic models for 3d medical image generation. Sci Rep 13(1):7303
53. Kingma DP, Welling M (2013) Auto-encoding variational bayes. arXiv:1312.6114
54. Kuijf HJ, Biesbroek JM, De Bresser J, Heinen R, Andermatt S, Bento M, Berseth M, Belyaev M, Cardoso MJ, Casamitjana A, et al (2019) Standardized assessment of automatic segmentation of white matter hyperintensities and results of the WMH segmentation challenge. IEEE Trans Med Imag 38(11):2556–2568
55. Kumar N, Verma R, Sharma S, Bhargava S, Vahadane A, Sethi A (2017) A dataset and a technique for generalized nuclear segmentation for computational pathology. IEEE Trans Med Imag 36(7):1550–1560
56. Kumar V, Abbas A, Aster JC (2017) Robbins basic pathology. Elsevier, Amsterdam

57. Laeseke PF, Chen R, Jeffrey RB, Brentnall TA, Willmann JK (2015) Combining in vitro diagnostics with in vivo imaging for earlier detection of pancreatic ductal adenocarcinoma: challenges and solutions. Radiology 277(3):644–661
58. Lahouel K, Younes L, Danilova L, Giardiello FM, Hruban RH, Groopman J, Kinzler KW, Vogelstein B, Geman D, Tomasetti C (2020) Revisiting the tumorigenesis timeline with a data-driven generative model. Proc Natl Acad Sci 117(2):857–864
59. Lai Y, Chen X, Wang A, Yuille A, Zhou Z (2024) From pixel to cancer: cellular automata in computed tomography. arXiv:2403.06459. https://github.com/MrGiovanni/Pixel2Cancer
60. Lee K, O'Malley M, Haider M, Hanbidge A (2004) Triple-phase MDCT of hepatocellular carcinoma. Am J Roentgenol 182(3):643–649
61. Leveridge MJ, Bostrom PJ, Koulouris G, Finelli A, Lawrentschuk N (2010) Imaging renal cell carcinoma with ultrasonography, CT and MRI. Nat Rev Urol 7(6):311–325
62. Thompson H (1986) Tumors of the esophagus and stomach. J Clinical Pathol 39(3):351–351. BMJ Publishing Group. https://doi.org/10.1136/jcp.39.3.351-e. https://jcp.bmj.com/content/39/3/351.5. eprint: https://jcp.bmj.com/content/39/3/351.5.full.pdf. ISSN: 0021-9746
63. Li B, Chou YC, Sun S, Qiao H, Yuille A, Zhou Z (2023) Early detection and localization of pancreatic cancer by label-free tumor synthesis. In: MICCAI workshop on big task small data, 1001-AI. https://github.com/MrGiovanni/SyntheticTumors
64. Li C, Liu H, Liu Y, Feng BY, Li W, Liu X, Chen Z, Shao J, Yuan Y (2024) Endora: video generation models as endoscopy simulators. In: International conference on medical image computing and computer-assisted intervention
65. Li W, Qu C, Chen X, Bassi PR, Shi Y, Lai Y, Yu, Q, Xue H, Chen Y, Lin X, et al (2024) Abdomenatlas: a large-scale, detailed-annotated, & multi-center dataset for efficient transfer learning and open algorithmic benchmarking. Med Image Anal 97:103285. https://github.com/MrGiovanni/AbdomenAtlas
66. Li W, Yuille A, Zhou Z (2024) How well do supervised models transfer to 3d image segmentation? In: International conference on learning representations. https://github.com/MrGiovanni/SuPreM
67. Liu J, Zhang Y, Chen JN, Xiao J, Lu Y, A Landman B, Yuan Y, Yuille A, Tang Y, Zhou Z (2023) Clip-driven universal model for organ segmentation and tumor detection. In: Proceedings of the IEEE/CVF international conference on computer vision, pp. 21152–21164. https://github.com/ljwztc/CLIP-Driven-Universal-Model
68. Liu J, Zhang Y, Wang K, Yavuz MC, Chen X, Yuan Y, Li H, Yang Y, Yuille A, Tang Y, et al (2024) Universal and extensible language-vision models for organ segmentation and tumor detection from abdominal computed tomography. Med Image Anal 97:103226. https://github.com/ljwztc/CLIP-Driven-Universal-Model
69. Luo Y, Zhou L, Zhan B, Fei Y, Zhou J, Wang Y, Shen D (2022) Adaptive rectification based adversarial network with spectrum constraint for high-quality pet image synthesis. Med Image Anal 77:102335
70. Lyu F, Ye M, Ma AJ, Yip TCF, Wong GLH, Yuen PC (2022) Learning from synthetic ct images via test-time training for liver tumor segmentation. IEEE Trans Med Imag 41(9):2510–2520
71. Cunha GM, Fowler KJ, Roudenko A, Taouli B, Fung AW, Elsayes KM, Marks RM, Cruite I, Horvat N, Chernyak, V, et al (2021) How to use li-rads to report liver CT and MRI observations. RadioGraphics 41(5):1352–1367
72. Menze BH, Jakab A, Bauer S, Kalpathy-Cramer J, Farahani K, Kirby J, Burren Y, Porz N, Slotboom J, Wiest R, et al (2014) The multimodal brain tumor image segmentation benchmark (brats). IEEE Trans Med Imag 34(10):1993–2024
73. Mukherkjee D, Saha P, Kaplun D, Sinitca A, Sarkar R (2022) Brain tumor image generation using an aggregation of gan models with style transfer. Sci Rep 12(1):9141
74. Nerad E, Lahaye MJ, Maas M, Nelemans P, Bakers FC, Beets GL, Beets-Tan RG (2016) Diagnostic accuracy of ct for local staging of colon cancer: a systematic review and meta-analysis. Am J Roentgenol 207(5):984–995

75. Orbes-Arteaga M, Varsavsky T, Sudre CH, Eaton-Rosen Z, Haddow LJ, Sørensen L, Nielsen M, Pai A, Ourselin S, Modat M, et al (2019) Multi-domain adaptation in brain MRI through paired consistency and adversarial learning. In: Domain adaptation and representation transfer and medical image learning with less labels and imperfect data. Springer, Berlin, pp. 54–62
76. Özbey M, Dalmaz O, Dar SUH, Bedel HA, Özturk Ş, Güngör A, Çukur T (2023) Unsupervised medical image translation with adversarial diffusion models. IEEE Trans Med Imag 42(12):3524–3539. https://doi.org/10.1109/TMI.2023.3290149
77. Park S, Chu L, Fishman E, Yuille A, Vogelstein B, Kinzler K, Horton K, Hruban R, Zinreich E, Fouladi DF, et al (2020) Annotated normal CT data of the abdomen for deep learning: challenges and strategies for implementation. Diagnos Intervent Imag 101(1):35–44
78. Park JE, Eun D, Kim HS, Lee DH, Jang RW, Kim N (2021) Generative adversarial network for glioblastoma ensures morphologic variations and improves diagnostic model for isocitrate dehydrogenase mutant type. Sci Rep 11(1):9912
79. Qu C, Zhang T, Qiao H, Liu J, Tang Y, Yuille A, Zhou Z (2023) Abdomenatlas-8k: annotating 8,000 abdominal CT volumes for multi-organ segmentation in three weeks. In: Conference on neural information processing systems. https://github.com/MrGiovanni/AbdomenAtlas
80. Qu C, Zhang T, Qiao H, Tang Y, Yuille AL, Zhou Z, et al (2024) Abdomenatlas-8k: annotating 8,000 CT volumes for multi-organ segmentation in three weeks. Adv Neural Inf Process Syst 36:36620–36636
81. Ramesh A, Dhariwal P, Nichol A, Chu C, Chen M (2022) Hierarchical text-conditional image generation with clip latents. 1(2):3. arXiv:2204.06125
82. Reynolds AR, Furlan A, Fetzer DT, Sasatomi E, Borhani AA, Heller MT, Tublin ME (2015) Infiltrative hepatocellular carcinoma: what radiologists need to know. Radiographics 35(2):371–386
83. Roth K, Pemula L, Zepeda J, Schölkopf B, Brox T, Gehler P (2022) Towards total recall in industrial anomaly detection. In: Proceedings of the IEEE/CVF conference on computer vision and pattern recognition, pp. 14318–14328
84. Saar B, Kellner-Weldon F (2008) Radiological diagnosis of hepatocellular carcinoma. Liver Int 28(2):189–199
85. Sahani DV, Samir AE (2016) Abdominal imaging e-book: expert radiology series. Elsevier, Amsterdam
86. Schlegl T, Seeböck P, Waldstein SM, Langs G, et al (2019) f-AnoGAN: fast unsupervised anomaly detection with generative adversarial networks. Med Image Anal 54:30–44. https://doi.org/10.1016/j.media.2019.01.010. ISSN: 13618423
87. Setio AAA, Traverso A, De Bel T, Berens MS, van den Bogaard C, Cerello P, Chen H, Dou Q, Fantacci ME, Geurts B, et al (2017) Validation, comparison, and combination of algorithms for automatic detection of pulmonary nodules in computed tomography images: the luna16 challenge. Med Image Anal 42:1–13
88. Sharan L, Romano G, Koehler S, Kelm H, Karck M, De Simone R, Engelhardt S (2021) Mutually improved endoscopic image synthesis and landmark detection in unpaired image-to-image translation. IEEE J Biomed Health Inf 26(1):127–138
89. Silverman PM (2012) Oncologic imaging: a multidisciplinary approach. Elsevier, Amsterdam
90. Skarin AT (2015) Atlas of diagnostic oncology e-book. Elsevier, Amsterdam
91. Smaldone MC, Kutikov A, Egleston BL, Canter DJ, Viterbo R, Chen DY, Jewett MA, Greenberg RE, Uzzo RG (2012) Small renal masses progressing to metastases under active surveillance: a systematic review and pooled analysis. Cancer 118(4):997–1006
92. Soga J (2005) Early-stage carcinoids of the gastrointestinal tract: an analysis of 1914 reported cases. Cancer Interdiscip Int J Am Cancer Soc 103(8):1587–1595
93. Stout AP (1953) Tumors of the stomach. Armed Forces Institute of Pathology, Washington
94. Stout AP, Lattes R (1957) Tumors of the esophagus. Armed Forces Institute of Pathology, Washington
95. Tanase M, Waliszewski P (2015) On complexity and homogeneity measures in predicting biological aggressiveness of prostate cancer; implication of the cellular automata model of tumor growth. J Surg Oncol 112(8):791–801

96. Tang Y, Liu J, Zhou Z, Yu X, Huo Y (2024) Efficient 3D representation learning for medical image analysis. World Sci Ann Rev Artif Intell 02:2450002. https://doi.org/10.1142/S2811032324500024. eprint: https://doi.org/10.1142/S2811032324500024
97. Teixeira B, Singh V, Chen T, Ma K, Tamersoy B, Wu Y, Balashova E, Comaniciu D (2018) Generating synthetic x-ray images of a person from the surface geometry. In: Proceedings of the IEEE conference on computer vision and pattern recognition, pp. 9059–9067
98. Turing AM (2009) Computing machinery and intelligence. Springer, Berlin
99. Van Griethuysen JJ, Fedorov A, Parmar C, Hosny A, Aucoin N, Narayan V, Beets-Tan RG, Fillion-Robin JC, Pieper S, Aerts HJ (2017) Computational radiomics system to decode the radiographic phenotype. Cancer Res 77(21):e104–e107
100. Veeling BS, Linmans J, Winkens J, Cohen T, Welling M (2018) Rotation equivariant CNNs for digital pathology. In: Medical image computing and computer assisted intervention, pp. 210–218. Springer, Berlin
101. Waheed A, Goyal M, Gupta D, Khanna A, Al-Turjman F, Pinheiro PR (2020) CovidGAN: data augmentation using auxiliary classifier GAN for improved covid-19 detection. IEEE Access 8:91916–91923
102. Wang H, Zhou Z, Li Y, Chen Z, Lu P, Wang W, Liu W, Yu L (2017) Comparison of machine learning methods for classifying mediastinal lymph node metastasis of non-small cell lung cancer from 18F-FDG PET/CT images. EJNMMI Res 7(1):1–11
103. Wang Y, Zhou L, Wang L, Yu B, Zu C, Lalush DS, Lin W, Wu X, Zhou J, Shen D (2018) Locality adaptive multi-modality gans for high-quality PET image synthesis. In: Medical image computing and computer assisted intervention. Springer, Berlin, pp. 329–337
104. Wang ZJ, Westphalen AC, Zagoria RJ (2018) CT and MRI of small renal masses. Br J Radiol 91(1087):20180131
105. Wei Z, Chen Y, Guan Q, Hu H, Zhou Q, Li Z, Xu X, Frangi A, Chen F (2022) Pancreatic image augmentation based on local region texture synthesis for tumor segmentation. In: International conference on artificial neural networks. Springer, Berlin, pp. 419–431
106. Wong KC, Summers RM, Kebebew E, Yao J (2015) Pancreatic tumor growth prediction with multiplicative growth and image-derived motion. In: International conference on information processing in medical imaging. Springer, Berlin, pp. 501–513
107. Wu E, Wu K, Cox D, Lotter W (2018) Conditional infilling GANS for data augmentation in mammogram classification. In: Image analysis for moving organ, breast, and thoracic images: third international workshop. Springer, Berlin, pp. 98–106
108. Xia Y, Yu Q, Chu L, Kawamoto S, Park S, Liu F, Chen J, Zhu Z, Li B, Zhou Z, et al (2022) The felix project: deep networks to detect pancreatic neoplasms. medRxiv
109. Xiao J, Yu L, Zhou Z, Bai Y, Xing L, Yuille A, Zhou Y (2022) Catenorm: categorical normalization for robust medical image segmentation. In: MICCAI workshop on domain adaptation and representation transfer. Springer, Berlin, pp. 129–146. https://github.com/lambert-x/CateNorm
110. Xue Y, Ye J, Zhou Q, Long LR, Antani S, Xue Z, Cornwell C, Zaino R, Cheng KC, Huang X (2021) Selective synthetic augmentation with histogan for improved histopathology image classification. Med Image Anal 67:101816
111. Yan W, Huang L, Xia L, Gu S, Yan F, Wang Y, Tao Q (2020) MRI manufacturer shift and adaptation: increasing the generalizability of deep learning segmentation for MR images acquired with different scanners. Radiol Artif Intell 2(4):e190195
112. Yang X, He X, Zhao J, Zhang Y, Zhang S, Xie P (2020) Covid-CT-dataset: a CT scan dataset about covid-19. arXiv:2003.13865
113. Yao Q, Xiao L, Liu P, Zhou SK (2021) Label-free segmentation of COVID-19 lesions in lung CT. IEEE Trans Med Imag 40(10):2808–2819. https://doi.org/10.1109/TMI.2021.3066161
114. Yao Y, Liu F, Zhou Z, Wang Y, Shen W, Yuille A, Lu Y (2022) Unsupervised domain adaptation through shape modeling for medical image segmentation. arXiv:2207.02529
115. Yee PP, Li W (2021) Tumor necrosis: a synergistic consequence of metabolic stress and inflammation. Bioessays 43(7):2100029

116. Yoon D, Kong HJ, Kim BS, Cho WS, Lee JC, Cho M, Lim MH, Yang SY, Lim SH, Lee J, et al (2022) Colonoscopic image synthesis with generative adversarial network for enhanced detection of sessile serrated lesions using convolutional neural network. Sci Rep 12(1):261
117. Yu B, Zhou L, Wang L, Fripp J, Bourgeat P (2018) 3d CGAN based cross-modality MR image synthesis for brain tumor segmentation. In: 2018 IEEE 15th international symposium on biomedical imaging (ISBI 2018). IEEE, Piscataway, pp. 626–630
118. Zhang Y, Li X, Chen H, Yuille AL, Liu Y, Zhou Z (2023) Continual learning for abdominal multi-organ and tumor segmentation. In: International conference on medical image computing and computer-assisted intervention. Springer, Berlin, pp. 35–45. https://github.com/MrGiovanni/ContinualLearning
119. Zhao J, Li D, Kassam Z, Howey J, Chong J, Chen B, Li S (2020) Tripartite-GAN: synthesizing liver contrast-enhanced mri to improve tumor detection. Med Image Anal 63:101667
120. Zhou Z (2021) Towards annotation-efficient deep learning for computer-aided diagnosis. Ph.D. Thesis, Arizona State University. https://github.com/MrGiovanni/Dissertation
121. Zhou Z, Gotway MB, Liang J (2022) Interpreting medical images. In: Intelligent systems in medicine and health. Springer, Berlin, pp. 343–371
122. Zhou, Z, Sodha V, Siddiquee MMR, Feng R, Tajbakhsh N, Gotway MB, Liang J (2019) Models genesis: generic autodidactic models for 3d medical image analysis. In: International conference on medical image computing and computer-assisted intervention. Springer, Berlin, pp. 384–393. https://github.com/MrGiovanni/ModelsGenesis
123. Zhu Z, Kang M, Yuille A, Zhou Z (2022) Assembling and exploiting large-scale existing labels of common thorax diseases for improved covid-19 classification using chest radiographs. In: Radiological society of north america (RSNA). https://github.com/MrGiovanni/LabelAssemble

Chapter 6
Vision-Language Pre-training from Synthetic Data

Che Liu

Abstract Recent advancements in Medical Vision-Language Pre-training (MedVLP) demonstrate significant potential, leveraging extensive datasets of medical images and accompanying reports to deliver impressive performance across a wide range of downstream tasks, including both visual-based challenges and those integrating vision and language. However, MedVLP systems require substantial datasets with matched image-text pairs, which are often challenging to procure due to their labor-intensive and costly nature. Additionally, real-world datasets frequently encounter issues such as imbalanced concepts, unpaired image-text samples, and corrupted images. Recent progress in deep generative models, notably from Variational Autoencoders (VAEs) and Generative Adversarial Networks (GANs) to Stable Diffusion (SD)-based models, has been significant. SD-based models, in particular, excel in conditional generation, a crucial capability for synthesizing medical images with high fidelity. Moreover, the generation of medical reports can be enhanced using language models, especially large language models (LLMs) such as Llama, utilizing conditional generation driven by extensive medical concept definitions sourced from clinical peer-reviewed databases. This article introduces the principal MedVLP methodologies, the role of generative models, and the techniques of conditional generation, alongside an exploration of various downstream tasks employed to assess the effectiveness of MedVLP.

6.1 Introduction

Significant advancements in machine learning, particularly deep learning (DL), have revolutionized the processing and analysis of medical images [4, 15]. While traditional machine learning methods in medical imaging require extensive labeled datasets, deep learning approaches have somewhat alleviated this burden by employing sophisticated feature extraction capabilities. Despite these advancements, deep

C. Liu (✉)
Imperial College London, London, UK
e-mail: che.liu21@imperial.ac.uk

L. Zhang et al. (eds.), *Generative Machine Learning Models in Medical Image Computing*, https://doi.org/10.1007/978-3-031-80965-1_6

learning models still depend heavily on large annotated datasets [35, 46]. Self-supervised learning (SSL) methods have attempted to reduce the need for extensive annotations but often fail to capture nuanced features critical for medical applications [4, 12, 13, 15]. Vision-Language Pre-training (VLP) has emerged as a potent solution in this context, requiring fewer expert annotations by learning robust features from available paired image-text data [23, 34, 52, 55, 57].

However, acquiring such high-quality paired datasets is rare and typically involves significant financial and logistical challenges, necessitating innovative solutions like generative models [8, 18, 30]. Variational Autoencoders (VAEs) [31], Generative Adversarial Networks (GANs) [19], and more recently, Stable Diffusion (SD) models [45], have been pivotal in this regard. VAEs [31] are foundational in generating new data samples by learning the distribution of input data, making them ideal for tasks where modeling the underlying data distribution is crucial. GANs [19], by employing a dual-network architecture involving a generator and a discriminator, excel in generating high-fidelity images, making them particularly useful for creating realistic medical images. Stable Diffusion [45] models have taken this a step further by effectively conditioning the generation process on textual descriptions, thus providing a mechanism for creating detailed and specific medical imagery based on textual prompts.

The concept of conditional generation, especially text-conditioned, has become increasingly relevant. This approach utilizes detailed clinical descriptions from peer-reviewed medical databases to generate corresponding medical images, offering a promising avenue for enriching training datasets without the need for real-world data acquisition. This capability not only enhances the diversity of medical images but also aligns them more closely with specific clinical findings and annotations [10].

In addition to image synthesis, the generation of medical reports using large language models (LLMs) [41, 44, 51, 61] represents a transformative application within MedVLP. LLMs such as Llama [51] have shown exceptional capabilities in understanding and generating complex, domain-specific text. By leveraging vast amounts of medical literature and clinical case reports, these models are trained to produce detailed medical reports that are both clinically relevant and contextually accurate. The process involves conditioning the language models on specific medical imagery findings, allowing them to generate coherent and detailed descriptions akin to those written by healthcare professionals [20, 38]. This not only enhances the training datasets for MedVLP by providing paired image-text data but also serves as a tool for assisting medical practitioners in drafting diagnostic reports more efficiently. Such advancements hold the potential to significantly streamline the workflow in medical settings, reducing the cognitive load on radiologists and increasing the accuracy of diagnostic interpretations. This integration of LLMs into MedVLP platforms demonstrates the potential of combining advanced image and text generation technologies to improve the comprehensiveness and utility of medical imaging studies.

This article delves into the dynamics of Medical Vision-Language Pre-training (MedVLP), examining the integration of various generative models for synthesizing both medical images and accompanying reports. We explore different generative models tailored for medical imagery and text generation, evaluating their efficacy in contributing to the MedVLP paradigm. Moreover, we discuss the downstream tasks that serve as benchmarks for evaluating the performance of MedVLP systems. Finally, the article addresses the current challenges faced in deploying MedVLP with synthetic data, focusing on how these models cope with the nuanced complexities of medical data and their implications for clinical practice. Through this comprehensive analysis, we aim to shed light on the transformative potential of generative models in enhancing medical image analysis and the development of more effective and nuanced medical diagnostic tools.

6.2 Vision-Language Pre-training in Medical Image Computing

In the rapidly evolving field of Medical Vision-Language Pre-training (MedVLP), recent developments have marked significant achievements, particularly in learning clinically relevant visual and textual features from paired image-text datasets [23, 34–37, 39, 43, 52, 57]. This capability allows MedVLP systems to effectively interpret and analyze medical imagery alongside corresponding textual reports, thereby enhancing both the precision and breadth of medical diagnostics.

Most MedVLP architectures employ a dual-stream approach: an image encoder and a text encoder [48]. The image encoder is tasked with processing and analyzing visual data from medical images, while the text encoder concurrently processes the paired medical reports, extracting semantic and contextual latent features that relate to the visual data (Table 6.1).

Upon extracting visual and textual features, MedVLP systems generally adopt one of three mainstream approaches to integrate and utilize these features: alignment, reconstruction, and entity-based methods. The alignment approach focuses on maximizing the similarity of the paired image and text features to ensure that they correspond closely to one another. The reconstruction approach, on the other hand, involves either partially masking data (image or text) and then attempting to reconstruct the missing parts, which aids in strengthening the model's predictive and interpretative capabilities. Lastly, the entity-based approach prioritizes the extraction of specific clinical entities from the text, using them to guide the learning process of visual features. This method aims to refine the model's focus on clinically relevant features in the images, fostering a deeper understanding of the nuances in medical diagnostics. Together, these approaches form the backbone of MedVLP systems, each contributing uniquely to the advancement of medical image understanding and analysis. We have shown three such approaches in Fig. 6.1.

Table 6.1 Overview of various public datasets for MedVLP

Dataset	Patients	X-rays	Labels	Reports	DICOM	Metadata
MIMIC-CXR [27]	65,379	377,095	14	✓	✓	✓
OpenI [11]	3,996	8,121	–	✓	–	–
CandidPTX [17]	13,744	19,234	3	–	✓	–
PadChest [3]	67,625	160,861	–	✓[a]	✓	✓
CheXpert Plus [6]	64,725	223,462	14	✓	✓	✓

[a] The reports are in Spanish

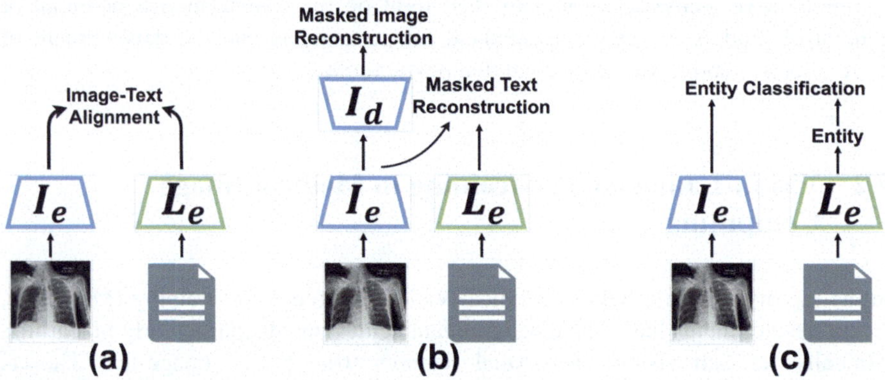

Fig. 6.1 Recent advancements in MedVLP have leveraged various architectures to improving both the learning process and prediction accuracy in medical imaging applications. The notation I_e represents the image encoder, I_d denotes the image decoder, and L_e signifies the language encoder. **(a)** Alignment-based method: Image-text alignment using contrastive loss (CLIP loss) to pull the features of paired image-text close together while pushing unpaired features apart, enhancing the model's ability to correlate relevant medical images and texts. **(b)** Reconstruction-based approaches: Masked reconstruction using reconstruction loss, where either masked image tokens or text tokens are reconstructed. This method focuses on recovering the original content, thus enabling the model to better understand and generate detailed components of both medical images and texts. **(c)** Entity-based approaches: This method uses extracted entities to supervise the visual feature learning. Unlike the other two methods that utilize the medical report directly, this style extracts entities from the report first and then aims to learn visual features from the entity classification task, thereby enhancing specific medical knowledge representation

6.2.1 Alignment-Based Approaches

The alignment-based approaches in MedVLP focus on aligning image and text features to enhance the model's understanding and interpretation of medical data [34, 52, 55, 57]. Utilizing CLIP loss, these methods aim to synchronize features at various levels of granularity—global, regional, and token. This multifaceted approach ensures a comprehensive alignment that covers the overall context of the images and texts, specific areas of interest within the images, and even the smallest units of information represented by individual tokens. Such detailed alignment supports the model in developing a robust understanding of the relationships between different modalities of medical data.

Moreover, some methods in alignment-based MedVLP incorporate multiscale visual features to align with different parts of medical reports, accommodating the varying levels of detail and information contained in clinical texts [23, 35]. By matching these multiscale visual features with corresponding segments of text, the model can learn high-level semantics more effectively, maximizing the similarity of paired image-text data while simultaneously distancing unpaired samples. This approach primarily focuses on high-level semantic alignment, which is crucial for understanding complex medical scenarios described in reports. However, it may overlook fine-grained features and low-level visual patterns, as the image encoder primarily learns from the medical report directly, potentially missing out on visual invariants that are critical for detailed medical analysis. Such trade-offs highlight the need for careful consideration in the deployment of alignment-based methods in clinical settings, ensuring that they capture both the broad semantic contexts and the detailed visual cues necessary for accurate medical diagnostics.

6.2.2 Reconstruction-Based Approaches

Reconstruction-based approaches in MedVLP primarily involve masking portions of image tokens or text tokens and then reconstructing them, leveraging both image and text features [7, 24, 32, 58, 60]. This method helps models learn the intricate interplay between visual and textual data, crucial for interpreting medical content. By deliberately obscuring parts of the input and challenging the model to fill in the missing information, these approaches encourage a deeper understanding of the underlying structures and relationships within the data. This process not only enhances the model's predictive capabilities but also improves its ability to integrate and synthesize information from both visual and textual sources effectively.

However, the technique of random masking can introduce complications, such as masking significant portions of normal or unremarkable areas, potentially leading the model to learn shortcuts or irrelevant features. To address these challenges, some studies have introduced guided masking strategies. These methods utilize attention maps to selectively obscure parts of the data that are deemed most informative for learning, thereby helping the model develop more robust and meaningful features. While this method excels in capturing low-level patterns and detailed visual-textual alignments, it can be somewhat limited when it comes to tasks requiring high-level conceptual understanding, such as classification. These limitations highlight the need for balanced approaches in MedVLP that can effectively bridge the gap between detailed feature extraction and high-level semantic comprehension.

6.2.3 Entity-Based Approaches

Entity-based approaches in MedVLP represent a distinct methodology where features are not learned directly from the medical report in its entirety. Instead, this method begins by extracting clinical entities, such as disease names and abnormal patterns, from the report, often relying on expert knowledge to guide the extraction process. This preliminary step focuses on identifying key medical terms and concepts that are crucial for understanding the underlying medical conditions depicted in the images [9, 16, 42, 56, 59].

Once these entities are extracted, the MedVLP task is transformed into a classification challenge, where the primary objective for the model is to classify the image based on the entities included in the medical report. This approach leverages a portion of supervised information during the pre-training phase, which can enhance model performance and provide greater interpretability. The use of expert knowledge in the extraction process ensures that the entities are clinically relevant and accurately represent significant aspects of the medical condition being analyzed.

However, there are inherent limitations to this approach. The extracted entities represent only a fraction of the information contained in the entire medical report, potentially omitting crucial details that could be important for a comprehensive understanding of the case. Moreover, the robustness of the entity extraction process is heavily dependent on the quality and scope of the knowledge database used, which can vary significantly. Additionally, this approach may struggle with newly identified diseases or rare conditions that are not yet well-represented in existing databases, limiting the model's effectiveness in handling emerging medical challenges.

6.3 Generating Synthetic Medical Images

The creation of synthetic medical images is spearheaded by key generative models such as VAEs, GANs, and Stable Diffusion (SD) [19, 31, 45], each serving distinct roles in medical imaging technology. VAEs and GANs are geared primarily towards unconditional generation, producing images in one step from input noise. VAEs function through an encoder-decoder architecture that models the input data distribution [14], while GANs employ a dual structure of a generator that creates images and a discriminator that evaluates them, training the system to generate increasingly realistic images [28].

Conversely, SD adopts a multi-step approach to image generation. Starting with random Gaussian noise, SD refines this input through several denoising steps, unlike the single-step generation of VAEs and GANs [29]. This methodical enhancement process allows SD to produce higher quality images, crucial for medical imaging where detail is paramount. However, the superior image quality comes with

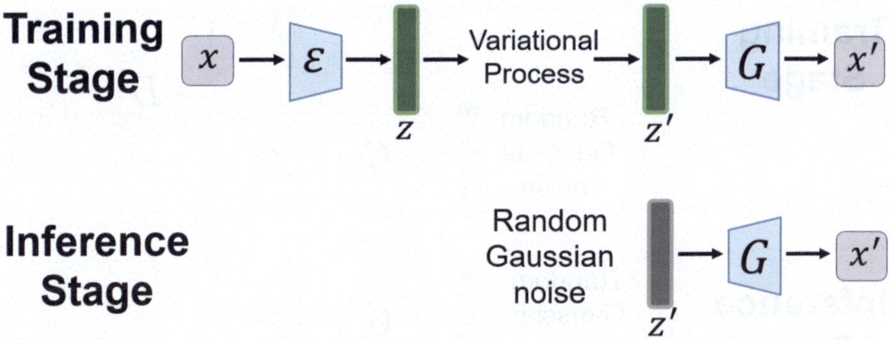

Fig. 6.2 The framework of a VAE is depicted, where x represents the original image input, and x' is the generated image output. The latent feature z of the input image is transformed through a variational process into z', a feature vector following a Gaussian distribution. $\mathcal{E}$ denotes the image encoder, and G is the image generator. The top panel illustrates the training stage, where the encoder $\mathcal{E}$ maps x to a latent representation z, which is then processed to produce z' that follows a Gaussian distribution through a variational process. This transformed latent vector z' is subsequently used by the generator G to produce the reconstructed image x'. The bottom panel shows the inference stage, where random Gaussian noise z' is input into the generator G to synthesize the image x'

increased computational demands, as each image requires multiple inference steps to achieve the final output, making SD both computationally intensive and effective for high-fidelity applications.

6.3.1 Variational Autoencoder

A VAE employs a unique generative model framework, as shown in Fig. 6.2, that utilizes an autoencoder architecture with a probabilistic approach. Unlike traditional autoencoders, which aim to minimize reconstruction error by directly encoding and decoding data, VAEs introduce a probabilistic twist to the encoding process. The encoder in a VAE transforms the input x into a latent feature space z, but instead of encoding to a fixed point, it outputs parameters that define a probability distribution, typically characterized by mean and variance. This distributional approach allows the model to handle the complex, varied nature of input data more effectively.

From the probabilistically defined latent space, a specific representation z is sampled based on the Gaussian distribution parameters provided by the encoder. This sampled latent feature is then passed to the decoder, which attempts to reconstruct the input by generating a new image x'. The capability to sample latent representations allows the VAE not only to reconstruct input images but also to generate new ones by feeding random Gaussian noise into the decoder. This process results in the generation of new images that are variations on the learned data distribution. However, since the generative aspect of VAEs is largely unconditional,

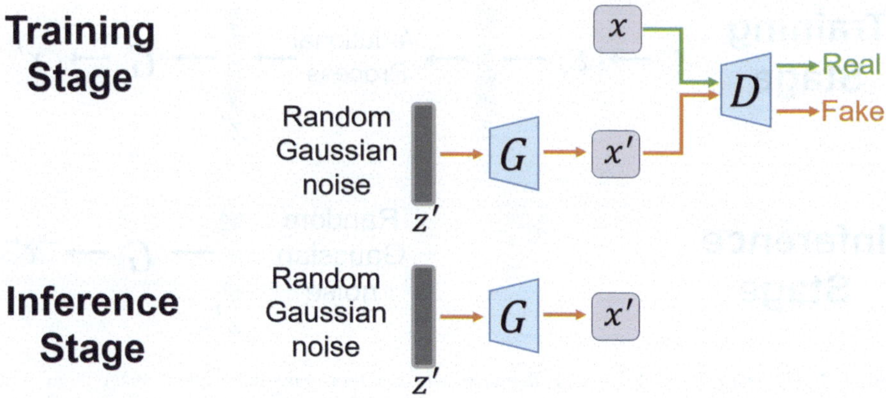

Fig. 6.3 The framework of a GAN is illustrated, where x represents the original image input and x' denotes the generated image output. The latent feature vector z', subject to a Gaussian distribution, is utilized to generate images. G denotes the generator that creates images from the latent vector z', and D is the discriminator tasked with distinguishing between real images x and synthetic images x'. The top panel shows the training stage, where G generates an image x' from z' which, along with real images x, is evaluated by D to train G to produce increasingly realistic images. The bottom panel depicts the inference stage, where random Gaussian noise z' is input into G to synthesize the image x', independent of the discriminator

the model generates images based on the distribution characteristics of the latent space rather than on explicit, controllable semantic content, positioning VAEs as versatile tools in image synthesis but less so for tasks requiring precise semantic consistency.

6.3.2 *Generative Adversarial Network*

GAN, illustrated in Fig. 6.3, represent a novel and powerful class of generative models distinguished by their use of two neural network components: the generator (G) and the discriminator (D). This architecture enables GANs to generate highly realistic data by effectively learning the distribution of the input data through adversarial processes. The generator is tasked with creating data that is indistinguishable from genuine data, while the discriminator evaluates whether the data it receives (either from the generator or the real dataset) is real or synthetic. This adversarial interaction pushes the generator to produce increasingly sophisticated outputs, thereby enhancing the realism and quality of the generated data.

The training process for a GAN is framed as a game between G and D, where G learns to produce data that D cannot distinguish from real data, and D simultaneously sharpens its ability to identify the fakes. Initially, the generator produces data based on random noise input, which the discriminator evaluates. Feedback from the discriminator guides the generator in refining its subsequent

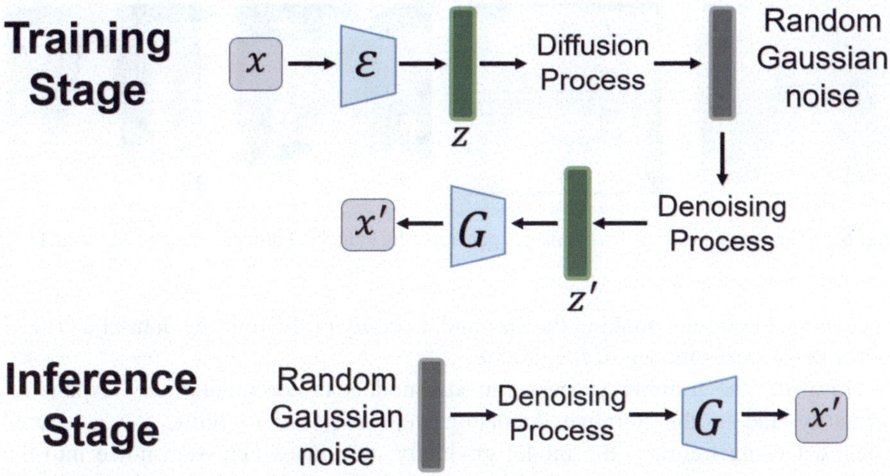

Fig. 6.4 The framework of a Stable Diffusion (SD) model is illustrated, where x represents the original image input, and x' denotes the generated image output. $\mathcal{E}$ is the image encoder that transforms x into the latent feature z. The diffusion process involves adding Gaussian noise to z, transforming it into z' through a denoising process aimed at predicting and removing the added noise. G, the image generator, then uses the denoised latent feature z' to generate the image x'. During the inference stage, random Gaussian noise is input into the denoising block, which processes the noise to refine z', and then G uses z' to produce the final image output x'

outputs. The discriminator's training on both real and generated data enables it to provide accurate assessments, which in turn train the generator to mimic the real data distribution closely.

GANs excel in generating high-quality images, making them ideal for applications requiring photorealistic rendering. However, training GANs can be challenging due to issues such as mode collapse, where the generator learns to produce only a limited variety of outputs, or non-convergence, where the generator and discriminator do not reach a stable state.

6.3.3 Stable Diffusion

Stable Diffusion, the framework of which is shown in Fig. 6.4, represents a significant advancement in generative modeling, requiring extensive datasets for effective training. For example, SD models are often trained on massive datasets such as LAION-5B, which contains billions of images. This extensive training set enables SD models to learn a diverse array of features and styles, contributing to their ability to generate high-fidelity and highly diverse synthetic images. The complexity and variety of the dataset directly influence the quality and versatility of

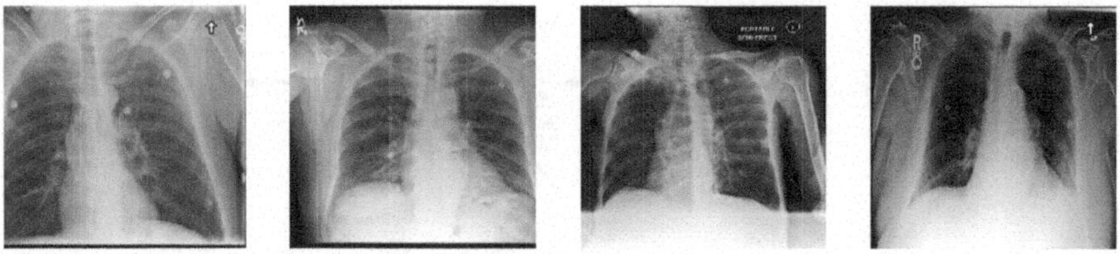

Fig. 6.5 The synthetic chest X-ray images generated by a medical domain-specific SD model [5]

the generated outputs, making the size and diversity of the training dataset a critical factor in the performance of SD models.

However, the training process for SD models is computationally expensive, primarily due to the iterative denoising steps required to refine the generated images. During training, the model gradually introduces Gaussian noise into the data and then learns to reverse this process, effectively 'denoising' to recreate the original input or generate new, high-quality images from noisy inputs. This step-by-step denoising process, though resource-intensive, allows SD models to achieve remarkable levels of detail and realism in the generated images, setting them apart from other generative models that might use less computationally demanding processes. The fidelity and quality of images produced by Stable Diffusion are notably high, making it a preferred choice in applications where visual detail and authenticity are paramount (Fig. 6.5).

6.3.4 Generating Medical Images Conditioned on Text

Although the previously mentioned methods can generate high-quality images, they do so without specific conditions guiding the output. This unconditioned approach, while useful for general purposes, does not necessarily meet the needs of MedVLP, where the generated image must be paired specifically with corresponding textual data to ensure meaningful learning and applicability in medical contexts [2, 29, 49].

To generate images for MedVLP effectively, it's crucial that the images not only exhibit high fidelity but also align semantically with text descriptions. This necessity gives rise to the need for conditional generation, where the synthesis of images is directly influenced by textual conditions [21]. Among the architectures capable of this, SD stands out as both popular and powerful. SD incorporates conditions during the denoising stage through a cross-attention mechanism. This method allows the integration of text conditions to constrain and guide the image generation process, ensuring that the synthetic images are semantically consistent with the accompanying text.

By utilizing text prompts to guide the synthesis, SD enables the creation of synthetic medical images that are tightly coupled with textual descriptions [5, 33, 38]. This capability is crucial for building robust image-text pairs that are indispensable for effective MedVLP training. Through conditional generation, SD not only enhances the relevance of the generated images but also significantly boosts the potential of MedVLP systems in learning and applying nuanced medical knowledge from integrated image-text data.

6.4 Generating Synthetic Medical Text

In the context of MedVLP, generating synthetic medical text, typically in the form of medical reports, is equally crucial as image synthesis. These generated texts serve as detailed descriptions or diagnostic reports that complement synthetic images, thereby enabling comprehensive training of MedVLP systems. The process begins by using advanced language models to craft medical reports that can mirror the complexity and specificity required in actual medical documentation [20, 25, 40]. This capability significantly enhances the dataset used for training MedVLP models by providing contextually relevant textual data.

Once these synthetic medical reports are generated, they are utilized as textual conditions to guide the generation of corresponding medical images. This integrative approach ensures that the synthetic images not only exhibit high fidelity but also align accurately with the medical scenarios described in the text. This methodological synergy between generated text and images fosters a more effective training environment for MedVLP systems, allowing them to better understand and interpret the nuanced interplay between medical imagery and textual data.

The generation of structured medical reports is largely facilitated by mainstream LLMs such as Llama3 [1] and GPT [41], which utilize transformer-based architectures. These models are adept at processing natural language inputs and generating coherent and contextually appropriate outputs. They employ an autoregressive method of text generation, where each word is predicted based on the sequence of words that came before it, as demonstrated in Fig. 6.6. For instance, when provided with a prompt such as "Now you are a professional radiologist, please generate a standard medical report including pneumonia in the right upper lobe," these models can produce precise and clinically relevant reports like: "Right upper lobe pneumonia or mass. However, given right hilar fullness, a mass resulting in post-obstructive pneumonia is within the differential."

After generating the synthetic medical text, this text is then used to condition the process of generating medical images through models such as SD. This ensures that the images not only visually represent the described medical conditions but also correspond precisely to the clinical details outlined in the synthetic reports. After preparing the synthetic text and synthetic images, both can be utilized for MedVLP using purely synthetic data, employing the VLP approaches described in Sect. 6.2.

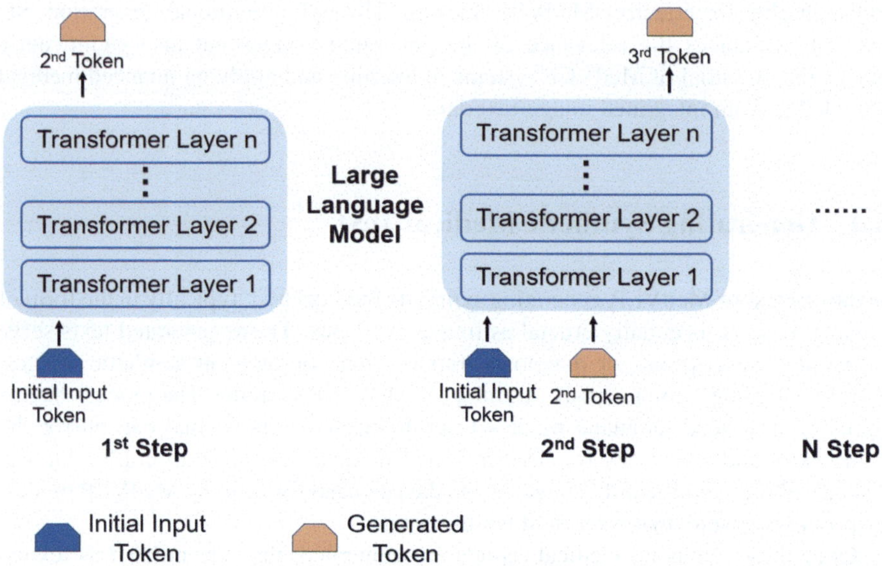

Fig. 6.6 The figure illustrates the autoregressive text generation process using a transformer-based LLM. In the first step, the initial input token is processed through multiple transformer layers to generate the second token. Subsequently, each step incorporates the previously generated token as input, which is again processed through the same transformer layers to produce the next token. This sequence continues iteratively through 'N' steps, with each step generating a subsequent token until the completion of the sequence

6.5 Downstream Tasks for Evaluating Medical Vision-Language Pre-training

After the development and pretraining phases of MedVLP, it is crucial to evaluate the quality and efficacy of the pre-trained models. This evaluation typically involves various downstream tasks that test different aspects of the models, focusing particularly on their ability to handle cross-modal tasks that involve both images and textual data. We have listed various public datasets for downstream tasks in Table 6.2.

6.5.1 Zero-Shot Tasks

Zero-shot tasks are key for assessing the cross-modal feature quality of pre-trained models. These tasks do not require traditional training with labeled examples specific to the task at hand; instead, they use the general understanding and features learned during the MedVLP phase to make inferences about unseen data.

Table 6.2 Overview of various public datasets for downstream tasks: The symbol '/' denotes that training/validation data is not required for zero-shot tasks

Task	Dataset	Train	Valid	Test
Fine-tune Classification	CheXpert [26]	186,027	5,000	202
	RSNA [47]	16,010	5,337	5,337
	COVIDx [54]	23,988	5,998	400
	CXR14 [53]	77,872	8,652	25,596
Fine-tune Segmentation	RSNA [47]	16,010	5,337	5,337
	SIIM [50]	8,433	1,807	1,807
Fine-tune Object Detection	RSNA [47]	16,010	5,337	5,337
	Object-CXR [22]	6,400	1,600	1,000
Zero-shot Classification	RSNA [47]	/	/	5,337
	SIIM [50]	/	/	1,807
	CXR14 [53]	/	/	25,596
	CheXpert [26]	/	/	500
Zero-shot Grounding	RSNA [47]	/	/	5,337
	SIIM [50]	/	/	1,807

- **Zero-shot Classification (Fig. 6.7a):** This task evaluates the ability of the model to classify images based on textual descriptions that were not part of the training set. For instance, a model might be given an image of a lung and a text description "pneumonia" and would need to classify whether the image fits the description based solely on the learned embeddings.
- **Zero-shot Grounding (Fig. 6.7b):** Here, the model must localize objects or areas within an image that correspond to a given textual description. This task checks how well the model understands the spatial relationships and details within the image that relate to the descriptions.

6.5.2 *Fine-Tuning Tasks*

In addition to zero-shot tasks, fine-tuning tasks are employed to further refine and evaluate the visual feature quality of the models. These tasks involve adjusting the model on a specific dataset or for a particular task to improve performance, thereby assessing how effectively the pre-trained model adapts to new visual information.

- **Fine-tune Classification (Fig. 6.8 a)** This task involves retraining the model to classify medical images into predefined categories, such as differentiating between types of lung diseases, based on their visual content. It uses disease labels and cross-entropy loss to fine-tune the model.
- **Fine-tune Segmentation (Fig. 6.8b):** Segmentation tasks require the model to outline specific structures within an image, such as tumors or other pathological

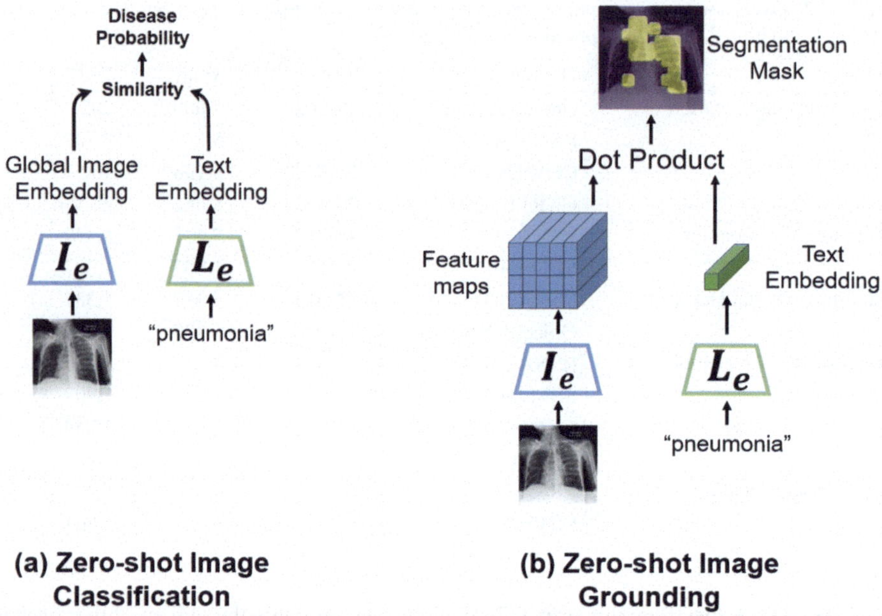

Fig. 6.7 Zero-shot downstream tasks utilizing disease names as prompts. (**a**) Zero-shot Image Classification: The process involves using the disease name as a prompt to extract global image features and text prompt features. The similarity between these features is then computed and used as the probability of the disease mentioned in the prompt. (**b**) Zero-shot Image Grounding: This task also starts with the disease name as a prompt but focuses on extracting regional image features and a global text feature. The similarity between the text feature and each regional image feature is calculated, resulting in a similarity score for each image region relative to the disease. This similarity map is then used as the final segmentation result to compute metrics

features. This is crucial for applications like automated diagnostics where precise anatomical segmentation is necessary.

- **Fine-tune Object Detection (Fig. 6.8c):** Finally, object detection tasks challenge the model to identify and localize multiple objects within medical images, which is essential for applications such as detecting abnormalities across different scans.

Based on the comprehensive evaluation provided by these downstream tasks, we can effectively assess the capabilities and performance of MedVLP systems across a range of critical dimensions. These tasks allow us to determine not only how well the models handle specific visual recognition tasks post-training but also their ability to integrate and interpret cross-modal information from both textual and visual inputs. As such, the outcomes of zero-shot and fine-tuning tasks provide essential metrics that reflect the robustness, adaptability, and overall utility of MedVLP systems in practical, clinical settings.

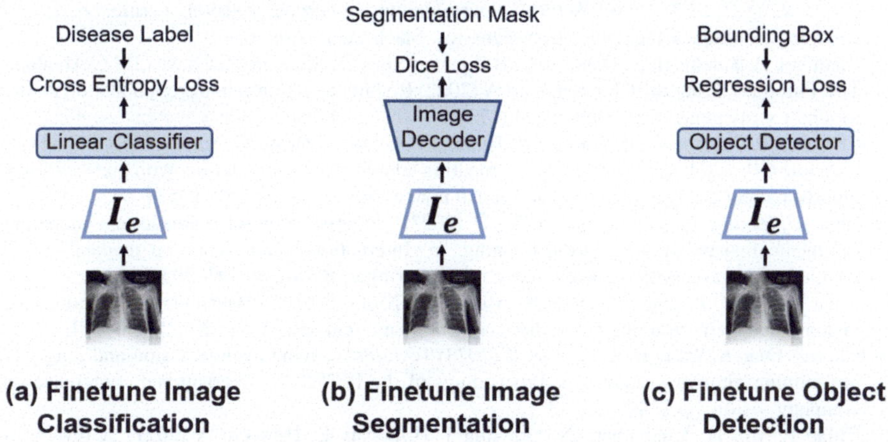

Fig. 6.8 Figure illustrates three finetuning tasks using image embeddings. (**a**) Finetune Image Classification: This process involves a linear classifier that uses the global image embedding derived from medical images. The classifier is trained with a cross-entropy loss function to predict the disease label based on the image features. (**b**) Finetune Image Segmentation: An image decoder utilizes the global image embedding to reconstruct segmentation masks of anatomical or pathological features, trained via a Dice loss to enhance the metric of the segmentation. (**c**) Finetune Object Detection: In this task, an object detector processes the image embedding to identify and locate objects within medical images, using bounding box coordinates adjusted through regression loss to refine the detection performance

6.6 Conclusion

In this chapter, we explored the use of synthetic data and its impact on MedVLP. We highlighted various MedVLP methods and discussed the utilization of public real image-text datasets for MedVLP. We detailed the generative models used for synthesizing images and LLMs for generating medical text. We also demonstrated how text can be used as a condition for generating medical images. Finally, we discussed the evaluation of MedVLP on various downstream tasks using a wide range of datasets.

References

1. AI@Meta (2024) Llama 3 model card. https://github.com/meta-llama/llama3/blob/main/MODEL_CARD.md
2. AlAmir M, AlGhamdi M (2022) The role of generative adversarial network in medical image analysis: an in-depth survey. ACM Comput Surv 55(5):1–36
3. Bustos A, Pertusa A, Salinas JM, de la Iglesia-Vayá M (2020) Padchest: a large chest x-ray image dataset with multi-label annotated reports. Med Image Anal 66:101797

4. Chai J, Zeng H, Li A, Ngai EW (2021) Deep learning in computer vision: a critical review of emerging techniques and application scenarios. Mach Learn Appl 6:100134
5. Chambon P, Bluethgen C, Delbrouck JB, Van der Sluijs R, Połacin M, Chaves JMZ, Abraham TM, Purohit S, Langlotz CP, Chaudhari A (2022) Roentgen: vision-language foundation model for chest x-ray generation. arXiv:221112737
6. Chambon P, Delbrouck JB, Sounack T, Huang SC, Chen Z, Varma M, Truong SQ, Chuong CT, Langlotz CP (2024) CheXpert Plus: augmenting a large chest x-ray dataset with text radiology reports, patient demographics and additional image formats. arXiv:240519538
7. Chen C, Zhong A, Wu D, Luo J, Li Q (2023) Contrastive masked image-text modeling for medical visual representation learning. In: International conference on medical image computing and computer-assisted intervention. Springer, Berlin, pp 493–503
8. Chen Y, Liu C, Huang W, Cheng S, Arcucci R, Xiong Z (2023) Generative text-guided 3d vision-language pretraining for unified medical image segmentation. arXiv:230604811
9. Chen Z, Diao S, Wang B, Li G, Wan X (2023) Towards unifying medical vision-and-language pre-training via soft prompts. In: Proceedings of the IEEE/CVF international conference on computer vision, pp 23403–23413
10. Chlap P, Min H, Vandenberg N, Dowling J, Holloway L, Haworth A (2021) A review of medical image data augmentation techniques for deep learning applications. J Med Imag Rad Oncol 65(5):545–563
11. Demner-Fushman D, Kohli MD, Rosenman MB, Shooshan SE, Rodriguez L, Antani S, Thoma GR, McDonald CJ (2016) Preparing a collection of radiology examinations for distribution and retrieval. J Am Med Inf Assoc 23(2):304–310
12. Denize J, Rabarisoa J, Orcesi A, Hérault R, Canu S (2023) Similarity contrastive estimation for self-supervised soft contrastive learning. In: Proceedings of the IEEE/CVF winter conference on applications of computer vision, pp 2706–2716
13. Devlin J, Chang MW, Lee K, Toutanova K (2018) Bert: pre-training of deep bidirectional transformers for language understanding. arXiv:181004805
14. Ehrhardt J, Wilms M (2022) Autoencoders and variational autoencoders in medical image analysis. In: Biomedical image synthesis and simulation. Elsevier, Amsterdam, pp 129–162
15. Esteva A, Chou K, Yeung S, Naik N, Madani A, et al (2021) Deep learning-enabled medical computer vision. NPJ Digi Med 4(1):1–9
16. Fan W, Suvon MNI, Zhou S, Liu X, Alabed S, Osmani V, Swift A, Chen C, Lu H (2024) Medslip: medical dual-stream language-image pre-training for fine-grained alignment. arXiv:240310635
17. Feng S, Liu Q, Patel A, Bazai SU, Jin CK, Kim JS, Sarrafzadeh M, Azzollini D, Yeoh J, Kim E, et al (2022) Automated pneumothorax triaging in chest x-rays in the new zealand population using deep-learning algorithms. J Med Imag Rad Oncol 66(8):1035–1043
18. Ficek J, Wang W, Chen H, Dagne G, Daley E (2021) Differential privacy in health research: a scoping review. J Am Med Inf Assoc 28(10):2269–2276
19. Goodfellow I, Pouget-Abadie J, Mirza M, Xu B, Warde-Farley D, Ozair S, Courville A, Bengio Y (2014) Generative adversarial nets. Adv Neural Inf Process Syst 27:139–144
20. Guan J, Li R, Yu S, Zhang X (2018) Generation of synthetic electronic medical record text. In: 2018 IEEE international conference on bioinformatics and biomedicine (BIBM). IEEE, Piscataway, pp 374–380
21. Havaei M, Mao X, Wang Y, Lao Q (2021) Conditional generation of medical images via disentangled adversarial inference. Med Image Anal 72:102106
22. Healthcare J (2020) Object-CXR - automatic detection of foreign objects on chest X-rays. https://web.archive.org/web/20201127235812/; https://jfhealthcare.github.io/object-CXR/
23. Huang SC, Shen L, Lungren MP, Yeung S (2021) Gloria: a multimodal global-local representation learning framework for label-efficient medical image recognition. In: Proceedings of the IEEE/CVF international conference on computer vision, pp 3942–3951
24. Huang W, Zhou H, Li C, Yang H, Liu J, Wang S (2023) Enhancing representation in radiography-reports foundation model: a granular alignment algorithm using masked contrastive learning. arXiv:230905904

25. Hüske-Kraus D (2003) Text generation in clinical medicine–a review. Methods Inf Med 42(01):51–60
26. Irvin J, Rajpurkar P, Ko M, Yu Y, Ciurea-Ilcus S, Chute C, Marklund H, Haghgoo B, Ball R, Shpanskaya K, et al (2019) Chexpert: a large chest radiograph dataset with uncertainty labels and expert comparison. In: Proceedings of the AAAI conference on artificial intelligence, vol 33, pp 590–597
27. Johnson AEW, Pollard TJ, Berkowitz SJ, Greenbaum NR, Lungren MP, Ying Deng C, Mark RG, Horng S (2019) Mimic-cxr: a large publicly available database of labeled chest radiographs. ArXiv abs/1901.07042
28. Kazeminia S, Baur C, Kuijper A, van Ginneken B, Navab N, Albarqouni S, Mukhopadhyay A (2020) Gans for medical image analysis. Artif Intell Med 109:101938
29. Kazerouni A, Aghdam EK, Heidari M, Azad R, Fayyaz M, Hacihaliloglu I, Merhof D (2023) Diffusion models in medical imaging: a comprehensive survey. Med Image Anal 88:102846
30. Khokhar RH, Chen R, Fung BC, Lui SM (2014) Quantifying the costs and benefits of privacy-preserving health data publishing. J Biomed Inf 50:107–121
31. Kingma DP, Welling M (2013) Auto-encoding variational bayes. arXiv:13126114
32. Li M, Meng M, Fulham M, Feng DD, Bi L, Kim J (2024) Enhancing medical vision-language contrastive learning via inter-matching relation modelling. arXiv:240110501
33. Liu G, Hsu TMH, McDermott M, Boag W, Weng WH, Szolovits P, Ghassemi M (2019) Clinically accurate chest x-ray report generation. In: Machine learning for healthcare conference. Proceedings of machine learning research, pp 249–269
34. Liu C, Cheng S, Chen C, Qiao M, Zhang W, Shah A, Bai W, Arcucci R (2023) M-flag: medical vision-language pre-training with frozen language models and latent space geometry optimization. arXiv:230708347
35. Liu C, Cheng S, Shi M, Shah A, Bai W, Arcucci R (2023) Imitate: clinical prior guided hierarchical vision-language pre-training. arXiv:231007355
36. Liu C, Ouyang C, Chen Y, Quilodrán-Casas CC, Ma L, Fu J, Guo Y, Shah A, Bai W, Arcucci R (2023) T3d: towards 3d medical image understanding through vision-language pre-training. arXiv:231201529
37. Liu C, Ouyang C, Cheng S, Shah A, Bai W, Arcucci R (2023) G2d: from global to dense radiography representation learning via vision-language pre-training. arXiv:231201522
38. Liu C, Shah A, Bai W, Arcucci R (2023) Utilizing synthetic data for medical vision-language pre-training: bypassing the need for real images. arXiv:231007027
39. Liu C, Wan Z, Wang Y, Shen H, Wang H, Zheng K, Zhang M, Arcucci R (2024) Benchmarking and boosting radiology report generation for 3d high-resolution medical images. arXiv:240607146
40. Luo R, Sun L, Xia Y, Qin T, Zhang S, Poon H, Liu TY (2022) BioGPT: generative pre-trained transformer for biomedical text generation and mining. Brief Bioinf 23:bbac409
41. OpenAI (2023) Gpt-4 technical report. ArXiv abs/2303.08774
42. Phan VMH, Xie Y, Qi Y, Liu L, Liu L, Zhang B, Liao Z, Wu Q, To MS, Verjans JW (2024) Decomposing disease descriptions for enhanced pathology detection: a multi-aspect vision-language pre-training framework. In: Proceedings of the IEEE/CVF conference on computer vision and pattern recognition, pp 11492–11501
43. Qin J, Liu C, Cheng S, Guo Y, Arcucci R (2024) Freeze the backbones: a parameter-efficient contrastive approach to robust medical vision-language pre-training. In: ICASSP 2024–2024 IEEE international conference on acoustics, speech and signal processing (ICASSP). IEEE, Piscataway, pp 1686–1690
44. Radford A, Wu J, Child R, Luan D, Amodei D, Sutskever I, et al (2019) Language models are unsupervised multitask learners. OpenAI Blog 1(8):9
45. Rombach R, Blattmann A, Lorenz D, Esser P, Ommer B (2022) High-resolution image synthesis with latent diffusion models. In: Proceedings of the IEEE/CVF conference on computer vision and pattern recognition, pp 10684–10695

46. Ronneberger O, Fischer P, Brox T (2015) U-net: convolutional networks for biomedical image segmentation. In: Medical image computing and computer-assisted intervention–MICCAI 2015: 18th international conference, Munich, October 5–9. Proceedings, Part III 18, Springer, Berlin, pp 234–241
47. Shih G, Wu CC, Halabi SS, Kohli MD, Prevedello LM, Cook TS, Sharma A, Amorosa JK, Arteaga V, Galperin-Aizenberg M, et al (2019) Augmenting the national institutes of health chest radiograph dataset with expert annotations of possible pneumonia. Radiol Artif Intell 1(1):e180041
48. Shrestha P, Amgain S, Khanal B, Linte CA, Bhattarai B (2023) Medical vision language pretraining: a survey. arXiv:231206224
49. Singh NK, Raza K (2021) Medical image generation using generative adversarial networks: a review. In: Health informatics: a computational perspective in healthcare, pp 77–96
50. Langer SG, Shih G (2019) SIIM-ACR pneumothorax segmentation. Available link: https://www.kaggle.com/competitions/siim-acr-pneumothorax-segmentation/data. Access time: 08-06-2020
51. Touvron H, Martin L, Stone K, Albert P, Almahairi A, Babaei Y, Bashlykov N, Batra S, Bhargava P, Bhosale S, et al (2023) Llama 2: open foundation and fine-tuned chat models. arXiv:230709288
52. Wan Z, Liu C, Zhang M, Fu J, Wang B, Cheng S, Ma L, Quilodrán-Casas C, Arcucci R (2023) Med-unic: unifying cross-lingual medical vision-language pre-training by diminishing bias. arXiv:230519894
53. Wang X, Peng Y, Lu L, Lu Z, Bagheri M, Summers RM (2017) Chestx-ray8: hospital-scale chest x-ray database and benchmarks on weakly-supervised classification and localization of common thorax diseases. In: Proceedings of the IEEE conference on computer vision and pattern recognition, pp 2097–2106
54. Wang L, Lin ZQ, Wong A (2020) Covid-net: a tailored deep convolutional neural network design for detection of covid-19 cases from chest x-ray images. Sci Rep 10(1):1–12
55. Wang F, Zhou Y, Wang S, Vardhanabhuti V, Yu L (2022) Multi-granularity cross-modal alignment for generalized medical visual representation learning. arXiv:221006044
56. Wu C, Zhang X, Zhang Y, Wang Y, Xie W (2023) Medklip: medical knowledge enhanced language-image pre-training for x-ray diagnosis. In: Proceedings of the IEEE/CVF International Conference on Computer Vision, pp 21372–21383
57. Zhang Y, Jiang H, Miura Y, Manning CD, Langlotz CP (2020) Contrastive learning of medical visual representations from paired images and text. arXiv:201000747
58. Zhang K, Yang Y, Yu J, Jiang H, Fan J, Huang Q, Han W (2023) Multi-task paired masking with alignment modeling for medical vision-language pre-training. IEEE Trans Multimedia 26:4706–4721
59. Zhang X, Wu C, Zhang Y, Xie W, Wang Y (2023) Knowledge-enhanced visual-language pre-training on chest radiology images. Nat Commun 14(1):4542
60. Zhou HY, Lian C, Wang L, Yu Y (2023) Advancing radiograph representation learning with masked record modeling. arXiv:230113155
61. Zhu D, Chen J, Shen X, Li X, Elhoseiny M (2023) Minigpt-4: Enhancing vision-language understanding with advanced large language models. arXiv preprint arXiv:2304.10592

Chapter 7
Diffusion Models for Inverse Problems in Medical Imaging

Hyungjin Chung and Jong Chul Ye

Abstract Diffusion model is a class of generative models that learns the gradient of the unnormalized log prior density. Diffusion models are easy to train, as the training amounts to training a denoiser on multiple noise levels. Equipped with a powerful generative prior that is modeled with a diffusion model, one can solve inverse problems through posterior sampling, leveraging the principles of Bayesian inference. In this chapter, we review the principles of diffusion models and study how they can be used to solve inverse problems that arise in medical imaging, focusing on MRI and CT reconstruction tasks.

7.1 Introduction

Let us consider the following linear inverse problem, which, despite its simplicity, can be used to model the measurement process of diverse medical imaging modalities (e.g. MRI, CT)

$$\boldsymbol{y} = \boldsymbol{A}\boldsymbol{x} + \boldsymbol{n}, \quad \boldsymbol{y} \in \mathbb{R}^m, \quad \boldsymbol{x} \in \mathbb{R}^n, \quad \boldsymbol{A} \in \mathbb{R}^{m \times n}, \quad \boldsymbol{n} \sim \mathcal{N}(\boldsymbol{0}, \sigma_y^2 \boldsymbol{I}) \tag{7.1}$$

where typically $m < n$, making the problem ill-posed. The problem is to reconstruct a clean signal $\boldsymbol{x}$ from the deficient and noisy measurement $\boldsymbol{y}$. In a probabilistic sense, this can be represented as the following *likelihood* model

$$p(\boldsymbol{y}|\boldsymbol{x}) = \mathcal{N}(\boldsymbol{y}; \boldsymbol{A}\boldsymbol{x}, \sigma_y^2 \boldsymbol{I}) = Z \exp\left(-\frac{\|\boldsymbol{y} - \boldsymbol{A}\boldsymbol{x}\|_2^2}{2\sigma_y^2}\right), \tag{7.2}$$

where Z is a normalizing constant. On the other hand, we are interested in the *posterior* distribution, which is achieved by Bayes rule

H. Chung (✉) · J. C. Ye
KAIST, Daejeon, South Korea
e-mail: hj.chung@kaist.ac.kr; jong.ye@kaist.ac.kr

L. Zhang et al. (eds.), *Generative Machine Learning Models in Medical Image Computing*, https://doi.org/10.1007/978-3-031-80965-1_7

$$\underbrace{p(\boldsymbol{x}|\boldsymbol{y})}_{\text{posterior}} \propto \underbrace{p(\boldsymbol{x})}_{\text{prior}} \underbrace{p(\boldsymbol{y}|\boldsymbol{x})}_{\text{likelihood Eq. (7.2)}} . \tag{7.3}$$

To access the posterior, one needs to define a suitable prior $p(\boldsymbol{x})$, which can be thought of as the **naturalness** of the signal.

Intuitive Meaning of Prior and the Likelihood
High posterior probability requires high prior probability conjugated with a high likelihood value. A high prior probability means that the image is **realistic**, while a low prior probability means that the image is **unrealistic**. However, in order to also achieve a high likelihood, $\boldsymbol{x}$ should not be just *any* realistic image. It should adhere to the measurement information contained in $\boldsymbol{y}$. This is often denoted as data consistency, measurement consistency, fidelity, etc.

The advances in inverse problem-solving can be attributed to the advancements in devising a better prior. Traditional methods used hand-crafted priors: total variation [2, 14], sparsity [12, 23] are two of the most widely used priors that are used in the context of medical imaging. Once we define a prior, we can choose to either find $\boldsymbol{x}$ that maximizes the posterior (i.e. maximum a posteriori; MAP), or to sample from the posterior (i.e. posterior sampling). For instance, performing MAP can be done in the following way. From Eq. (7.3), we can take the log on both sides to have

$$\log p(\boldsymbol{x}|\boldsymbol{y}) = \log p(\boldsymbol{x}) + \log p(\boldsymbol{y}|\boldsymbol{x}) - \log p(\boldsymbol{y}). \tag{7.4}$$

We can equivalently minimize the negative log posterior, leading to

$$\boldsymbol{x}^* = \arg\min_{\boldsymbol{x}} -\log p(\boldsymbol{x}) - \log p(\boldsymbol{y}|\boldsymbol{x}) \tag{7.5}$$

$$= \arg\min_{\boldsymbol{x}} f(\boldsymbol{x}) + \frac{1}{2\sigma_y^2}\|\boldsymbol{y} - \boldsymbol{A}\boldsymbol{x}\|_2^2, \tag{7.6}$$

where $f(\boldsymbol{x}) = \exp(p(\boldsymbol{x}))$ defines our implicit prior. Taking $f(\boldsymbol{x}) := \|\boldsymbol{T}(\boldsymbol{x})\|_1$ regularizes so that the reconstructed signal is sparse in some transform domain acquired through $\boldsymbol{T}(\cdot) : \mathbb{R}^n \mapsto \mathbb{R}^n$, and setting $f(\boldsymbol{x}) := \|\boldsymbol{D}\boldsymbol{x}\|_1$ where $\boldsymbol{D}$ is the finite difference operator regularizes so that the signal is smooth.

In the modern deep learning era, we can *learn* the prior from the data itself, rather than hand-crafting it. That is, we can train a deep generative model [15, 21, 25] to approximate $p_\theta(\boldsymbol{x}) \approx p_{\text{data}}(\boldsymbol{x})$, where θ is the parameter of our generative model. Different from the MAP formulation in Eq. (7.5), we can define a constrained optimization problem where we constrain $\boldsymbol{x}$ to be in the range space of our generative model, i.e.

$$x^* = \arg\min_{x} \|y - Ax\|_2^2 \quad \text{subject to} \quad x \sim p_\theta(x). \tag{7.7}$$

As deep generative models typically learn a mapping from the reference distribution (typically a standard normal distribution, denoted as $z \sim p_z(z)$) to the data distribution, a natural way to solve Eq. (7.7) is to optimize for this latent variable z. A method proposed in CSGM [3] can be succinctly represented as

$$z^* = \arg\min_{z} \|AG_\theta(z) - y\|^2, \tag{7.8}$$

which is possible as we can effectively take the gradient w.r.t. z by backpropagation, and G_θ is a direct mapping that requires a single neural network forward pass. Once the optimization of Eq. (7.8) is solved, the final reconstruction is given as $x^* = G_\theta(z^*)$. It was shown that the same paradigm applies to GANs, VAEs [3], and normalizing flows [33]. We will see in the following sections that this is not directly applicable to diffusion models.

7.2 Background: Diffusion Models

Let us define a random variable $x_0 \sim p(x_0) = p_{\text{data}}(x)$, where p_{data} denotes the data distribution. In diffusion models, we construct a continuous Gaussian perturbation kernel

$$p(x_t|x_0) = \mathcal{N}(x_t; s_t x_0, s_t^2 \sigma_t^2 I), \quad t \in [0, 1], \tag{7.9}$$

which smooths out the distribution. As $t \to 1$, the marginal distribution $p_t(x_t)$ is smoothed such that it approximates the Gaussian distribution, which becomes our reference distribution to sample from. Using the reparametrization trick, one can directly sample

$$x_t = s_t x_0 + s_t \sigma_t z, \quad z \sim \mathcal{N}(0, I). \tag{7.10}$$

Diffusion models aim to revert the data noising process. Remarkably, it was shown that the data noising process and the denoising process can both be represented as a stochastic differential equation (SDE), governed by the score function $\nabla_{x_t} \log p(x_t)$ [19, 28].

Variance Preserving (VP)/Variance Exploding (VE) Diffusion Models
In the diffusion literature, one of the two different forward processes is used. VE diffusion [19, 28] sets the signal coefficient $s_t = 1$, and only scales the noise coefficient σ_t to very high values as $t \to 1$, making the signal coefficient negligible after enough diffusion. On the other hand, VP diffusion [11, 16] scales both the signal and the noise coefficient $s_t \to 0$, $\sigma_t \to 1$ as $t \to 1$. Choosing which diffusion process to use is often a design choice. Moreover, these two processes can be thought of as equivalent, as one can redefine a scaled variable $\tilde{x}$ by dividing x with its signal coefficient [19, 20]. In this chapter, we typically set $s_t = 1$ for simplicity, unless specified otherwise.

Namely, the forward/reverse diffusion SDE can be succinctly represented as

$$d\boldsymbol{x}_{\pm} = -\dot{\sigma}_t\sigma_t\nabla_{\boldsymbol{x}_t}\log p(\boldsymbol{x}_t)\,dt \pm \dot{\sigma}_t\sigma_t\nabla_{\boldsymbol{x}_t}\log p(\boldsymbol{x}_t)\,dt + \sqrt{\dot{\sigma}_t\sigma_t}d\boldsymbol{w}_t, \tag{7.11}$$

where $\boldsymbol{w}_t$ is the standard Wiener process. Here, the $+$ sign denotes the forward process, where Eq. (7.11) collapses to a Brownian motion. With the $-$ sign, the process runs backward, and we see that the score function $\nabla_{\boldsymbol{x}_t}\log p(\boldsymbol{x}_t)$ governs the reverse SDE. In other words, in order to run reverse diffusion sampling (i.e. generative modeling), we need access to the score function of the data distribution.

The procedure called score matching, where one tries to train a parametrized model $\boldsymbol{s}_\theta$ to approximate $\nabla_{\boldsymbol{x}_t}\log p(\boldsymbol{x}_t)$ can be done through score matching [17]. As explicit and implicit score matching methods are costly to perform, the most widely used training method in the modern sense is the so-called denoising score matching (DSM) [32]

$$\min_\theta \mathbb{E}_{\boldsymbol{x}_t,\boldsymbol{x}_0,\boldsymbol{\epsilon}}\left[\|\boldsymbol{s}_\theta^{(t)}(\boldsymbol{x}_t) - \nabla_{\boldsymbol{x}_t}\log p(\boldsymbol{x}_t|\boldsymbol{x}_0)\|_2^2\right], \tag{7.12}$$

which is easy to train as our perturbation kernel is Gaussian. Once $\boldsymbol{s}_{\theta^*}$ is trained, we can use it as a plug-in approximation of the score function to plug into Eq. (7.11).

7.2.1 Detour: Score Function, Posterior Mean, and DDPM

7.2.1.1 Score Function and Posterior Mean

The score function has close relation to the posterior mean $\mathbb{E}[\boldsymbol{x}_0|\boldsymbol{x}_t]$, which can be formally linked through Tweedie's formula [13]

Lemma 7.1 (Tweedie's Formula) *Given a Gaussian perturbation kernel defined in Eq. (7.9), the posterior mean is given by*

$$\mathbb{E}[\boldsymbol{x}_0|\boldsymbol{x}_t] = \frac{1}{s_t}(\boldsymbol{x}_t + \sigma_t^2 \nabla_{\boldsymbol{x}_t} \log p(\boldsymbol{x}_t)) \tag{7.13}$$

In other words, having access to the score function is equivalent to having access to the posterior mean $\mathbb{E}[\boldsymbol{x}_0|\boldsymbol{x}_t]$. The posterior mean is the minimum-mean-squared-error (MMSE) estimate of the Gaussian-noisy $\boldsymbol{x}_t$. This shouldn't come as a surprise, as rearranging Eq. (7.12) with $s_t = 1$ and defining

$$D_\theta(\boldsymbol{x}_t) := \boldsymbol{x}_t + \sigma_t^2 s_\theta(\boldsymbol{x}_t), \tag{7.14}$$

Equation (7.12) is equivalent to a denoising autoencoder (DAE).

$$\min_\theta \mathbb{E}_{\boldsymbol{x}_t, \boldsymbol{x}_0, \boldsymbol{\epsilon}} \left[\frac{1}{\sigma_t} \|D_\theta^{(t)}(\boldsymbol{x}_t) - \boldsymbol{x}_0\|_2^2 \right]. \tag{7.15}$$

This means that running the reverse diffusion in Eq. (7.11) by using a plug-in estimate $\nabla_{\boldsymbol{x}_t} \log p(\boldsymbol{x}_t) \approx s_{\theta*}^{(t)}(\boldsymbol{x}_t)$ is essentially refining the posterior mean $\mathbb{E}[\boldsymbol{x}_0|\boldsymbol{x}_t]$ through the process. Under this view, diffusion models always keep a *dual* representation: the noisy variable $\boldsymbol{x}_t$, and the empirical posterior mean $\hat{\boldsymbol{x}}_{0|t}^\theta := \boldsymbol{x}_t + \sigma_t^2 D_\theta^{(t)}(\boldsymbol{x}_t)$. The relation between the posterior mean, score function, and the dual representation will come in handy later on.

7.2.1.2 Denoising Diffusion Probabilistic Models (DDPM)

DDPM is a diffusion model, where the forward and the reverse diffusion are defined by discrete Markov Gaussian transition kernels

$$p_\theta(\boldsymbol{x}_0) = \int p_\theta(\boldsymbol{x}_T) \prod_{t=1}^{T} p_\theta^{(t)}(\boldsymbol{x}_{t-1}|\boldsymbol{x}_t)\, d\boldsymbol{x}_{1:T}, \tag{7.16}$$

where $\boldsymbol{x}_{\{1,\ldots,T\}} \in \mathbb{R}^d$ are *noisy* latent variables that have the same dimension as the data random vector $\boldsymbol{x}_0 \in \mathbb{R}^d$, defined by the Markovian forward conditional densities

$$q(\boldsymbol{x}_t|\boldsymbol{x}_{t-1}) = \mathcal{N}(\boldsymbol{x}_t|\sqrt{\beta_t}\boldsymbol{x}_{t-1}, (1-\beta_t)\boldsymbol{I}), \tag{7.17}$$

$$q(\boldsymbol{x}_t|\boldsymbol{x}_0) = \mathcal{N}(\boldsymbol{x}_t|\sqrt{\bar{\alpha}_t}\boldsymbol{x}_0, (1-\bar{\alpha}_t)\boldsymbol{I}). \tag{7.18}$$

Here, the noise schedule β_t is an increasing sequence of t, with $\bar{\alpha}_t := \prod_{i=1}^t \alpha_t$, $\alpha_t := 1 - \beta_t$. Training of diffusion models amounts to training a multi-noise level residual denoiser (i.e. epsilon matching)

$$\min_\theta \mathbb{E}_{\boldsymbol{x}_t \sim q(\boldsymbol{x}_t|\boldsymbol{x}_0), \boldsymbol{x}_0 \sim p_{\text{data}}(\boldsymbol{x}_0), \boldsymbol{\epsilon} \sim \mathcal{N}(0, \boldsymbol{I})} \left[\|\boldsymbol{\epsilon}_\theta^{(t)}(\boldsymbol{x}_t) - \boldsymbol{\epsilon}\|_2^2 \right],$$

such that $\boldsymbol{\epsilon}_{\theta^*}^{(t)}(\boldsymbol{x}_t) \simeq \frac{\boldsymbol{x}_t - \sqrt{\bar{\alpha}_t}\boldsymbol{x}_0}{\sqrt{1-\bar{\alpha}_t}}$. Interestingly, this training objective is equivalent to denoising score matching up to a multiplicative constant, similar to the relation between DSM and DAE. Indeed, it can be seen that the score function approximating $\nabla_{\boldsymbol{x}_t} \log q(\boldsymbol{x}_t|\boldsymbol{x}_0)$ has the following relation

$$\boldsymbol{s}_{\theta^*}^{(t)}(\boldsymbol{x}_t) \approx -\frac{\boldsymbol{x}_t - \sqrt{\bar{\alpha}_t}\boldsymbol{x}_0}{1-\bar{\alpha}_t} = -\boldsymbol{\epsilon}_{\theta^*}^{(t)}(\boldsymbol{x}_t)/\sqrt{1-\bar{\alpha}_t}. \tag{7.19}$$

Sampling from Eq. (7.16) can be implemented by ancestral sampling, which iteratively performs

$$\boldsymbol{x}_{t-1} = \frac{1}{\sqrt{\alpha_t}}\left(\boldsymbol{x}_t - \frac{1-\alpha_t}{\sqrt{1-\bar{\alpha}_t}}\boldsymbol{\epsilon}_{\theta}^{(t)}(\boldsymbol{x}_t)\right) + \tilde{\beta}_t\boldsymbol{\epsilon}, \tag{7.20}$$

where $\tilde{\beta}_t := \frac{1-\bar{\alpha}_{t-1}}{1-\bar{\alpha}_t}\beta_t$. One can also view ancestral sampling Eq. (7.20) as solving the reverse VP-SDE [28]. Due to the equivalence revealed in Sect. 7.2.1, we simply use the term "diffusion models" regardless of the specifics of the model.

7.2.1.3 Denoising Diffusion Implicit Models (DDIM) [28]

Seen either from the variational or the SDE perspective, diffusion models are inevitably slow to sample from. To overcome this issue, DDIM [27] proposes another method of sampling which only requires matching the marginal distributions $q(\boldsymbol{x}_t|\boldsymbol{x}_0)$. Specifically, the update rule is given as follows

$$\begin{aligned} \boldsymbol{x}_{t-1} &= \sqrt{\bar{\alpha}_{t-1}}\hat{\boldsymbol{x}}_t + \sqrt{1-\bar{\alpha}_{t-1}-\eta^2\tilde{\beta}_t^2}\boldsymbol{\epsilon}_{\theta^*}^{(t)}(\boldsymbol{x}_t) + \eta\tilde{\beta}_t\boldsymbol{\epsilon}, \\ &= \sqrt{\bar{\alpha}_{t-1}}\hat{\boldsymbol{x}}_t + \tilde{\boldsymbol{w}}_t \end{aligned} \tag{7.21}$$

where $\hat{\boldsymbol{x}}_t$ is the *denoised* estimate

$$\hat{\boldsymbol{x}}_t := \boldsymbol{x}_{\theta^*}^{(t)}(\boldsymbol{x}_t) := \frac{1}{\sqrt{\bar{\alpha}_t}}(\boldsymbol{x}_t - \sqrt{1-\bar{\alpha}_t}\boldsymbol{\epsilon}_{\theta^*}^{(t)}(\boldsymbol{x}_t)), \tag{7.22}$$

which can also be equivalently derived from Tweedie's formula [13], and $\tilde{\boldsymbol{w}}_t$ denotes the total noise given by

$$\tilde{\boldsymbol{w}}_t := \sqrt{1-\bar{\alpha}_{t-1}-\eta^2\tilde{\beta}_t^2}\boldsymbol{\epsilon}_{\theta^*}^{(t)}(\boldsymbol{x}_t) + \eta\tilde{\beta}_t\boldsymbol{\epsilon} \tag{7.23}$$

In Eq. (7.21), $\eta \in [0, 1]$ is a parameter controlling the stochasticity of the update rule: $\eta = 0.0$ leads to fully deterministic sampling, whereas $\eta = 1.0$ with $\tilde{\beta}_t = \sqrt{(1-\bar{\alpha}_{t-1})/(1-\bar{\alpha}_t)}\sqrt{1-\bar{\alpha}_t/\bar{\alpha}_{t-1}}$ recovers the ancestral sampling of DDPMs.

It is important to note that the noise component $\tilde{\boldsymbol{w}}_t$ properly matches the forward marginal [27]. The direction $\tilde{\boldsymbol{w}}_t$ of this transition is determined by the vector sum of the deterministic and the stochastic directional component. Accordingly, assuming optimality of $\boldsymbol{\epsilon}_{\theta*}^{(t)}$, the total noise $\tilde{\boldsymbol{w}}_t$ in Eq. (7.23) can be represented by

$$\tilde{\boldsymbol{w}}_t = \sqrt{1 - \bar{\alpha}_{t-1}}\tilde{\boldsymbol{\epsilon}} \tag{7.24}$$

for some $\tilde{\boldsymbol{\epsilon}} \sim \mathcal{N}(\boldsymbol{0}, \boldsymbol{I})$. In other words, Eq. (7.21) is equivalently represented by $\boldsymbol{x}_{t-1} = \sqrt{\bar{\alpha}_{t-1}}\hat{\boldsymbol{x}}_t + \sqrt{1 - \bar{\alpha}_{t-1}}\tilde{\boldsymbol{\epsilon}}$ for some $\tilde{\boldsymbol{\epsilon}} \sim \mathcal{N}(\boldsymbol{0}, \boldsymbol{I})$. Therefore, it can be seen that the difference between DDIM and DDPM lies only in the degree of dependence on the deterministic estimate of the noise component with feasible intermediate values $\eta \in (0, 1)$.

7.3 Solving Medical Imaging Inverse Problems with Diffusion Models

7.3.1 Iterative Projection Approach

Recall the problem formulation for using generative models to solve inverse problems in Eq. (7.7), and the canonical CSGM approach in Eq. (7.8). Directly trying to adopt the CSGM approach to the diffusion model framework would yield the following formulation

$$z^* = \arg\min_{z} \|A\hat{\boldsymbol{x}} - \boldsymbol{y}\|, \quad \text{where} \quad \hat{\boldsymbol{x}} \sim p_\theta(\boldsymbol{x}), \tag{7.25}$$

where the sampling $\hat{\boldsymbol{x}} \sim p_\theta(\boldsymbol{x})$ would have to be done through solving Eq. (7.11) numerically. This would require at least few tens of neural function evaluations (NFE) just for sampling. However, in order to optimize the problem given in Eq. (7.25), one would have to *backpropagate* the long chain, which would be infeasible.[1] In the following, we discuss ways in which we can use an alternative approach to try to solve for Eq. (7.25).

The first canonical approach of solving inverse problems following the formulation presented in Eq. (7.7) is to perform iterative projections to impose data consistency while leveraging the stochastic samples from the generative diffusion model. Note that numerically solving the reverse VE-SDE of Eq. (7.11) can be done through Euler-Maruyama discretization

$$\boldsymbol{x}_i \leftarrow (\sigma_{i+1}^2 - \sigma_i^2)\boldsymbol{s}_\theta(\boldsymbol{x}_{i+1}, \sigma_{i+1}) + \sqrt{\sigma_{i+1}^2 - \sigma_i^2}\boldsymbol{z}, \quad \boldsymbol{z} \sim \mathcal{N}(0, \boldsymbol{I}) \tag{7.26}$$

[1] In practice, even on a 40GB VRAM A100 GPU, trying to backpropagate more than 2 NFE would result in out-of-memory errors.

While iteratively applying Eq. (7.26) would lead to samples from the prior distribution, we can project the intermediate samples $\boldsymbol{x}_i$ so that they meet the measurement condition $\boldsymbol{y} = \boldsymbol{A}\boldsymbol{x}$

$$\boldsymbol{x}'_i \leftarrow (\boldsymbol{I} - A^* A)\boldsymbol{x}_i + A^* \boldsymbol{y}, \tag{7.27}$$

where $\boldsymbol{A}^*$ is the Hermitian transpose of the operator $\boldsymbol{A}$. Moreover, it was proposed in [28] that applying some Langevin dynamics corrector steps in between the numerical SDE solve steps in Eq. (7.26) leads to better sample quality (denoted as PC sampler, short for predictor-corrector sampling). Applying the same logic, the update rule now reads

$$\begin{aligned} \boldsymbol{x}_i &\leftarrow \boldsymbol{x}_{i+1} + \epsilon_i \boldsymbol{s}_\theta(\boldsymbol{x}_{i+1}, \sigma_{i+1}) + \sqrt{2\epsilon_i}\boldsymbol{z} \\ \boldsymbol{x}'_i &\leftarrow (\boldsymbol{I} - A^* A)\boldsymbol{x}_i + A^* \boldsymbol{y}, \end{aligned} \tag{7.28}$$

where ϵ_i is some step size at the i-th iteration. So far, we have not discussed how the prior $p(\boldsymbol{x})$ was trained. There are two ways to go about this, as MRI signals are inherently complex. The first choice, which would be the easiest way to train a diffusion model in a large-scale fashion, would be to train the model with DICOM images. DICOM images are magnitude values of the originally complex-valued MRI, and in most cases, medical images are saved in this form, with raw, heavy k-space being discarded. The second choice would be to train the prior to model the complex-valued distribution (in the standard two-channel way) of the minimum variance unbiased estimate (MVUE) images [18]. Here, let us consider the first case (which is the harder case), as for the second case, additional care is not necessary.

When the model is trained with real-valued (magnitude) images, we cannot reconstruct the complex-valued MRI directly. A surprisingly simple fix that enables this is presented in Algorithm 7.1. Here, we run two parallel reverse diffusion processes, one for the real part, and another for the imaginary part of the image. The denoising (i.e. Predictor or Corrector) steps are done independently, and the cross-talk between them is enforced through the data consistency step in Eq. (7.27).

Extending to Multi-Coil MRI While the complex-valued MRI reconstruction algorithm presented in Algorithm 7.1 is useful, most modern MRI scanners [34] have multiple receiver coils, which capture the signal with different sensitivities. Can we apply the same logic to parallel imaging? The answer is yes, where the idea is presented in Algorithm 7.2. The algorithm essentially states that all we have to do is run Algorithm 7.1 individually for each coil image. Notably, although the score function has never seen individual coil images, thanks to the high generalization capacity of diffusion models, we observe that the individual coil images are reconstructed with high accuracy, and the final merge can be obtained through a simple sum-of-root-sum-of-squares (SSOS). Observe that the coil components are easily parallelizable as there exists no cross-talk. Interested readers are pointed towards the original work of score-MRI [4].

Algorithm 7.1 Score-MRI (single-coil; complex-valued)

Require: $s_\theta, N, M, \{\epsilon_i\}$ ▷ step size, $\{\sigma_i\}$ ▷ noise schedule

if parallel imaging (PI) **then**
  $A := \mathcal{P}_\Omega \mathcal{F} \mathcal{S}$
else
  $A := \mathcal{P}_\Omega \mathcal{F}$
end if
$\boldsymbol{x}_N \sim \mathcal{N}(\mathbf{0}, \sigma_T^2 \mathbf{I})$
for $i = N-1 : 0$ **do**
  $\mathrm{Re}(\boldsymbol{x}_i) \leftarrow \mathrm{Predictor}(\mathrm{Re}(\boldsymbol{x}_{i+1}), \sigma_i, \sigma_{i+1})$
  $\mathrm{Im}(\boldsymbol{x}_i) \leftarrow \mathrm{Predictor}(\mathrm{Im}(\boldsymbol{x}_{i+1}), \sigma_i, \sigma_{i+1})$
  $\boldsymbol{x}_i = \mathrm{Re}(\boldsymbol{x}_i) + \iota\, \mathrm{Im}(\boldsymbol{x}_i)$
  $\boldsymbol{x}_i \leftarrow \boldsymbol{x}_i + A^*(y - A\boldsymbol{x}_i)$
  for $j = 1 : M$ **do**
    $\mathrm{Re}(\boldsymbol{x}_i) \leftarrow \mathrm{Corrector}(\mathrm{Re}(\boldsymbol{x}_i), \sigma_i, \epsilon_i)$
    $\mathrm{Im}(\boldsymbol{x}_i) \leftarrow \mathrm{Corrector}(\mathrm{Im}(\boldsymbol{x}_i), \sigma_i, \epsilon_i)$
    $\boldsymbol{x}_i = \mathrm{Re}(\boldsymbol{x}_i) + \iota\, \mathrm{Im}(\boldsymbol{x}_i)$
    $\boldsymbol{x}_i \leftarrow \boldsymbol{x}_i + A^*(y - A\boldsymbol{x}_i)$
  end for
end for
return $\boldsymbol{x}_0$

Algorithm 7.2 Score-MRI (multi-coil)

Require: $s_\theta, N, \{\epsilon_i\}$ ▷ step size, $\{\sigma_i\}$ ▷ noise schedule

Define $A := \mathcal{P}_\Omega \mathcal{F}$
$\boldsymbol{x}_N^{(k)} \sim \mathcal{N}(\mathbf{0}, \sigma_T^2 \mathbf{I})$
for $i = N-1 : 0$ **do**
  for $k = 1 : c$ **do (parallel)**
    $\mathrm{Re}(\boldsymbol{x}_i^{(k)}) \leftarrow \mathrm{Predictor}(\mathrm{Re}(\boldsymbol{x}_{i+1}^{(k)}), \sigma_i, \sigma_{i+1})$
    $\mathrm{Im}(\boldsymbol{x}_i^{(k)}) \leftarrow \mathrm{Predictor}(\mathrm{Im}(\boldsymbol{x}_{i+1}^{(k)}), \sigma_i, \sigma_{i+1})$
    $\boldsymbol{x}_i^{(k)} = \mathrm{Re}(\boldsymbol{x}_i^{(k)}) + \iota\, \mathrm{Im}(\boldsymbol{x}_i^{(k)})$
    $\boldsymbol{x}_i^{(k)} \leftarrow \boldsymbol{x}_i^{(k)} + A^*(y^{(k)} - A\boldsymbol{x}_i^{(k)})$
    $\mathrm{Re}(\boldsymbol{x}_i^{(k)}) \leftarrow \mathrm{Corrector}(\mathrm{Re}(\boldsymbol{x}_i^{(k)}), \sigma_i, \epsilon_i)$
    $\mathrm{Im}(\boldsymbol{x}_i^{(k)}) \leftarrow \mathrm{Corrector}(\mathrm{Im}(\boldsymbol{x}_i^{(k)}), \sigma_i, \epsilon_i)$
    $\boldsymbol{x}_i^{(k)} = \mathrm{Re}(\boldsymbol{x}_i^{(k)}) + \iota\, \mathrm{Im}(\boldsymbol{x}_i^{(k)})$
    $\boldsymbol{x}_i^{(k)} \leftarrow \boldsymbol{x}_i^{(k)} + A^*(y^{(k)} - A\boldsymbol{x}_i^{(k)})$
  end for
end for
$\boldsymbol{x}_0 = \sqrt{\sum_{k=1}^{c} |\boldsymbol{x}_0^{(c)}|^2}$ ▷ SSOS
return $\boldsymbol{x}_0$

Using the score function trained as the second case (i.e. with complex images) is a trivial extension. The two parallel denoising steps that were applied independently can now be merged into a single stream of complex-valued denoising, with the same data consistency steps. For the rest of the chapter, for simplicity, we will only consider this second case.

Up until now, we only discussed MRI reconstruction. For CT reconstruction, the same idea of using iterative projections can be applied, but the problem is actually easier as now there is no need to consider complex values. For further reference, consult [6, 29].

7.3.2 *Direct Bayesian Approach*

Recall that solving the reverse SDE in Eq. (7.11) led to sampling from $p(\boldsymbol{x})$. When solving for inverse problems, what we would instead want is to sample from the posterior. All we would have to change would be to switch the gradient of the log prior $\nabla_{\boldsymbol{x}_t} \log p(\boldsymbol{x}_t)$ to the gradient of the log posterior $\nabla_{\boldsymbol{x}_t} \log p(\boldsymbol{x}_t|\boldsymbol{y})$. Using Bayes rule, we see that

$$\nabla_{\boldsymbol{x}_t} \log p(\boldsymbol{x}_t|\boldsymbol{y}) = \nabla_{\boldsymbol{x}_t} \log p(\boldsymbol{x}_t) + \nabla_{\boldsymbol{x}_t} \log p(\boldsymbol{y}|\boldsymbol{x}_t). \tag{7.29}$$

As usual, the gradient of the log prior can be approximated with the diffusion model. But what about the time-dependent likelihood? At first sight, this may seem trivial, as it was stated in Eq. (7.2) that for many measurement models in inverse imaging, the likelihood term is known. However, care must be taken as we now have an additional dependence on the diffusion time t. Writing out explicitly, we have

$$p(\boldsymbol{y}|\boldsymbol{x}_t) = \int p(\boldsymbol{y}|\boldsymbol{x}_0)p(\boldsymbol{x}_0|\boldsymbol{x}_t)d\boldsymbol{x}_0. \tag{7.30}$$

Notice that $p(\boldsymbol{y}|\boldsymbol{x}_0)$ is tractable, but $p(\boldsymbol{x}_0|\boldsymbol{x}_t)$ is not. Hence, one has to make *some* approximation to it. In this section, we will review some of the canonical approaches. Before we begin this section, it should be noted that when we consider MRI reconstruction, we will always be referring to the multi-coil case here after, and hence the sensitivity coil maps estimated through e.g. ESPiRiT [31].

7.3.2.1 Score-ALD [18]

$\boldsymbol{x}_t$ is intuitively a noiser version of $\boldsymbol{x}_0$. One straightforward approximation, hence, is to treat it as if the excessive noise exists on the measurement $\boldsymbol{y}$. The approximation then reads

$$\nabla_{\boldsymbol{x}_t} \log p(\boldsymbol{y}|\boldsymbol{x}_t) \approx A^\top \frac{\boldsymbol{A}\boldsymbol{x}_t - \boldsymbol{y}}{\sigma_y^2 + \gamma_t^2}, \tag{7.31}$$

where γ_t is a hyperparameter that is correlated with the noise level at time t. Score-ALD was one of the earliest works to show the effectiveness of using diffusion models for MRI reconstruction. However, it required designing an effective choice of the hyperparameter γ_t, which is often non-trivial.

7.3.2.2 Diffusion Posterior Sampling (DPS) [8]

Observe that Eq. (7.30) can be rewritten in terms of expectation

$$p(\boldsymbol{y}|\boldsymbol{x}_t) = \mathbb{E}_{\boldsymbol{x}_0 \sim p(\boldsymbol{x}_0|\boldsymbol{x}_t)}[p(\boldsymbol{y}|\boldsymbol{x}_0)]. \tag{7.32}$$

However, even when we consider Monte Carlo samples, running the reverse diffusion to sample $\boldsymbol{x}_0$ from the reverse distribution for all timesteps t would be computationally extremely heavy. In DPS, the authors propose an effective approximation by pushing the expectation inside

$$p(\boldsymbol{y}|\boldsymbol{x}_t) \approx p(\boldsymbol{y}|\hat{\boldsymbol{x}}_t), \quad \text{where} \quad \hat{\boldsymbol{x}}_t := \mathbb{E}[\boldsymbol{x}_0|\boldsymbol{x}_t] \tag{7.33}$$

Notice that the posterior mean can be obtained thanks to Tweedie's formula in Lemma 7.13. Further details and the approximation error (i.e. Jensen gap) induced by this process can be found in [8]. While DPS was shown to be effective for image restoration tasks, it did not scale well to medical image reconstruction tasks, as taking the gradient with respect to $\boldsymbol{x}_t$ involves taking backpropagation through the score function, which is often unstable and slow, especially combined with the forward operators used in medical imaging.

7.3.2.3 Decomposed Diffusion Sampler (DDS) [10]

Let us consider the case where we are using the DDIM sampler in Eq. (7.21) for our reverse diffusion with DPS. One iteration of the diffusion step can be rewritten as

$$\boldsymbol{x}_{t-1} = \sqrt{\bar{\alpha}_{t-1}}\left(\hat{\boldsymbol{x}}_t - \gamma_t \nabla_{\boldsymbol{x}_t} \ell(\hat{\boldsymbol{x}}_t)\right) + \tilde{\boldsymbol{w}}_t, \tag{7.34}$$

where $\ell(\boldsymbol{x}) = \|\boldsymbol{y} - \boldsymbol{A}\boldsymbol{x}\|^2/2\sigma_y^2$ for the Gaussian case. By applying chain rule for the gradient term, we have

$$\nabla_{\boldsymbol{x}_t} \ell(\hat{\boldsymbol{x}}_t) = \frac{\partial \hat{\boldsymbol{x}}_t}{\partial \boldsymbol{x}_t} \nabla_{\hat{\boldsymbol{x}}_t} \ell(\hat{\boldsymbol{x}}_t).$$

Here, the main computational complexity, and the instability arise from the network Jacobian term $\frac{\partial \hat{\boldsymbol{x}}_t}{\partial \boldsymbol{x}_t}$. Interestingly, it was shown in [10] that if the data manifold $\mathcal{M}$ in which the signal resides is assumed to be an affine subspace, then the Jacobian term is an orthogonal projection onto the clean manifold up to a scale factor. Formally, we have the following result

Proposition 7.1 (Manifold Constrained Gradient [10]) *Suppose the clean data manifold $\mathcal{M}$ is represented as an affine subspace and assumes the uniform distribution on $\mathcal{M}$. Then,*

$$\frac{\partial \hat{\boldsymbol{x}}_t}{\partial \boldsymbol{x}_t} = \frac{1}{\sqrt{\bar{\alpha}_t}} \mathcal{P}_{\mathcal{M}} \tag{7.35}$$

$$\hat{\boldsymbol{x}}_t - \gamma_t \nabla_{\boldsymbol{x}_t} \ell(\hat{\boldsymbol{x}}_t) = \mathcal{P}_{\mathcal{M}} \left(\hat{\boldsymbol{x}}_t - \zeta_t \nabla_{\hat{\boldsymbol{x}}_t} \ell(\hat{\boldsymbol{x}}_t) \right) \tag{7.36}$$

for some $\zeta_t > 0$*, where* $\mathcal{P}_{\mathcal{M}}$ *denotes the orthogonal projection to* $\mathcal{M}$.

Notably, the DPS gradient update step can be achieved by taking the standard gradient update step with the Tweedie estimate $\hat{\boldsymbol{x}}_t$, and projecting onto the manifold $\mathcal{M}$. Nonetheless, a notable limitation is the use of a single projected gradient step for each ancestral steps. A natural question arises: can we explore extensions that allow computationally efficient multi-step optimization steps?

Let $\mathcal{T}_t$ denote the tangent space of the clean manifold at a denoised sample $\hat{\boldsymbol{x}}_t$. Suppose, furthermore, that there exists the l-th order Krylov subspace

$$\mathcal{K}_{t,l} := \text{Span}(\boldsymbol{b}, A\boldsymbol{b}, \cdots, A^{l-1}\boldsymbol{b}), \quad \boldsymbol{b} := \boldsymbol{y} - A\hat{\boldsymbol{x}}_t \tag{7.37}$$

such that

$$\mathcal{T}_t = \hat{\boldsymbol{x}}_t + \mathcal{K}_{t,l}.$$

Then, we can use the conjugate gradient (CG) update steps, as it can be guaranteed that the updates will not leave the Krylov subspace. Using the properties of CG, it is easy to see that M-step CG update with $M \leq l$ starting from $\hat{\boldsymbol{x}}_t$ are confined in $\mathcal{T}_t$ since it corresponds to the solution of

$$\min_{\boldsymbol{x} \in \hat{\boldsymbol{x}}_t + \mathcal{K}_M} \|\boldsymbol{y} - A\boldsymbol{x}\|^2 \tag{7.38}$$

and $\mathcal{K}_M \subset \mathcal{K}_l$ when $M \leq l$. In other words, we have shown that if the tangent space at each denoised sample is representable by a Krylov subspace, there is no need to compute the DPS gradient. Rather, CG suffices to guarantee that the updated samples stay within the tangent space. To sum up, DDS can be summarized as follows

$$\boldsymbol{x}_{t-1} = \sqrt{\bar{\alpha}_{t-1}} \hat{\boldsymbol{x}}_t' + \tilde{\boldsymbol{w}}_t, \tag{7.39}$$

$$\hat{\boldsymbol{x}}_t' = \mathsf{CG}(A^*A, A^*\boldsymbol{y}, \hat{\boldsymbol{x}}_t, M), \quad M \leq l \tag{7.40}$$

where $\mathsf{CG}(\cdot)$ denotes the M-step CG for the normal equation starting from $\hat{\boldsymbol{x}}_t$.

7.3.3 Properties

In this section, we discussed several different approaches for solving inverse problems with diffusion models. There are many meanings to *solving* an inverse problem, and in the context of doing so with diffusion models, it often means performing (approximate) posterior sampling. In the literature, these approaches are often called **Di**ffusion model-based **I**nverse problem **S**olvers (DIS). In DIS, we keep the prior diffusion model fixed and leverage the likelihood function

7.4 Experiments

In the experiments section, we will first focus on showing the intriguing properties of acquiring stochastic posterior samples through the Score-MRI approach introduced in Sect. 7.3.1, although the results will not be specific to this approach. Then, the later parts will be focused more on presenting the accelerated results through the DDS approach introduced in Sect. 7.3.2.3. For the MRI case, the fastMRI knee public dataset [34] is used. For the CT case, AAPM 256×256 dataset is used [24].

7.4.1 DIS Are Agnostic to the Sampling Pattern

Diffusion models are agnostic to the forward model, as it is leveraged as a plug-and-play prior. The likelihood (i.e. information about the measurement, and in the case of MRI, sampling pattern) information is only used during the inference phase to guide the sampling. In Fig. 7.1, we show that this is indeed the case by comparing score-MRI against strong supervised deep learning-based methods: U-Net [34] and E2E-varnet [30] trained on 1D sampling patterns. Notice that while the supervised methods show strong performance on the in-domain measurements (i.e. 1D sampling patterns), the performance degrades heavily when OOD measurements are used for reconstruction (i.e. 2D sampling patterns such as Gaussian or VD poisson disk). In contrast, score-MRI is agnostic to the variations in the sampling pattern, and produces superior reconstructions. Note that this not only holds for MRI reconstruction but also for CT reconstruction. Traditionally, sparse-view CT reconstruction (SV-CT) and limited-angle CT reconstruction (LA-CT) have often been studied separately, and one had to re-train a new network for a new level of sparsity. This is not the case for DIS.

7.4.2 Pathology Detection

Supervised learning leads to MMSE reconstructions. These minimize the distortion while sacrificing the perceptual quality by yielding blurry reconstructions [1]. On the other hand, by leveraging diffusion models, we can generate high perceptual quality reconstructions, while they may compromise the distortion metric. In medical imaging, which is better? At first thought, it might seem like the answer

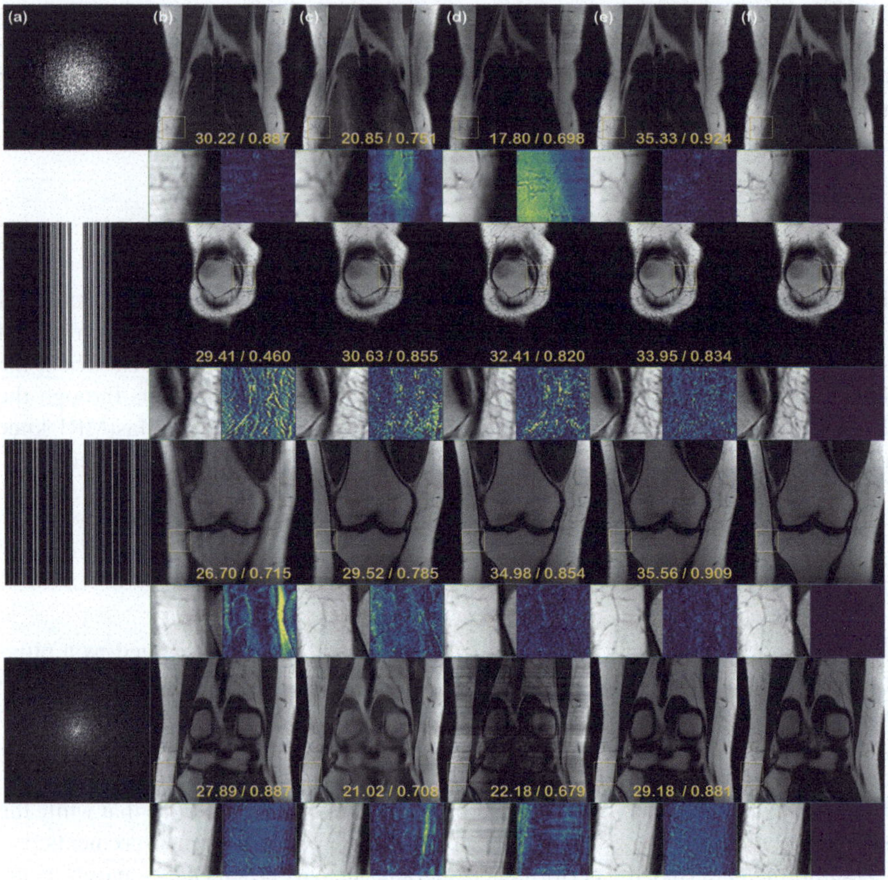

Fig. 7.1 Multi-coil reconstruction results. (**a**) Sub-sampling mask used to generate under-sampled image, (**b**) TV, (**c**) supervised learning (U-Net), (**d**) E2E-varnet [30], (**e**) score-MRI, and (**f**) the ground truth. First row: 2D $\times 8$ Gaussian random sampling, second row: 1D $\times 4$ Gaussian random sampling, third row: 1D $\times$ 4 uniform random sampling, fourth row: $\times 8$ variable density (VD) poisson disk sampling. Green box: Zoom in version of the indicated yellow box, Blue box: Difference magnitude of the inset. Yellow numbers in the upper right corner indicate PSNR [db], and SSIM, respectively

is obviously the former, as one would want to minimize any hallucinations and be conservative. Nonetheless, recall that the objective of medical imaging is to make an accurate diagnosis. Which case would be more favorable? To show this, we fine-tuned an object detection model, YOLO v5[2] on fastMRI+ [35] with fully-sampled MRI images, and ran inference with different reconstructions obtained through various methods (including the test-set of the fully-sampled MRI images).

[2] https://github.com/ultralytics/yolov5.

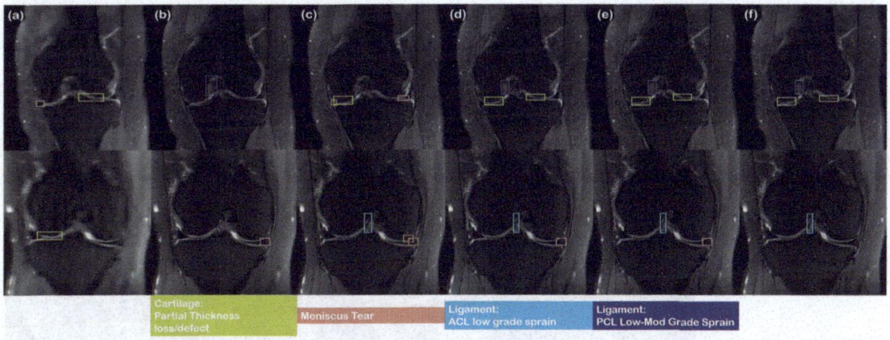

Fig. 7.2 Results of pathology detection. Detection using (**a**) TV reconstruction, (**b**) supervised U-Net, (**c**) DuDoRNet, (**d**) proposed method, (**e**) fully-sampled images. Ground-truth label for the pathologies are shown in (**f**). (Yellow green box): Cartilage partial thickness loss/defect, (Pink box): Meniscus tear, (Purple box): Ligament PCL Low-Mod grade sprain, (Skyblue box): Ligament ACL low grade sprain

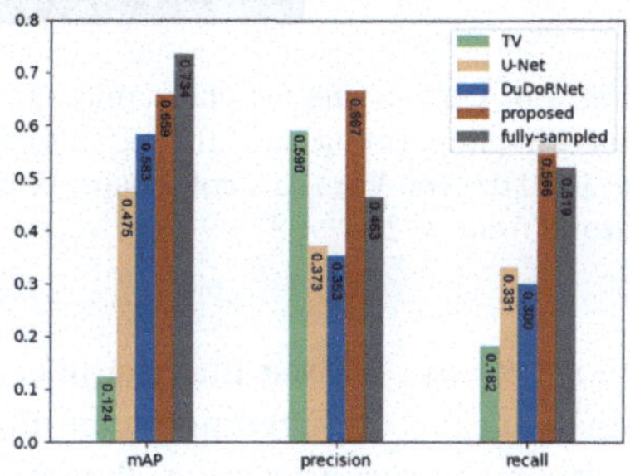

Fig. 7.3 Quantitative metrics of pathology detection

Overall results on the pathology detection task is illustrated in Fig. 7.2, and the quantitative metric is shown in Fig. 7.3. From the results, we immediately see, rather surprisingly, that the best-performing method is score-MRI, lending weight to the strengths of DIS even for medical imaging.

7.4.3 *Quantifying Uncertainty of the Prediction*

Score-MRI, and generally all DIS are *generative* posterior sampling algorithms, with two sources of stochasticity (i.e. initial point, noise along the sampling process). Due to the stochastic nature, we can run multiple reconstructions in parallel, and quantify the uncertainty of the prediction, as depicted in Fig. 7.4. At low acceleration factors ($\times$ 2), we see little variation between the different reconstructions. This indicates high confidence in the model, and hence we can conclude that the reconstruction is relatively exact in all parts of the image. As the acceleration factor is increased, and the degree of aliasing artifacts becomes

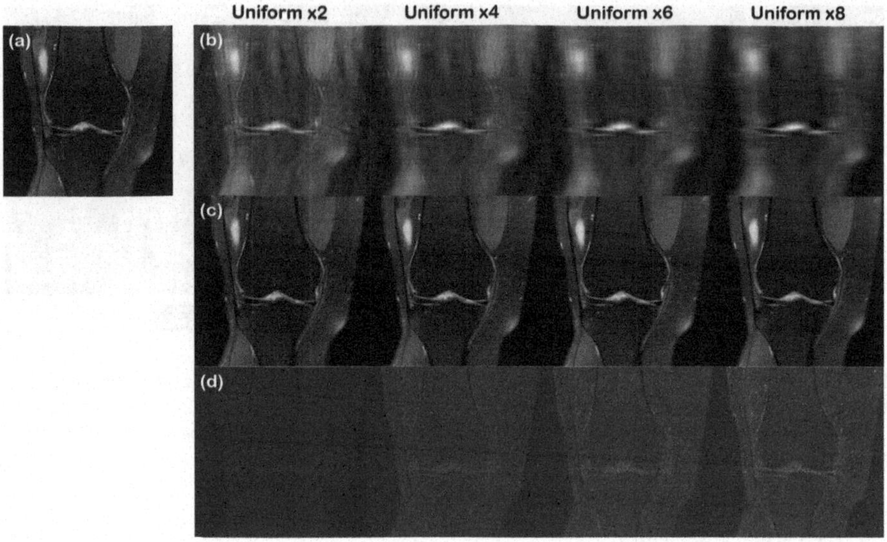

Fig. 7.4 Quantifying the uncertainty of reconstruction. (**a**) Ground truth, (**b**) aliased image from sub-sampling, (**c**) mean of the reconstruction, (**d**) standard deviation of the samples: range is set to [0, 0.02] (on `Viridis` colormap). From the first row to the fourth row, the acceleration factor grows from $\times 2$ to $\times 8$

more severe, we see that the uncertainty increase in specific regions. Potentially, this measure of uncertainty can inform the practitioners on how much they should rely on the reconstruction, thereby deciding whether to use a different diagnostic tool.

7.4.4 Accelerated Sampling with DDS

A downside of score-MRI was the slow inference time. Four thousand neural function evaluations (NFE; the number of forward passes through the diffusion model) lead to several minutes of reconstruction time even for a moderately-sized image. This is note a downside unique for score-MRI, but also a downside for the direct Bayesian approaches such as score-ALD (Sect. 7.3.2.1) and DPS (Sect. 7.3.2.2). We can alleviate this downside by using a fast sampler called DDS, introduced in Sect. 7.3.2.3. In Fig. 7.5, we see that DDS is capable achieving fast sampling with under 50 NFEs and yield even *better* results.

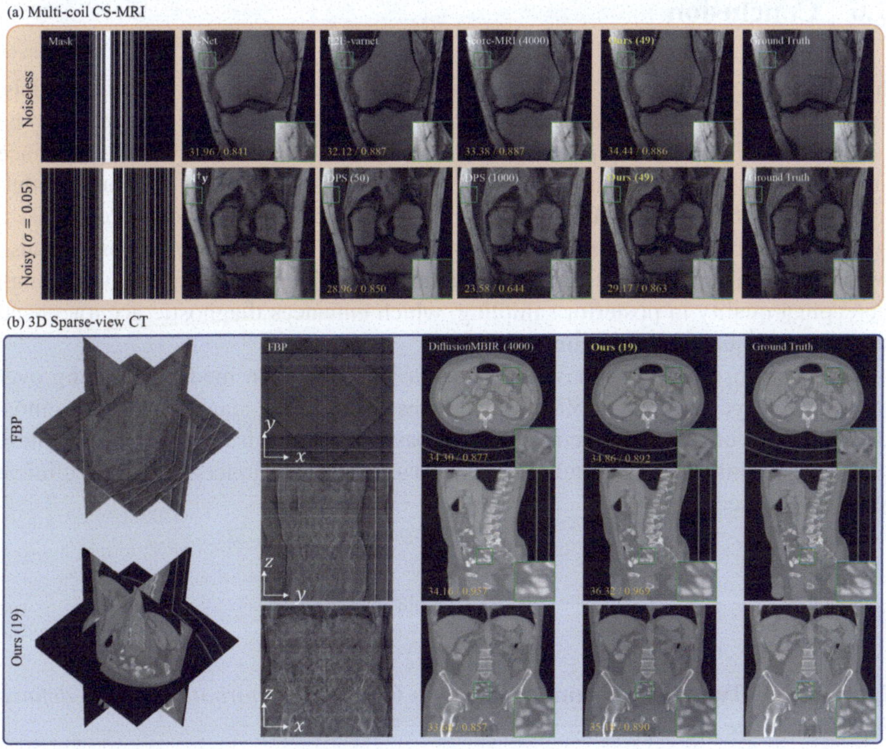

Fig. 7.5 Representative reconstruction results. (**a**) Multi-coil MRI reconstruction, (**b**) 3D sparse-view CT. Numbers in parenthesis: NFE. Yellow numbers in bottom left corner: PSNR/SSIM

7.5 Discussion

The methods described in the chapter were designed mostly for the most basic 2D imaging cases. However, it should be noted that there is much more to medical image reconstruction that is out of the scope of this work. For different applications, while the fundamental theory remains the same, one often needs to adapt the specifics of the algorithm for the suitable application. For instance, using shortcut sampling and using regularization introduced in CCDF [7] was shown to be useful in MRI denoising [5]. Methods for compensation of high dynamic range and variance in positron emission tomography (PET) [26] was used for PET reconstruction. Orthogonal to the developments specific to the imaging modalities at hand, extension of 2D reconstruction-oriented methods to 3D imaging situations were also proposed [9, 22], enabling direct adoption of 2D priors even for 3D cases.

7.6 Conclusion

In this chapter, we explored methods for employing unconditional diffusion models, originally trained to sample from the prior (data) distribution, to sample from the posterior distribution using measurement information provided only at the inference stage. This complete separation of the two factors allows for forward model-agnostic application of diffusion models across a wide range of downstream tasks, a capability unattainable with traditional supervised learning approaches. We also highlighted the benefits of Diffusion Inference Sampling (DIS), including high perceptual quality in posterior sampling, which enhances diagnostic accuracy, and the ability to quantify uncertainty.

While diffusion models have seen increasing interest in medical imaging over the past few years, their application remains in the early stages. Currently, most deep learning engines in practical use are based on supervised methods. For these emerging techniques to gain reliable traction among practitioners, extensive clinical validation is necessary.

Appendix

Lemma 7.1 (Tweedie's Formula) *Given a Gaussian perturbation kernel defined in Eq. (7.9), the posterior mean is given by*

$$\mathbb{E}[\boldsymbol{x}_0|\boldsymbol{x}_t] = \frac{1}{s_t}(\boldsymbol{x}_t + \sigma_t^2 \nabla_{\boldsymbol{x}_t} \log p(\boldsymbol{x}_t)) \tag{7.13}$$

Proof

$$\nabla_{\boldsymbol{x}_t} \log p(\boldsymbol{x}_t) = \frac{\nabla_{\boldsymbol{x}_t} p(\boldsymbol{x}_t)}{p(\boldsymbol{x}_t)} \tag{7.41}$$

$$= \frac{1}{p(\boldsymbol{x}_t)} \nabla_{\boldsymbol{x}_t} \int p(\boldsymbol{x}_t|\boldsymbol{x}_0) p(\boldsymbol{x}_0)\, d\boldsymbol{x}_0 \tag{7.42}$$

$$= \frac{1}{p(\boldsymbol{x}_t)} \int \nabla_{\boldsymbol{x}_t} p(\boldsymbol{x}_t|\boldsymbol{x}_0) p(\boldsymbol{x}_0)\, d\boldsymbol{x}_0 \tag{7.43}$$

$$= \frac{1}{p(\boldsymbol{x}_t)} \int p(\boldsymbol{x}_t|\boldsymbol{x}_0) \nabla_{\boldsymbol{x}_t} \log p(\boldsymbol{x}_t|\boldsymbol{x}_0) p(\boldsymbol{x}_0)\, d\boldsymbol{x}_0 \tag{7.44}$$

$$= \int p(\boldsymbol{x}_0|\boldsymbol{x}_t) \nabla_{\boldsymbol{x}_t} \log p(\boldsymbol{x}_t|\boldsymbol{x}_0)\, d\boldsymbol{x}_0 \tag{7.45}$$

$$= \int p(\boldsymbol{x}_0|\boldsymbol{x}_t) \frac{s_t \boldsymbol{x}_0 - \boldsymbol{x}_t}{s_t^2 \sigma_t^2}\, d\boldsymbol{x}_0 \tag{7.46}$$

$$= \frac{s_t \mathbb{E}[\boldsymbol{x}_0|\boldsymbol{x}_t] - \boldsymbol{x}_t}{s_t^2 \sigma_t^2}. \tag{7.47}$$

□

References

1. Blau Y, Michaeli T (2018) The perception-distortion tradeoff. In: Proceedings of the IEEE conference on computer vision and pattern recognition, pp 6228–6237
2. Block KT, Uecker M, Frahm J (2007) Undersampled radial MRI with multiple coils. Iterative image reconstruction using a total variation constraint. Magn Reson Med 57(6):1086–1098
3. Bora A, Jalal A, Price E, Dimakis AG (2017) Compressed sensing using generative models. In: International conference on machine learning, PMLR, pp 537–546
4. Chung H, Ye JC (2022) Score-based diffusion models for accelerated MRI. Med Image Anal 80:102479
5. Chung H, Lee ES, Ye JC (2022) Mr image denoising and super-resolution using regularized reverse diffusion. IEEE Trans Med Imaging 42(4):922–934
6. Chung H, Sim B, Ryu D, Ye JC (2022) Improving diffusion models for inverse problems using manifold constraints. In: Oh AH, Agarwal A, Belgrave D, Cho K (eds) Advances in neural information processing systems. https://openreview.net/forum?id=nJJjv0JDJju
7. Chung H, Sim B, Ye JC (2022) Come-closer-diffuse-faster: accelerating conditional diffusion models for inverse problems through stochastic contraction. In: Proceedings of the IEEE/CVF conference on computer vision and pattern recognition
8. Chung H, Kim J, Mccann MT, Klasky ML, Ye JC (2023) Diffusion posterior sampling for general noisy inverse problems. In: International conference on learning representations. https://openreview.net/forum?id=OnD9zGAGT0k
9. Chung H, Ryu D, Mccann MT, Klasky ML, Ye JC (2023) Solving 3d inverse problems using pre-trained 2d diffusion models. In: IEEE/CVF conference on computer vision and pattern recognition
10. Chung H, Lee S, Ye JC (2024) Decomposed diffusion sampler for accelerating large-scale inverse problems. In: International conference on learning representations
11. Dhariwal P, Nichol AQ (2021) Diffusion models beat GANs on image synthesis. In: Beygelzimer A, Dauphin Y, Liang P, Vaughan JW (eds) Advances in neural information processing systems
12. Donoho DL (2006) Compressed sensing. IEEE Trans Inf Theory 52(4):1289–1306
13. Efron B (2011) Tweedie's formula and selection bias. J Am Stat Assoc 106(496):1602–1614
14. Ehrhardt MJ, Betcke MM (2016) Multicontrast MRI reconstruction with structure-guided total variation. SIAM J Imaging Sci 9(3):1084–1106
15. Goodfellow I, Pouget-Abadie J, Mirza M, Xu B, Warde-Farley D, Ozair S, Courville A, Bengio Y (2014) Generative adversarial nets. In: Advances in neural information processing systems 27
16. Ho J, Jain A, Abbeel P (2020) Denoising diffusion probabilistic models. In: Advances in neural information processing systems 33, pp 6840–6851
17. Hyvärinen A, Dayan P (2005) Estimation of non-normalized statistical models by score matching. J Mach Learn Res 6(4):695
18. Jalal A, Arvinte M, Daras G, Price E, Dimakis AG, Tamir J (2021) Robust compressed sensing MRI with deep generative priors. In: Advances in neural information processing systems 34
19. Karras T, Aittala M, Aila T, Laine S (2022) Elucidating the design space of diffusion-based generative models. In: Proc. NeurIPS

20. Kawar B, Elad M, Ermon S, Song J (2022) Denoising diffusion restoration models. In: Oh AH, Agarwal A, Belgrave D, Cho K (eds) Advances in neural information processing systems. https://openreview.net/forum?id=kxXvopt9pWK
21. Kingma DP, Welling M (2013) Auto-encoding variational bayes. Preprint. arXiv:13126114
22. Lee S, Chung H, Park M, Park J, Ryu WS, Ye JC (2023) Improving 3D imaging with pre-trained perpendicular 2D diffusion models. Preprint. arXiv:230308440
23. Lustig M, Donoho D, Pauly JM (2007) Sparse MRI: The application of compressed sensing for rapid MR imaging. Magn Reson Med 58(6):1182–1195
24. McCollough CH, Bartley AC, Carter RE, Chen B, Drees TA, Edwards P, Holmes III DR, Huang AE, Khan F, Leng S, et al (2017) Low-dose CT for the detection and classification of metastatic liver lesions: results of the 2016 low dose CT grand challenge. Med Phys 44(10):e339–e352
25. Rezende D, Mohamed S (2015) Variational inference with normalizing flows. In: International conference on machine learning, PMLR, pp 1530–1538
26. Singh IR, Denker A, Barbano R, Kereta Ž, Jin B, Thielemans K, Maass P, Arridge S (2023) Score-based generative models for pet image reconstruction. Preprint. arXiv:230814190
27. Song J, Meng C, Ermon S (2021) Denoising diffusion implicit models. In: 9th International conference on learning representations, ICLR
28. Song Y, Sohl-Dickstein J, Kingma DP, Kumar A, Ermon S, Poole B (2021) Score-based generative modeling through stochastic differential equations. In: 9th International conference on learning representations, ICLR
29. Song Y, Shen L, Xing L, Ermon S (2022) Solving inverse problems in medical imaging with score-based generative models. In: International conference on learning representations. https://openreview.net/forum?id=vaRCHVj0uGI
30. Sriram A, Zbontar J, Murrell T, Defazio A, Zitnick CL, Yakubova N, Knoll F, Johnson P (2020) End-to-end variational networks for accelerated MRI reconstruction. In: International conference on medical image computing and computer-assisted intervention, pp 64–73. Springer
31. Uecker M, Lai P, Murphy MJ, Virtue P, Elad M, Pauly JM, Vasanawala SS, Lustig M (2014) ESPIRiT—an eigenvalue approach to autocalibrating parallel MRI: where SENSE meets GRAPPA. Magn Reson Med 71(3):990–1001
32. Vincent P (2011) A connection between score matching and denoising autoencoders. Neural Comput 23(7):1661–1674
33. Whang J, Lei Q, Dimakis A (2021) Solving inverse problems with a flow-based noise model. In: International conference on machine learning, PMLR, pp 11146–11157
34. Zbontar J, Knoll F, Sriram A, Murrell T, Huang Z, Muckley MJ, Defazio A, Stern R, Johnson P, Bruno M, et al (2018) fastMRI: An open dataset and benchmarks for accelerated MRI. Preprint. arXiv:181108839
35. Zhao R, Yaman B, Zhang Y, Stewart R, Dixon A, Knoll F, Huang Z, Lui YW, Hansen MS, Lungren MP (2022) fastmri+, clinical pathology annotations for knee and brain fully sampled magnetic resonance imaging data. Sci Data 9(1):152

Chapter 8
Virtual Elastography Ultrasound via Generative Adversarial Network and Its Application to Breast Cancer Diagnosis

Zhao Yao, Yuanyuan Wang, Min Liu, Jianqiao Zhou, and Jinhua Yu

Abstract Elastography ultrasound (EUS) imaging is a vital ultrasound imaging modality. The current use of EUS faces many challenges, such as vulnerability to subjective manipulation, echo signal attenuation, and unknown risks of elastic pressure in certain delicate tissues. The hardware requirement of EUS also hinders the trend of miniaturization of ultrasound equipment. Here we show a cost-efficient solution by designing an improved generative adversarial model (GAN) to synthesize virtual EUS (V-EUS) from conventional B-mode images. Specifically, a bi-discriminator structure and a color prior module are designed to model the intrinsic attributes of the EUS. A total of 4580 cases were collected from 15 medical centers and extensive experiments were designed to demonstrate the validity of the proposed model. In the task of differentiating benign and malignant breast tumors, there is no significant difference between V-EUS and real EUS on high-end ultrasound, while the diagnostic performance of pocket-sized ultrasound can be improved by about 5% after V-EUS is equipped.

8.1 Introduction

Ultrasound imaging (US) is an essential component of modern medical imaging technology. Elastography ultrasound imaging (EUS), as a widely used ultrasound imaging modality, can be used to assess the biomechanical properties of soft tissues. EUS provides distinctive information different from other ultrasound (US)

Z. Yao · M. Liu
National Engineering Research Center for Robot Visual Perception and Control Technology, College of Electrical and Information Engineering, Hunan University, Hunan, China

Y. Wang · J. Yu (✉)
Department of Electronic Engineering, Fudan University, Shanghai, China
e-mail: jhyu@fudan.edu.cn

J. Zhou
Department of Ultrasound, Ruijin Hospital, Shanghai Jiaotong University School of Medicine, Shanghai, China

L. Zhang et al. (eds.), *Generative Machine Learning Models in Medical Image Computing*, https://doi.org/10.1007/978-3-031-80965-1_8

modalities and plays an increasingly important role in diagnosing many diseases, especially tumors, with significant clinical value [1, 2].

With the rapid development of integrated circuits, an important trend in US equipment is towards miniaturization and portability to take full advantage of real-time, non-invasive, inexpensive, and easily accessible US [3, 4]. Due to the hardware requirements of EUS, none of the existing pocket-sized ultrasound instruments are able to provide elastography modality, which has become an obstacle to the widespread use of miniaturized ultrasound equipment [3, 5]. On the other hand, compared with B-mode US, EUS is more susceptible to subjective manipulation, including probe position, applied pressure, and frequency of compression, which dictates a higher operator dependence and longer learning curve [6]. In addition, EUS requires the calculation of tissue displacement based on ultrasound echo signals, and the accuracy of displacement calculation is strongly influenced by signal attenuation, with the consequence that the quality of EUS of deep tissues degrades significantly. Furthermore, as EUS relies on stress changes to capture the elasticity of tissue, and the biomechanical properties of delicate tissues, such as carotid plaque, eye, and brain tissue, are not well understood, leading to no clear conclusions about the safety of EUS in the diagnosis of these lesions.

Recently, deep learning-based medical image synthesis technology offers promising solutions to many data-driven clinical application challenges. For example, data synthesis technology can improve the imaging quality of low-end acquisition equipment and break through the limits of the original imaging methods in various aspects such as imaging speed [7], resolution [8], modality [9], and slice staining techniques [10].

To tackle the barriers mentioned above to use EUS in clinical applications, in this paper, we propose a cost-efficient solution by designing an image synthesis method based on deep learning. Specifically, a virtual EUS (V-EUS) reconstruction method based on generative adversarial network (GAN) is proposed to establish an end-to-end translation from B-mode US to EUS. To fully validate the clinical value of V-EUS, we choose the clinical problem of breast cancer diagnosis and validate it in 4580 breast tumor cases from 15 medical centers. In order to obtain an accurate elasticity assessment of the tumor region and to make the color distribution of V-EUS highly compatible with the one of real EUS, we propose to integrate a tumor discriminator module and a color balancing module in the GAN framework.

The remainder of this chapter is organized as follows. In Sect. 8.2, we present the design of the model structure and detailed description of the training and validation. In Sect. 8.3, we show the multi center experimental design and the corresponding analysis of the experimental results. Finally, in Sect. 8.4 we discuss the application of the model to the diagnosis of benign and malignant breast tumor. An earlier version of the main content of this chapter was published in [11].

8.2 Deep Neural Network Architecture, Training and Validation

8.2.1 Generator

Under the paradigm of the GAN model, the architecture of the generator follows the design of U-net [12], as shown in Fig. 8.1. It is pretty suitable to use U-net structure for this study. In addition to learning the overall mapping relationship between inputs and outputs, the encoder-decoder structure of the model is helpful to learn semantic information at different scale. The skip connection between encoder and decoder ensures that the decoder can integrate more low-level features which is essential for enriching the details of EUS image [13].

After data preprocess, the input B-mode US with a size of 256*256 were feed into the generator. In the encoder, it contains an input layer and 6 convolutional blocks. Each convolutional block is composed of a ReLU layer, a convolutional layer and a batch-normalization layer. Between each convolutional block, we used convolution with step size of 2 instead of down-sampling, which may decrease the information loss [14]. The output channels of each convolutional block in encoder was set to 64, 128, 256, 512, 512, 512, 512. In the decoder, it contains 6 convolutional blocks and an output layer. Different from the convolutional blocks in the encoder, the convolution operation in decoder is replaced by the deconvolution operation, which reconstructs the feature map back to the input image size. The input channels of each convolutional blocks in decoder was set to 512, 1024, 1024, 1024, 512, 256, 128. The last layer is a deconvolution operation followed by a Tanh activation layer, which mapping 128 channels feature maps into 3 channels EUS.

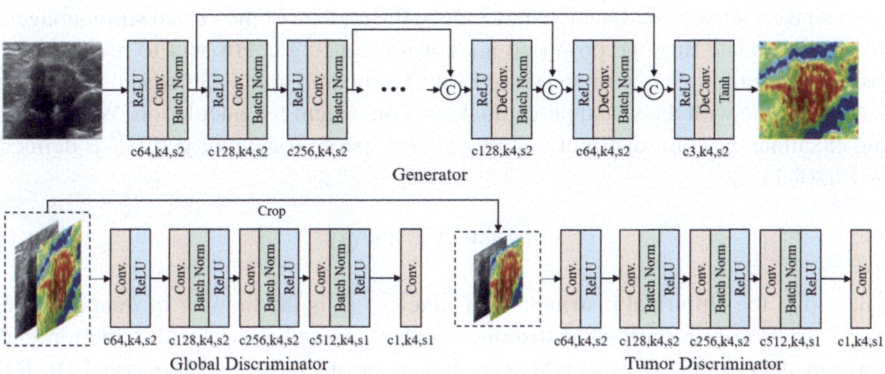

Fig. 8.1 Overview of the model architecture. The generator adopts a U-net design and the discriminator uses a fully convolutional network. The global and tumor discriminator uses the same network architecture. (In the figure, c, k and s represent the number of convolution kernels, convolution kernel size and stride, respectively)

8.2.2 Discriminator

The discriminator, as shown in Fig. 8.1, receives 4-channel composite image (concatenating 1-channel B-mode US and 3-channel EUS) as input. This is a paradigm of conditional GAN, which aims to expose the discriminator to more prior knowledge [15]. The 4 channels composite image is then feed into a convolutional layer followed by 4 convolutional blocks and an output layer. Each convolutional block is composed of a convolution layer, a batch-norm layer and a Leaky-ReLU activation layer. The output channels of each convolution layer in discriminator were set to 64, 128, 256, 512, 512 and 1. The local connection characteristic of convolution operation makes patch retain the spatial information of the input image, so the discriminator effectively models the input image as a Markov random field, which is crucial for high-frequencies reconstruction [16].

In addition to the global discriminator used to classify whether the input image is real or fake, we further designed a local discriminator to determine whether the tumor area is real or fake. Because the color distribution of the tumor region is different from the normal tissue on EUS, the local discriminator, by taking tumor area as input, can effectively distinguish between tumor tissue and normal tissue, thus improving the realism of the elastic reconstruction of the tumor region.

8.2.3 Color Rebalancing

A remarkable characteristic of EUS is the simple color distribution, with blue and red dominating most of the color distribution. Thus the output of the model has a tendency to be dominated by a large number of color types if distribution differences are not taken into account, which may reduce the realism of the virtual strain images. To accommodate this, we proposed a color-rebalancing coefficient to reweight L1 loss during training based on the color rarity. Compared with RGB space, *Lab* space is more in line with the visual perceptual and convenient for calculation. We statistic and calculate the color distribution in *Lab* color space. The factor $\gamma \in \mathbb{R}^Q$ is defined by Eq. (8.1):

$$\gamma_p = (\alpha p + (1 - \alpha)/Q)^{-1}, \tag{8.1}$$

where p is the empirical distribution of pixel p, Q is the number of quantized *ab* space, so $1/Q$ is a uniform distribution and we mixed the prior distribution and uniform distribution with weight $\alpha \in [0, 1]$. In our experiment, α equals to 0.8 works well.

The model training loss comes from two components, the generator and the discriminator. The loss function of the generator l_g s defined by Eq. (8.2):

$$l_g = \lambda * \gamma * \ell_{L1}(y_r, y_v) * \left[\ell_{CE}(1, D(x, y_v)) + \ell_{CE}(1, D(x_t, y_v^t))\right], \tag{8.2}$$

the loss function of the two discriminator l_d^{global} and l_d^{tumor} are defined by Eqs. (8.3) and (8.4):

$$l_d^{global} = \ell_{CE}(1, D(x, y_r)) + \ell_{CE}(0, D(x_t, y_v)), \tag{8.3}$$

$$l_d^{tumor} = \ell_{CE}(1, D(x, y_r^t)) + \ell_{CE}(0, D(x_t, y_v^t)), \tag{8.4}$$

where $\ell_{CE}(\cdot)$ denotes the cross-entropy loss, x denotes the input B-mode US, y_r and y_v refer to the V-EUS and the real EUS respectively, x_t, y_r^t and y_v^t denote tumor regions cropped from the B-mode US, the real EUS and the V-EUS, respectively. The factor λ is empirically set to 100 to accommodate ℓ_{L1} and ℓ_{CE} from discriminator.

Finally, the loss function is defined by Eq. (8.5):

$$loss = l_g + 0.5 * l_d^{global} + 0.5 * l_d^{tumor}. \tag{8.5}$$

8.3 Experimental Results

In this section, we first summarized the baseline characteristics of the enrolled patients and the evaluation methods of V-EUS, then we analyzed the robustness of V-EUS on multi center testing, after that we investigated the effect of tumor depth on V-EUS, and finally we elaborated on the application of V-EUS to portable US.

8.3.1 Patient and Breast Lesion Characteristics

This study, carried out from August 2016 to March 2021, was approved by the Ruijin Hospital Ethics Committee, Shanghai Jiao Tong University School of Medicine, and written informed consent to participate were acquired before examinations. All patients in the 15 centers underwent core needle biopsy or surgery after conventional US and elastography examination, and thus the histopathological findings were obtained for all breast lesions. The high-end US instrument used was the Resona 7 ultrasound system (Mindray Medical International, Shenzhen, China) equipped with L11-3 high-frequency probe, and the pocket-sized US device used was the Stork diagnostic ultrasound system (Stork Healthcare Co., Ltd. Chengdu, China) with L12-4 high-frequency probe.

All radiologists involved in the project at each sub-center had at least 3 years of experience in breast EUS and were uniformly trained in imaging methods prior to the start of the study. The acquired imaging data were stored on hard disks and sent to the study center for analysis. The mean age of 4580 cases was 48 ± 14 age, including 4578 women and 2 men. These included 2226 malignant tumors and

Table 8.1 Distribution of lesion according to BI-RADS

BI-RADS	Benign	Malignant	Total
2	7	1	8
3	905	64	969
4A	1047	234	1281
4B	259	448	707
4C	98	933	1031
5	38	546	584
Total	2354	2226	4580

2354 benign tumors, with the most common of the malignant tumors being invasive ductal carcinoma and the most common of the benign tumors being fibroadenoma. The distribution of the BI-RADS scores and the statistics of malignant and benign tumors are shown in Table 8.1.

8.3.2 Evaluation Metrics and Methods of V-EUS

In order to assess the quality of V-EUS comprehensively, we perform both quantitative and subjective evaluations. Quantitative evaluations are performed in following two aspects: similarity between V-EUS and real EUS and the efficacy of V-EUS in the diagnosis of breast cancer. We use structure similarity index measurement (SSIM), mean absolute percentage error (MAPE), and color histogram correlation (CHC) to quantitatively measure the reconstruction error between V-EUS and real EUS. These three indexes quantitatively compare V-EUS with EUS in terms of similarity of image structure, similarity of elasticity values, and similarity of color distribution, respectively. As an intuitive interpretation, large SSIM and CHC values indicate good agreement between V-EUS and real EUS, while large MAPE values indicate large synthetic errors. The calculation methods of these three indexes are detailed in Supplementary methods.

$$SSIM = \frac{(2\mu_{real}\mu_{virtual} + C_1)(2\sigma_{real,virtual} + C_2)}{(\mu_{real}^2 + \mu_{virtual}^2 + C_1)(\sigma_{real}^2 + \sigma_{virtual}^2 + C_1))}, \tag{8.6}$$

where μ_{real} and $\mu_{virtual}$ are the average of real EUS and V-EUS, respectively. σ_{real} and $\sigma_{virtual}$ are the variance of real EUS and V-EUS, respectively. $\sigma_{real,virtual}$ is the covariance of real EUS and V-EUS. C_1 and C_2 are constants.

$$MAPE = \frac{1}{m}\sum_{1}^{m}\frac{|p_i^{real} - p_i^{virtual}|}{p_i^{real}}, \tag{8.7}$$

where p_i^{real} and $p_i^{virtual}$ represents the strain scores of real EUS and V-EUS, respectively.

$$HC = 1 - \sqrt{1 - \frac{\sum Cnt_{real} \cdot Cnt_{virtual}}{\sqrt{\sum Cnt_{real} \cdot \sum Cnt_{virtual}}}}, \tag{8.8}$$

where the $\cdot Cnt_{real}$ and $\cdot Cnt_{virtual}$ are vectors containing the count of every bin in the histogram of real EUS and V-EUS respectively. Therefore, CHC is the mean of HC in hue and saturation color space.

We further quantify the stiffness of the tumor by calculating the strain ratio (SR), which is a semi-quantitative assessment method and defined as the ratio of the deformation of the normal breast tissue to the tumor tissue, and then analyze its diagnostic efficacy by using the receiver operating characteristic (ROC) curve.

In addition to the objective evaluation, we also conduct subjective blind evaluations on V-EUS. Both junior and senior US radiologists are required to perform visual Turing tests to evaluate the visual fidelity of V-EUS. The procedure of subjective evaluations is described in the corresponding results section.

8.3.3 V-EUS Evaluation in the Internal Validation Set

The overall values of SSIM, MAPE and CHC are 0.903, 0.304 and 0.849, respectively, which indicates a good agreement between V-EUS and real EUS.

An essential aspect of evaluating V-EUS is the application in the clinical practice, differentiating between benign and malignant breast tumors in our application. We calculate the SR values of real EUS and V-EUS, respectively, and use the SR values to calculate the AUCs for breast cancer diagnosis. The performance of SR values obtained from real EUS is similar to that of V-EUS, with AUC of 0.773 and 0.752, respectively ($p = 0.396$, Fig. 8.2a). In the task of breast cancer diagnosis, we usually choose a smaller diagnostic threshold to ensure high sensitivity, and it can be seen from the ROC that the diagnostic performance of real EUS and V-EUS is similar at this time. Further, we compared the diagnostic performance of V-EUS and real EUS stratified by tumor size (Fig. 8.2b) and location (Fig. 8.2c). The statistical results show that the performance of real EUS and V-EUS in the diagnosis of benign and malignant tumors in different groups is similar, without significant statistical difference. Several representative examples are shown in Fig. 8.2d.

8.3.4 Generalization to Multi-Center External Testing Sets

Due to differences in imaging parameters and clinical settings, US images can vary greatly among different medical centers. It is therefore important to verify that the model trained on the main cohort is robust to different cohorts from other medical centers. We collected 1730 cases from 14 medical centers as external test cohorts to

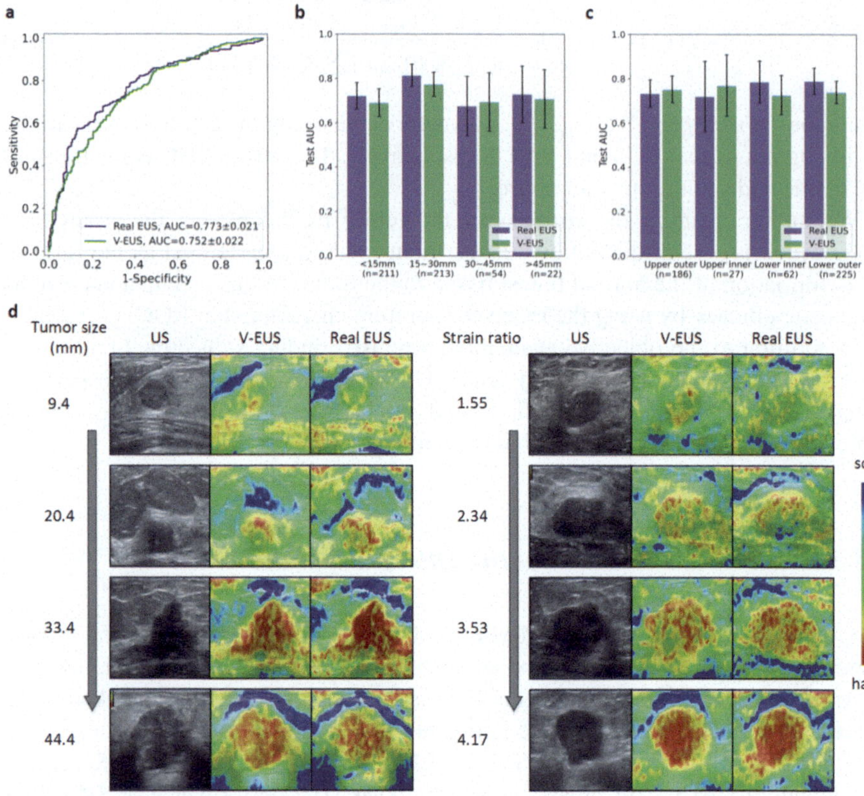

Fig. 8.2 Performance of the deep learning model on the internal validation set. (**a**) Comparison of ROCs between real EUS and V-EUS in determining breast tumor malignancy. (**b**) Comparison of diagnostic performance stratified by tumor size. n indicates the number of cases in the interval. Error bar indicates 95% confidence intervals of AUC. (**c**) Comparison of diagnostic performance stratified by tumor location. n indicates the number of cases in the interval. Error bar indicates 95% confidence intervals of AUC. (**d**) Results of several examples

evaluate the generalization performance of the model. Table 8.2 presents the number of samples of different centers and the corresponding numerical metrics.

For diagnosing breast cancer, the SR of real EUS and V-EUS were calculated, respectively, and the diagnostic AUCs of each center were analyzed (Fig. 8.3). It was found that the diagnostic AUC of V-EUS is not significant different from that of real UES in each centers. These results indicate that our model is capable of generalizing to diverse data sources.

Table 8.2 Comparison of multi center data distribution and numerical metrics

Center	Number	SSIM	MAPE	CHC
A	58	0.917	0.312	0.847
B	58	0.942	0.273	0.858
C	46	0.949	0.243	0.866
D	145	0.927	0.210	0.845
E	362	0.903	0.319	0.819
F	243	0.897	0.315	0.852
G	213	0.899	0.356	0.865
H	150	0.939	0.320	0.864
I	74	0.892	0.370	0.820
J	95	0.914	0.364	0.827
K	96	0.897	0.346	0.844
L	39	0.901	0.289	0.818
M	56	0.902	0.431	0.849
N	95	0.936	0.366	0.848

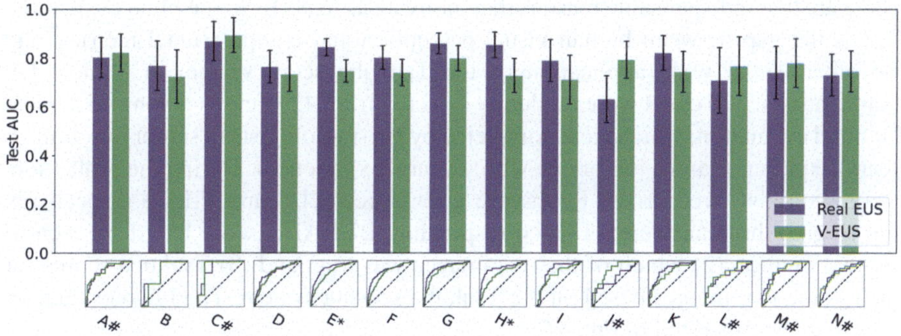

Fig. 8.3 AUC comparison of 14 medical centers. * indicates a significant difference ($p < 0.05$, the p-value for the center E is 0.0005 and the p-value for the center H is 0.0055). # indicates that the AUC of V-EUS is greater than that of real EUS. Error bar indicates 95% confidence intervals of AUC

8.3.5 Tumor Depth Dependence of Diagnostic Efficiency

EUS is strongly influenced by imaging attenuation and it was reported to show reduced sensitivity for diagnosing lesions at relatively deep locations [17–19]. With the reconstruction results we found that V-EUS rarely showed artefacts or loss of elastic pseudo-color in deeper tumors. We therefore design experiments to test whether V-EUS is robust to imaging depths. We mixed the main cohort and the multicenter cohort and then all 4231 cases were divided into training and testing datasets according to the depth of tumors. We set 15 mm as the threshold and get 2826 training cases with tumor depth less than 15 mm and 1405 testing cases. We use the AUCs of SR in determining breast malignancy to measure the effectiveness of EUS.

The diagnosis AUC of real EUS and V-EUS are 0.751 and 0.767 (Fig. 8.4a), respectively. The diagnostic performance of V-EUS is not significantly different from that of real EUS. From a more detailed perspective, we statistic the diagnosis AUC for samples of different tumor depth in the test set (Fig. 8.4b). With increasing tumor depth, the diagnostic performance of V-EUS progressively exceeds that of real EUS.

Representative examples of different tumor types with different tumor depths are shown in Fig. 8.4c. According to the statistics, we find when the tumor depth is greater than 20 mm, 25.9% (62 of 239) of real EUS exhibit artifacts caused by signal attenuation. It can be seen that V-EUS is more accurate in measuring the hardness of the lesion and can effectively avoid artifacts at the deep-located lesion.

8.3.6 Blind Evaluation on V-EUS

There are two indispensable reasons that motivate us to perform the blind evaluation. One is the gap between human visual perception and computational metrics, and the other is the wide application of the Tsukuba score system in clinical US examinations. 500 cases were randomly selected from 4231 cases among 15 centers for blind evaluation, which were completed by two radiologists (a senior one with 10 years' experience and a junior one with 4 years' experience). During the evaluation, two radiologists were asked to observe a set of real EUS and V-EUS respectively and to give three answers: (1) a corresponding BI-RADS score based on each of the two images, (2) which of the two images was true, and (3) Tsukuba scores for each of the two images based on the Tsukuba scoring system. The blind evaluation results are summarized in Fig. 8.5.

For the perceptual realism test, if the operator successfully picks out the real one from the two displayed EUS (one is real and the other is virtual), the model is considered to be failed and will score 0. Otherwise, the score will be 1. Therefore, if our model exactly reproduced real EUS, the perceptual score would be 0.5. Interestingly, in the blind test of junior radiologists, the perceptual score is 0.73, indicating our results are deemed more realistic than real EUS. In the blind test of senior US radiologists, the model score is 0.53, which also shows that V-EUS and real EUS are similar in visual authenticity (Fig. 8.5a).

In the experiment on the diagnosis of breast cancer, the Tsukuba scores of real EUS and V-EUS are used as a complement to the BI-RADS scores respectively, thus testing the extent to which they can contribute to the diagnostic performance (the combination method of Tsukuba scores and BI-RADS scores is described in Supplementary methods). In the junior radiologists group, the AUC of BI-RADS using the BUS is 0.754, while the AUCs are increased to 0.840 and 0.816 respectively when supplemented with the Tsukuba scoring system based on real EUS and V-EUS (Fig. 8.5b). In the senior radiologists group, the AUC using BUS is 0.789, while the AUCs are promoted to 0.890 and 0.862 respectively when incorporating with real EUS and V-EUS (Fig. 8.5c).

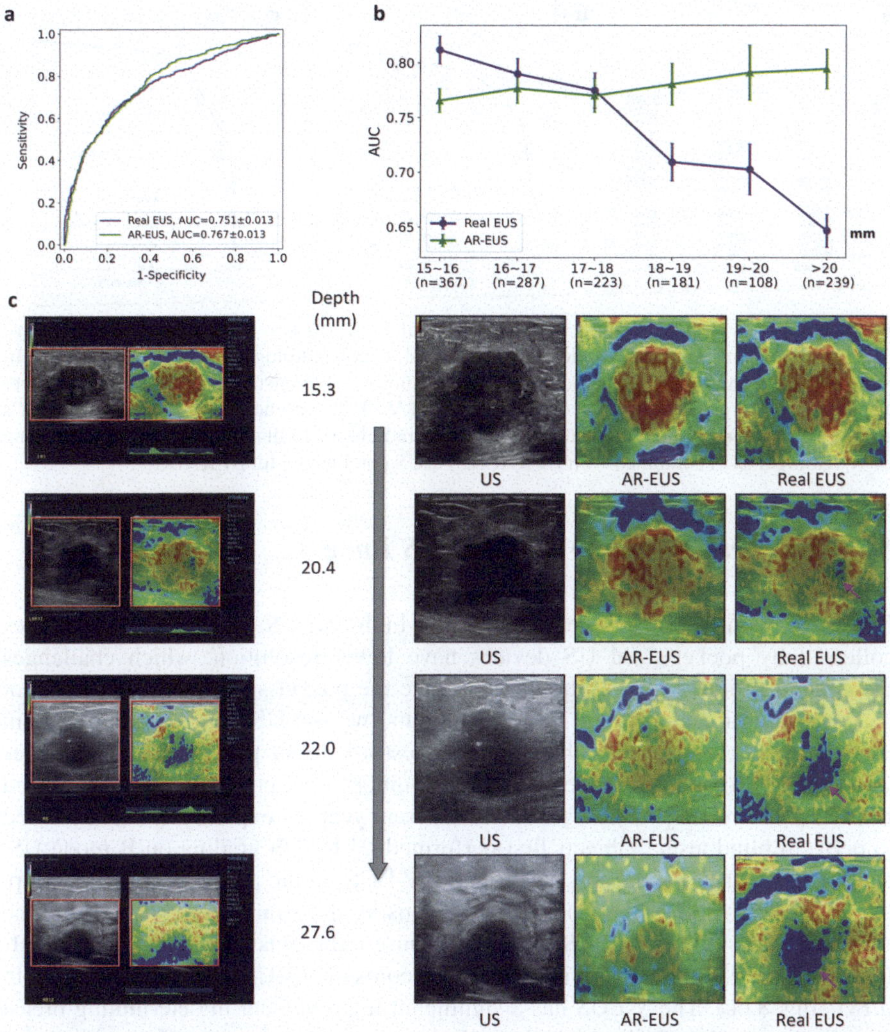

Fig. 8.4 Dependence of V-EUS on tumor depth in diagnosing breast cancer. (**a**) Comparison of ROCs in determining tumor malignancy on test set when dividing training and test set with 15 mm as the threshold. (**b**) The diagnostic performance of real EUS and V-EUS varies with the depth of tumor. For the real EUS, the centers of the error bar for each interval are 0.812, 0.790, 0.775, 0.709, 0.702, and 0.647, respectively. For the V-EUS, the centers of the error bar for each interval are 0.766, 0.777, 0.770, 0.781, 0.791 and 0.794 respectively. n indicates the number of cases in the interval. Error bar indicates 95% confidence intervals. (*$p<0.05$; **$p<0.01$, the p-values for the last three intervals are 0.0013, 0.0017, 0.0004 respectively). (**c**) Examples of typical case results. ROIs were cropped from the US images and displayed on the right together with V-EUS. We observe that for the deep-located tumor, V-EUS not only perform better than real EUS, but also avoid artifacts caused by US signal attenuation. Pink arrows highlight the US imaging at the signal attenuation

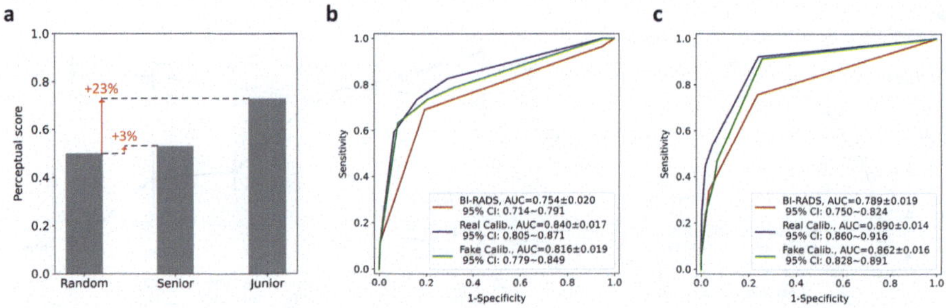

Fig. 8.5 Blind evaluation results of V-EUS and real EUS. (**a**) Perceptual score comparison of blind evaluation results of the junior radiologist and senior radiologist with random group. (**b**) ROCs comparison of blind evaluation results of the junior radiologist in diagnosing breast cancer using BI-RADS, real EUS combined with BI-RADS, V-EUS combined with BI-RADS. (**c**) ROCs comparison of blind evaluation results of the senior radiologist in diagnosing breast cancer using BI-RADS, real EUS combined with BI-RADS, V-EUS combined with BI-RADS

8.3.7 Generalization to Portable US Images

Compared with the US images collected by high-end US devices, the US images collected by pocket-sized US devices have lower resolution, which challenges the generalization ability of the model. Since the pocket-sized US devices cannot perform strain imaging to get the training data, we use US images collected from high-end US devices to train the model and test it with the pocket-sized US images (Fig. 8.6a). A total of 349 cases with breast tumors were collected by pocket-sized US devices. Similarly, radiologists with different years of experience were involved to perform blind tests. Subjects first performed BI-RADS grading on B-mode US, and then gave the strain scores according to V-EUS. In the junior radiologist group, the AUC of BI-RADS is 0.706, while after using the strain scores of V-EUS, the AUC increases to 0.755 (Fig. 8.6b). In the senior radiologist group, the AUC of BI-RADS is 0.729, while after using the strain scores of V-EUS, the AUC increases to 0.781 (Fig. 8.6c). The V-EUS has a significant improvement in determining breast malignancy ($p = 0.0001$ in the junior radiologist group and $p = 0.0012$ in the senior radiologist group). As shown in some examples, we can see that the proposed model can effectively capture the elastic information of the lesion (Fig. 8.6d).

8.4 Discussion

In this study, we propose a GAN-based model to directly translate US images into V-EUS, which is validated by comprehensive experiments to have good visual consistency and clinical value with real EUS. There are two main considerations in choosing the clinical task of breast cancer diagnosis. First, breast cancer accounts

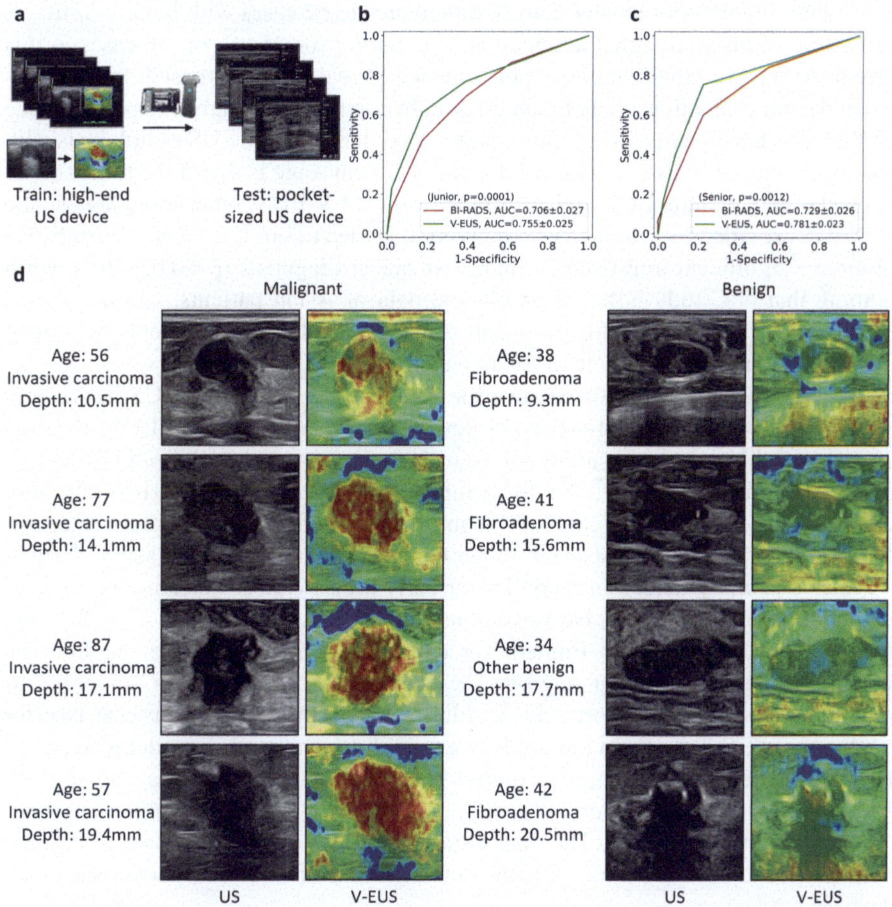

Fig. 8.6 Blind evaluation results of V-EUS and real EUS. (**a**) Adaptability to pocket-sized US images. (**a**) The deep learning model trained on high-quality US images is adapted to low-quality pocket-size US images. The photo of the pocket-sized device is from Stork Healthcare Co., Ltd. Chengdu, China. (**b**) ROCs comparison of blind evaluation results of the junior radiologist. (**c**) ROCs comparison of blind evaluation results of the senior radiologist in diagnosing breast cancer. (**d**) Examples of typical case results. For lesions with different tumor depth and different benign and malignant types, the model can capture the elastic information effectively

for 30% of malignancies in women, and its incidence continues to increase and result in noteworthy cancer death [20]. Breast cancer screening examinations prior to breast cancer diagnosis can reduce the mortality rate [21]. Second, conventional BUS combined with EUS is becoming the agenda operation and has improved the accuracy of identifying breast malignancies, both in diagnosis and screening.

Compared with the real EUS acquired by high-end US devices via signal processing, V-EUS avoids artifacts caused by attenuation of ultrasound signals in deep-located tumors. According to the statistical results, we find that among 239 cases with tumor depth greater than 20 mm, there are 62 cases with obvious artifacts caused by ultrasound signal attenuation, accounting for 25.9% of the cases in this group. As a result, the diagnostic performance of real EUS decreased dramatically when the tumor depth is greater than 20 mm. In contrast, the diagnostic performance of V-EUS is hardly affected by tumor depth. In order to provide US radiologists with the superiority of V-EUS in clinical diagnosis, an envisage is that if the tumor depth is greater than 20 mm, radiologists use the results of V-EUS, otherwise they use the real EUS provided by US devices. Applying this idea to our retrospective study, we observe a significant improvement in breast cancer diagnosis ($p < 0.05$). It is worth nothing that our study is based on clinical data of Asian patients, and the results may be more pronounced for European, American and African patients, who tend to have deeper breast tumor than Asian patients.

In addition to providing assistance for high-end US devices, V-EUS has a more profound impact on pocket-sized US devices that cannot perform EUS imaging. The current dilemma is that although the market share of pocketed-sized US devices is increasing in recent years due to its high flexibility and low cost, it is currently unable to perform EUS imaging for the limitation of imaging hardware. In resource-limited areas, portable US scanner, rather than standard high-end US scanner, could serve as a primary detection modality for early breast cancer detection because of its portability and low cost. However, due to cost and size limitations, the function of portable US scanner is limited, for example, it does not have the function of elastography, which can improve the accuracy of breast cancer screening as mentioned above. V-EUS provides a solution with almost hardware cost free for pocket-sized US devices. In this study, we train the deep learning model with paired B-mode US and EUS images acquired from high-end US devices and test the model with B-mode US acquired from pocket-sized US devices without any fine-tuning or domain adaption. The diagnostic results and examples shown in Fig. 8.6 demonstrate that V-EUS has a great potential to empower the pocket-sized US devices.

Although we have demonstrated that V-EUS performs well in the clinical task of breast cancer diagnosis, there are many aspects of future work that can be extended. From the perspective of clinical tasks, the effectiveness of V-EUS in the diagnosis of other breast diseases and the imaging of other organs, such as thyroid and liver, still need to be proved. In fact, the deep learning model proposed in this work is very convenient to transfer to other US image synthesis tasks. Using the shear wave elastography (SWE) images as training labels, the model can establish a mapping from B-mode US images to SWE images. If the clinical effectiveness of the synthesized SWE images can be proved, it will have a profound impact on the development and clinical application of US devices.

In conclusion, we present a deep learning framework for synthesizing V-EUS through B-mode US, and validate the clinical value of V-EUS in diagnosing breast cancer through comprehensive experiments. V-EUS can not only provide high-end US devices with accurate diagnostic results in examining deep located tumors, but more importantly, endow the pocket-sized US devices with the capability of performing EUS imaging.

References

1. Shen YQ et al (2021) Artificial intelligence system reduces false-positive findings in the interpretation of breast ultrasound exams. Nat Commun 12:5645
2. Zheng XY et al (2020). Deep learning radiomics can predict axillary lymph node status in early-stage breast cancer. Nat Commun 11:1236
3. Clevert A et al (2019) ESR statement on portable ultrasound devices. Insights Imaging 10:89
4. Bennett D et al (2021). Portable pocket-sized ultrasound scanner for the evaluation of lung involvement in coronavirus disease 2019 patients. Ultrasound Med Biol 47:19–24
5. Rykkje A, Carlsen JF, Nielsen MB (2019) Hand-held ultrasound devices compared with high-end ultrasound systems: a systematic review. Diagnostics 9:61
6. Sigrist RMS, Liau J, El Kaffas A, Chammas MC, Willmann JK (2017) Ultrasound elastography: review of techniques and clinical applications. Theranostics 7:1303–1329
7. Muckley MJ et al (2021) Results of the 2020 fastMRI challenge for machine learning MR image reconstruction. IEEE Trans Med Imaging 40:2306–2317
8. Qu LQ, Zhang YQ, Wang S, Yap PT, Shen DG (2020) Synthesized 7T MRI from 3T MRI via deep learning in spatial and wavelet domains. Med Image Anal 62:101663
9. Li ZJ et al (2021) DeepVolume: brain structure and spatial connection-aware network for brain MRI super-resolution. IEEE Trans Cybern 51:3441–3454
10. Rivenson Y et al (2019) Virtual histological staining of unlabelled tissue-autofluorescence images via deep learning. Nat Biomed Eng 3:466–477
11. Yao Z, Luo T, Dong Y et al (2023) Virtual elastography ultrasound via generative adversarial network for breast cancer diagnosis. Nat Commun 14:788
12. Ronneberger O, Fischer P, Brox T (2015) U-Net: convolutional networks for biomedical image segmentation. In: Proceedings of the international conference on medical image computing and computer assisted intervention, pp 234–241
13. He KM, Zhang XY, Ren SQ, Sun J (2016) Deep residual learning for image recognition. In: Proceedings of the IEEE conference on computer vision and pattern recognition, pp 770–778
14. Long J, Shelhamer E, Darrell T (2015) Fully convolutional networks for semantic segmentation. In: Proceedings of the IEEE conference on computer vision and pattern recognition, pp 3431–3440
15. Isola P, Zhu JY, Zhou TH, Efros AA (2017) Image-to-image translation with conditional adversarial networks. In: Proceedings of the IEEE conference on computer vision and pattern recognition, pp 5967–5976
16. Li C, Wand, M (2016) Precomputed real-time texture synthesis with Markovian generative adversarial networks. In: Computer vision – ECCV 2016. Springer, Cham, pp 702–716
17. Stachs A et al (2013) Differentiating between malignant and benign breast masses: factors limiting sonoelastographic strain ratio. Ultraschall Med 34:131–136
18. Barr RG et al (2015) Wfumb guidelines and recommendations for clinical use of ultrasound elastography: part 2: breast. Ultrasound Med Biol 41:1148–1160
19. Chang JM, Moon WK, Cho N, Kim SJ (2011) Breast mass evaluation: factors influencing the quality of US elastography. Radiology 259:59–64
20. Siegel RL, Miller KD, Fuchs HE, Jemal A (2021) Cancer statistics. CA-Cancer J Clin 71:7–33
21. Duffy SW et al (2021) Beneficial effect of consecutive screening mammography examinations on mortality from breast cancer: a prospective study. Radiology 299:541–547

Chapter 9
Generative Adversarial Networks for Brain MR Image Synthesis and Its Clinical Validation on Multiple Sclerosis

Hongwei Bran Li and Bene Wiestler

Abstract This chapter explores the application of generative adversarial networks (GANs) for synthesizing brain magnetic resonance imaging sequences in the context of multiple sclerosis (MS). It presents advanced MRI synthesis methods, including lesion-focused loss functions for improved lesion appearance and uncertainty quantification in synthetic images. It details the technical aspects of GANs, including their architecture, training, and optimization, and discusses their clinical applications from diagnostic enhancements to their integration into multi-center studies. Furthermore, the chapter assesses the validation of these models in clinical settings, showcasing their ability to enhance diagnostic accuracy, detecting and monitoring MS. Through extensive experiments and reader studies with experienced radiologists, it was demonstrated that synthetic images achieve high-quality clinical utility. Finally, the chapter discusses the limitations and future directions of generative MRI synthesis in MS, highlighting its potential to impact clinical practice and patient care.

9.1 Introduction

Magnetic Resonance Imaging (MRI) has long been a cornerstone in the diagnostic assessment of neurological disorders, notably Multiple Sclerosis (MS) [1]. Traditional MR imaging techniques, while effective, often face challenges—the acquisition of multiple MRI sequences can be time-consuming and costly, and some sequences may be missing or of poor quality due to various factors such as patient motion or differences in acquisition protocols across imaging centers [10].

H. B. Li (✉)
Athinoula A. Martinos Center for Biomedical Imaging, Massachusetts General Hospital, Harvard Medical School, Boston, MA, USA
e-mail: holi2@mgh.harvard.edu

B. Wiestler
AI for Image-Guided Diagnosis and Therapy, Technical University of Munich, Munich, Germany
e-mail: b.wiestler@tum.de

L. Zhang et al. (eds.), *Generative Machine Learning Models in Medical Image Computing*, https://doi.org/10.1007/978-3-031-80965-1_9

In recent years, generative models have been a transformative approach to medical imaging. These models, including Generative Adversarial Networks (GANs) [5] and diffusion models [15], have shown promising results in enhancing the capabilities of MRI by generating synthetic, high-quality images with diagnostic potentials.

The transition to generative models-driven methods to enhance image information marks a significant achievement in neuroradiology. Deep generative models can synthesize MRI data often indistinguishable from real scans [9]. This capability is not just a technological advancement but also a practical one, offering the potential to reduce scan times, decrease the necessity for repeat scans, and provide extensive data sets for medical training and research without additional patient exposure to MRI procedures.

The integration of generative models into MRI practices presents unique opportunities and challenges. On the one hand, these models can generate comprehensive synthetic datasets, facilitate enhanced diagnosis, and are instrumental in personalized medicine. On the other hand, challenges such as the risk of generating inaccurate images (e.g. images with false-positive lesions) and the necessity for robust validation and testing frameworks are critical considerations. The ongoing development of these technologies aims to address these challenges, ensuring that the benefits of AI-driven MRI can be fully realized in clinical settings. In the following section, we present the basics of GANs and their extension for neuroimaging, the evaluation strategy for synthetic images, and the clinical validation.

9.2 Generative Adversarial Networks for MRI Sequence Synthesis

The core of leveraging generative models in MRI lies in their ability to synthesize high-quality images that can significantly enhance the diagnostic process. This section explores GANs, focusing on the architectures, training mechanisms, and specific innovations tailored for neuroimaging.

9.2.1 Basics of Generative Adversarial Networks

GANs utilize a two-network architecture comprising a generator G and a discriminator D, engaged in a min-max adversarial game. This adversarial framework is formalized as:

$$\min_G \max_D V(D, G) = \mathbb{E}_{x\sim p_{data}(x)}[\log D(x)] + \mathbb{E}_{z\sim p_z(z)}[\log(1 - D(G(z)))] \quad (9.1)$$

where the generator G maps random noise z to synthetic images $G(z)$, while D differentiates between real samples x and generated samples $G(z)$. As shown in

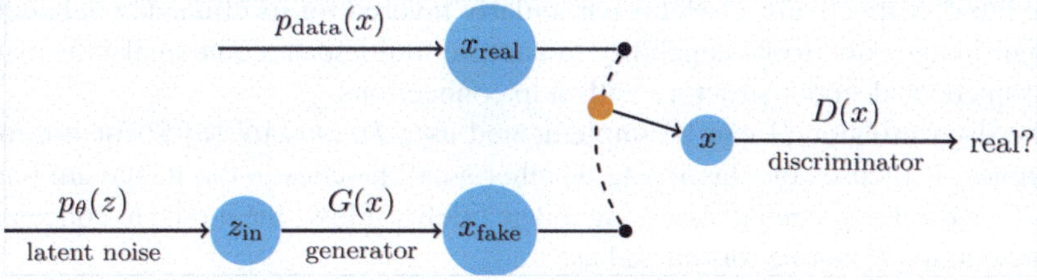

Fig. 9.1 A schematic view of GANs as a generative model that approximates the true data distribution in a min-max game

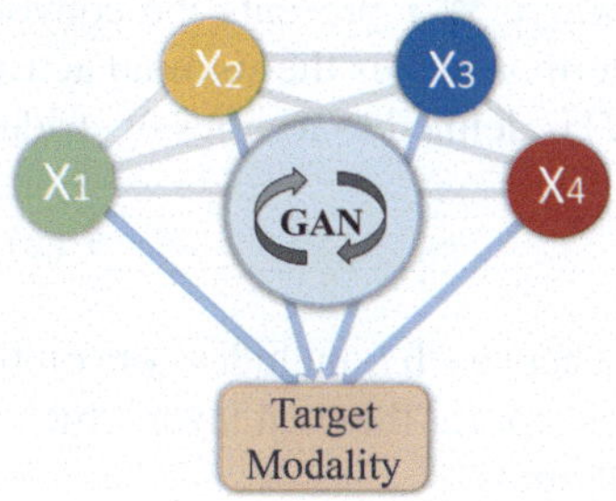

Fig. 9.2 The *DiamondGAN* [9] architecture for MRI modality synthesis, which learns a mapping between any subset of multiple input MRI modalities (X) to a target modality. Figure adapted courtesy of [9]

Fig. 9.1, the generator $G : \mathcal{Z} \rightarrow \mathcal{X}$ aims to learn a mapping from a latent space $\mathcal{Z}$ to the target MRI image space $\mathcal{X}$, approximating the true data distribution $p_{data}(x)$. Concurrently, the discriminator $D : \mathcal{X} \rightarrow [0, 1]$ estimates the probability that sample x is drawn from $p_{data}(x)$ rather than the generated distribution p_g.

9.2.2 *Image-to-Image Synthesis Using GANs*

In the context of MRI, GANs have been adapted for image-to-image synthesis, a task where the goal is to transform one modality or multiple modalities into another MRI modality while preserving underlying structural details. Instead of generating an image from random noise z, the generation is conditional on a source image (or its embedding). This is particularly useful for synthesizing different MRI sequences by taking multiple sequences as the input, to generate sequence-specific image features. One ideal framework is the *DiamondGAN* [9] setting that maps an arbitrary combination of source modalities to a target modality, as shown in Fig. 9.2.

9.2.2.1 Architectural Details

Practically, in an image-to-image synthesis task, the generator G could utilize an encoder-decoder architecture like U-Net [13], known as $\mathcal{U} : \mathbb{R}^{H \times W \times C} \rightarrow \mathbb{R}^{H \times W \times C'}$, where H, W, and C represent the height, width, and number of channels of the input, respectively. U-Net is particularly favored for its efficiency in handling medical images due to its capability to capture multi-scale contextual information via its encoder-decoder structure with skip connections.

The discriminator D can be implemented as a *PatchGAN* [8] $\mathcal{P}$ for improved coherence. It focuses on classifying whether small patches in the image are real or fake. This local approach to assessing image fidelity allows the model to concentrate on fine details. $\mathcal{P}$ can be formulated as:

$$\mathcal{P}(x)_{i,j} = \sigma((\mathbf{W} * x)_{i,j} + b) \tag{9.2}$$

where $\mathbf{W}$ represents the convolutional kernels, $*$ denotes convolution, b is a bias term, and σ is the sigmoid activation function. The architecture of the discriminator $\mathcal{P}$ is defined as a series of strided convolutional layers l_i:

$$\mathcal{P}(x) = l_m \circ l_{m-1} \circ \ldots \circ l_1(x) \tag{9.3}$$

where each l_i includes convolution, batch normalization, and *LeakyReLU* activation, except for the final layer which employs a *sigmoid* activation to produce probability outputs.

9.2.2.2 Training and Optimization

The training involves alternating updates to the discriminator and the generator. The generator learns to produce increasingly realistic images based on the feedback from the discriminator, which is trained to become more adept at distinguishing real images from synthesized ones, as well as a synthesis-specific loss objective. This form of training ensures that the generated images are realistic for diagnostic imaging. The optimization process is detailed in Algorithm 9.1.

9.2.3 *Loss Functions for MS-Specific MRI Synthesis*

To address the unique challenges of synthesizing MRI sequences for MS diagnosis and monitoring, specialized loss functions can be designed. These functions enhance the fidelity of MS lesion appearance and the overall quality of synthetic images.

9.2.3.1 Pixel-Wise Reconstruction Loss

One basic loss is to compute a pixel-wise reconstruction loss $\mathcal{L}_{rec}$. This loss is designed for a single generator that takes multiple input modalities and produces a single target modality. It can be formulated as:

Algorithm 9.1 Training of conditional GAN for synthetic image synthesis

Require: Real images dataset, number of epochs N, batch size
Ensure: Trained Generator G is capable of producing synthetic images based on input images

Initialize Generator G and Discriminator D with random weights
for each epoch in 1 to N **do**
  for each batch in dataset **do**
    $X_{real} \leftarrow$ sample_real_images(batch_size) // Sample real images
    $X_{condition} \leftarrow$ sample_condition_images(batch_size) // Sample condition images
    $X_{fake} \leftarrow G(X_{condition})$ // Generate fake images conditioned on $X_{condition}$
    // Train Discriminator D
    $D_{loss} \leftarrow -\text{mean}(\log(D(X_{real})) + \log(1 - D(X_{fake})))$
    Update D weights to minimize D_{loss}
    // Train Generator G
    $G_{loss} \leftarrow -\text{mean}(\log(D(X_{fake})))$
    Update G weights to minimize G_{loss}
  end for
  // Optionally evaluate the model performance on the validation set
  if epoch % evaluation_frequency == 0 **then**
    Evaluate G using qualitative and quantitative metrics
  end if
end for
return G

$$\mathcal{L}_{rec} = \mathbb{E}_{X,T}[\|T - G(X)\|_1] \tag{9.4}$$

where X are the source modalities after concatenation, T is the target modality, and G is the generator translating between source and target modalities. This loss minimizes the pixel-wise intensity difference between synthetic and acquired images.

9.2.3.2 Structural Similarity Index Measure Loss

To enhance the perceptual quality of synthetic images and ensure structural consistency with the target images, SSIM [18] is incorporated into the loss function. The SSIM between two image patches x and y is defined as:

$$SSIM(x, y) = \frac{(2\mu_x\mu_y + C_1)(2\sigma_{xy} + C_2)}{(\mu_x^2 + \mu_y^2 + C_1)(\sigma_x^2 + \sigma_y^2 + C_2)} \tag{9.5}$$

where μ_x and μ_y are the average intensities of x and y, σ_x^2 and σ_y^2 are the variances of x and y, σ_{xy} is the covariance of x and y, and C_1 and C_2 are constants to stabilize the division with weak denominator.

Hence, the SSIM loss to *minimize* the difference can be defined as:

$$\mathcal{L}_{SSIM} = 1 - SSIM(T, G(X)) \tag{9.6}$$

where T is the target image and $G(X)$ is the generated image. This formulation ensures that minimizing $\mathcal{L}_{SSIM}$ leads to maximizing the structural similarity between the synthetic and target images. Its differentiable implementation can be found in: https://github.com/VainF/pytorch-msssim.

9.2.3.3 Lesion-Targeting Loss

To place greater emphasis on accurately synthesizing MS lesions, a lesion-targeting loss $\mathcal{L}_{LT}$ is designed, which is critical for diagnosis and disease monitoring. This loss is defined as:

$$\mathcal{L}_{LT} = \|M \odot T - M \odot G(X)\|_1 \tag{9.7}$$

where M is the lesion segmentation mask, T is the target image, $G(X)$ is the generated image, and $\odot$ denotes element-wise multiplication. This loss encourages the generator to pay particular attention to lesion areas, which—though crucial for the clinical utility of the synthetic images—only make up a very small percentage of the image and thus contribute only little to the total loss.

9.2.3.4 Adversarial Loss

The adversarial loss, derived from the discriminator, plays a crucial role in our GAN framework. It encourages the generator to produce synthetic images that are indistinguishable from real MRI sequences. We adopt the *PatchGAN* [8] network mentioned in Sect. 9.2.2.1. The adversarial loss is formulated as:

$$\mathcal{L}_{adv}(G, D) = \mathbb{E}[\log D(T)] + \mathbb{E}[\log(1 - D(G(X)))] \tag{9.8}$$

9.2.3.5 Total Loss

All the loss components can be integrated into a total loss function as follows:

$$\mathcal{L}_{total} = \lambda_G \mathcal{L}_{adv} + \lambda_s \mathcal{L}_{SSIM} + \lambda_{LT} \mathcal{L}_{LT} + \lambda_r \mathcal{L}_{rec} \tag{9.9}$$

where λ_G, λ_s, λ_{LT}, and λ_r are weighting factors that balance the different loss components as shown in Fig. 9.3. These weights are crucial in determining the trade-off between overall image quality and local lesion accuracy of the synthesized MRI sequences.

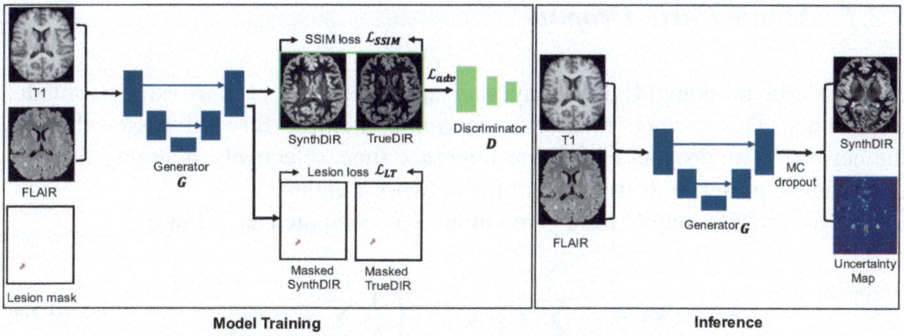

Fig. 9.3 Network architecture, training process, and inference stage task with GANs for the image synthesis task. The image Generator G takes the combination of FLAIR and T1w as input to generate synthetic double inversion recovery images (DIR). Additional supervision from the lesion maps during training enhances the synthesis of MS-specific lesions (such as lesion attention). The feedback on the similarity between synthetic DIR and true DIR is given by the Discriminator D and a structure similarity loss function and it updates the network weights. Figure adapted courtesy of [3]

9.3 Uncertainty Quantification in Synthetic MRI

Uncertainty quantification (UQ) is relevant to enhance the clinical utility of synthetic MRI images. It provides a measure of the model's confidence in its predictions, which is particularly crucial in medical imaging. In the realm of generative models, especially when applied to tasks like MRI sequence synthesis, UQ can be instrumental in assessing the reliability of generated images.

In theory, two primary types of uncertainty are typically considered: aleatoric uncertainty, which accounts for noise inherent in the data, and epistemic uncertainty, which stems from the model's lack of knowledge. Methods such as Bayesian neural networks [6] offer a framework for modeling epistemic uncertainty by placing priors over the network weights, thus enabling the model to express its confidence level regarding its outputs. Additionally, techniques like Monte Carlo dropout [4] can be employed during both training and inference to simulate the effect of randomness in neural network predictions, providing a quick estimation of uncertainty by running multiple forward passes and observing the variability in the outputs. Test-time augmentation is an effective method to quantify aleatoric uncertainty [19].

In clinical practice, quantifying uncertainty, either aleatoric or epistemic, can aid radiologists in making more informed decisions. For instance, high uncertainty in areas of an MRI scan might prompt additional testing or expert review, ensuring that diagnosis and treatment planning are based on reliable imaging data. Moreover, it helps in setting realistic expectations regarding the diagnostic capabilities of AI-driven tools in medical imaging, potentially leading to broader acceptance and trust among medical professionals. In the following section, we introduce the principle of Monte Carlo dropout.

9.3.1 Monte Carlo Dropout

Monte Carlo dropout [4] is a Bayesian approximation [11] to estimate model uncertainty. This method involves performing multiple forward passes through the network with dropout enabled at inference time, effectively sampling from an approximate posterior distribution of the network weights.

The uncertainty map U for a given input X is computed as follows:

$$U(X) = \frac{1}{N}\sum_{t=1}^{N} G_t(X)^2 - \left(\frac{1}{N}\sum_{t=1}^{N} G_t(X)\right)^2 \tag{9.10}$$

where $G_t(X)$ is the output of the t-th forward pass with dropout, and N is the total number of Monte Carlo samples.

9.3.2 Voxel-Wise Uncertainty Map

In the MRI image synthesis task, the resulting uncertainty map $U(X)$ provides a voxel-wise measure of the model's uncertainty. Higher values in $U(X)$ indicate areas where the model is less confident in its predictions, which often correspond to challenging regions such as lesion boundaries or areas with complex tissue interfaces. Notably, such an uncertainty map can be further leveraged to improve the image quality [17].

9.3.3 Clinical Implications of Uncertainty Maps

We argue that uncertainty maps may serve several important clinical functions:

1. **Reliability Assessment**: They provide clinicians with a visual guide to areas where the synthetic images may be less reliable, prompting closer examination or comparison with other modalities.
2. **Lesion Detection**: Areas of high uncertainty often correlate with regions of pathology, potentially aiding in the detection of subtle or early-stage lesions.
3. **Quality Control**: Uncertainty maps can be used as a quality control measure, flagging synthetic images with unusually high overall uncertainty for manual review.

9.4 Quantitative and Qualitative Evaluation of Synthetic Images

The evaluation of synthetic MRI sequences is crucial to validate their quality and clinical utility. This section presents a multi-faceted approach, combining quantitative metrics with qualitative assessments by expert radiologists.

9.4.1 *Quantitative Metrics*

When providing reference images, several established image quality metrics could be used to assess the synthetic images objectively:

- Peak Signal-to-Noise Ratio (PSNR): Measures the ratio between the maximum possible signal power and the power of distorted noise.
- SSIM: Assesses the perceived quality of the synthetic image compared to the real image, focusing on structural information, as defined in the previous section.
- Mean Absolute Error (MAE): Measures the average magnitude of the differences between predicted and actual values.

9.4.2 *Clinical Assessment by Lesion Counting*

In the MS context, the primary method for evaluating the clinical utility of our synthetic images is through lesion counting in three steps: (1) Two independent neuroradiologists, blinded to the image source (synthetic or real), count MS lesions in synthetic and real MRI sequences. (2) Lesions are categorized based on their location: juxtacortical, periventricular, infratentorial, and subcortical. (3) The lesion counts in synthetic images are compared to those in the corresponding real images to assess the ability of our method to represent MS pathology accurately.

9.5 Clinical Validation

Clinical validation forms the crux of transitioning generative models from theoretical constructs to practical tools in medical imaging, particularly in the diagnosis and monitoring of Multiple Sclerosis (MS). This section outlines the comprehensive validation process undertaken to ascertain the clinical utility and diagnostic accuracy of synthetic MRI sequences generated via GANs, originally presented in our two publications [2, 14].

9.5.1 *Validation Objectives*

Clinical validation was conducted through a series of structured experiments and collaborative studies across multiple imaging centers. The primary objectives were to (1) assess the diagnostic accuracy of synthetic MRI images compared to acquired MRI images and (2) evaluate the capability of synthetic images to accurately depict MS lesions and their progression over time.

9.5.2 *Experimental Design*

The validation involved a multi-center study with the following design:

- **Patient cohort:** A diverse cohort of MS patients, with varying degrees of disease progression, was selected to ensure comprehensive testing of the synthetic MRI images under different clinical scenarios.
- **Image assessment:** Both synthetic and conventional MRI images of the patients were evaluated by experienced neuroradiologists who were blinded to the image origin (synthetic or real).
- **Metrics used:** Diagnostic accuracy was quantified using metrics lesion-to-background ratio. Image quality was assessed using PSNR, SSIM, and MAE as outlined earlier.

9.5.3 *Reader Studies*

Reader studies were specifically designed to gauge the clinical acceptance and perceived image quality of synthetic MRI sequences:

- **Study participants:** A group of neuroradiologists from different centers participated, providing a broad base of expertise and opinion.
- **Study procedure:** Experts were asked to identify MS lesions from a set of anonymized images without knowing whether they were viewing synthetic or real MRI scans.
- **Feedback collection:** After the assessment, detailed feedback was collected regarding the perceived quality of the images, ease of lesion identification, and overall trust in the synthetic images for clinical decision-making.

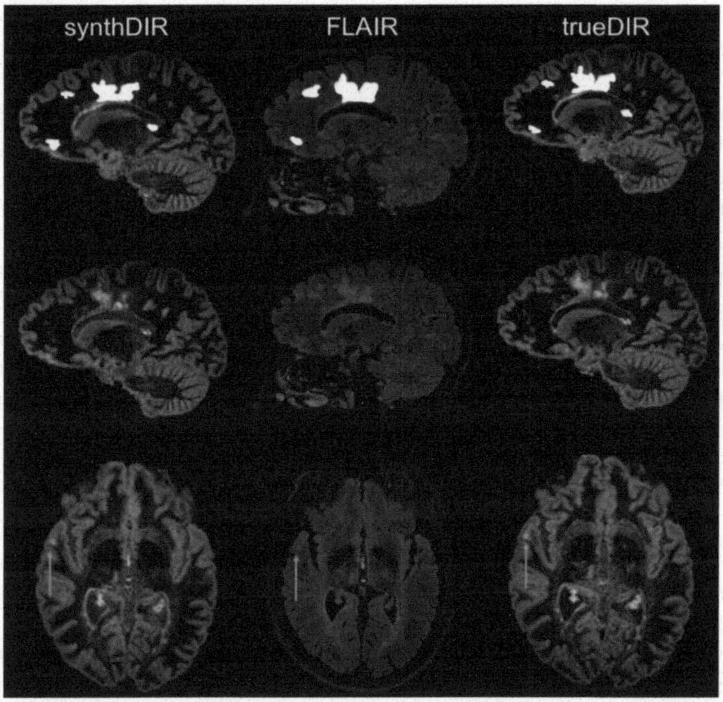

Fig. 9.4 Representative images of FLAIR, SynthDIR, and TrueDIR from the same patient [2]. Displayed are slices in both sagittal and axial planes along with their corresponding lesion segmentations. A notable enhancement in the detection of juxtacortical lesions (indicated by green arrows) is observed in SynthDIR compared to the input FLAIR images. Figure courtesy of [2]

9.5.4 Results and Findings

9.5.4.1 Synthetic DIR Images Enhanced Visualization of Juxtacortical Lesions

In a single-center study [2], the use of synthetic Double Inversion Recovery (synthDIR) images led to a statistically significant increase in lesion detection compared to conventional FLAIR images, with an average of 31.4 ± 20.7 lesions detected using synthDIR versus 22.8 ± 12.7 with FLAIR ($p < 0.001$), as shown in Fig. 9.4. This improvement was predominantly due to the enhanced visualization of juxtacortical lesions, where synthDIR detected 12.3 ± 10.8 lesions as opposed to 7.2 ± 5.6 lesions detected by FLAIR ($p < 0.001$).

Additionally, the contrast-to-noise ratio (CNR) in synthDIR images (22.0 ± 6.4) was superior to that in FLAIR images (16.7 ± 3.6, $p = 0.009$); however, it did not differ significantly from trueDIR images (22.0 ± 6.4 vs. 22.4 ± 7.9, $p = 0.87$), suggesting comparable performance with actual DIR images in terms of image contrast.

9.5.4.2 Uncertainty Maps Helped Discriminate Between Lesions and Artifacts

In another multi-center study [3], we observed that the utilization of synthDIR facilitated significantly more lesion detections compared to FLAIR images, with an average of 26.7 ± 2.6 lesions detected using synthDIR versus 22.5 ± 2.2 for FLAIR in Reader 1 ($p < 0.0001$), and 22.8 ± 2.2 versus 19.9 ± 2.0 in Reader 2 ($p = 0.0005$).

The use of uncertainty maps in the evaluation of synthDIR images helped to further discriminate between MS lesions and artifacts, enhancing the overall diagnostic utility of synthetic MRI, as shown in Fig. 9.5. The consistency of lesion detection improvements across internal and external data sets suggests that synthDIR can reliably reproduce critical diagnostic features across different scanners and patient cohorts.

9.5.4.3 Synthetic DIR Identified Disease Progression

In a longitudinal study, both readers identified a significantly higher number of newly formed, MS-specific lesions in the longitudinal subtractions from synthDIR compared to physical FLAIR. Reader 1 detected an average of 3.27 ± 0.60 lesions with synthDIR versus 2.50 ± 0.69 with FLAIR ($p = 0.0016$), and Reader 2 observed 3.31 ± 0.81 lesions versus 2.53 ± 0.72 ($p < 0.0001$). The enhancement in lesion detectability was particularly notable in juxtacortical lesions, showing a 36% relative gain in lesion counts, pooled across both readers. In 5% of the cases, synthDIR subtraction maps were instrumental in identifying disease progression that was missed on FLAIR subtraction maps, as shown in Fig. 9.6.

9.6 Conclusion and Future Directions

9.6.1 Clinical Validation and Implications

This chapter's exploration and clinical validation of GANs for synthesizing brain MRI sequences confirm their potential to transform neuroimaging. By enhancing diagnostic processes and potentially improving patient outcomes, these generative models promise to make significant clinical impacts. The integration of deep learning methods with clinical expertise paves the way for innovative, next-generation medical imaging solutions that are both effective and patient-centric.

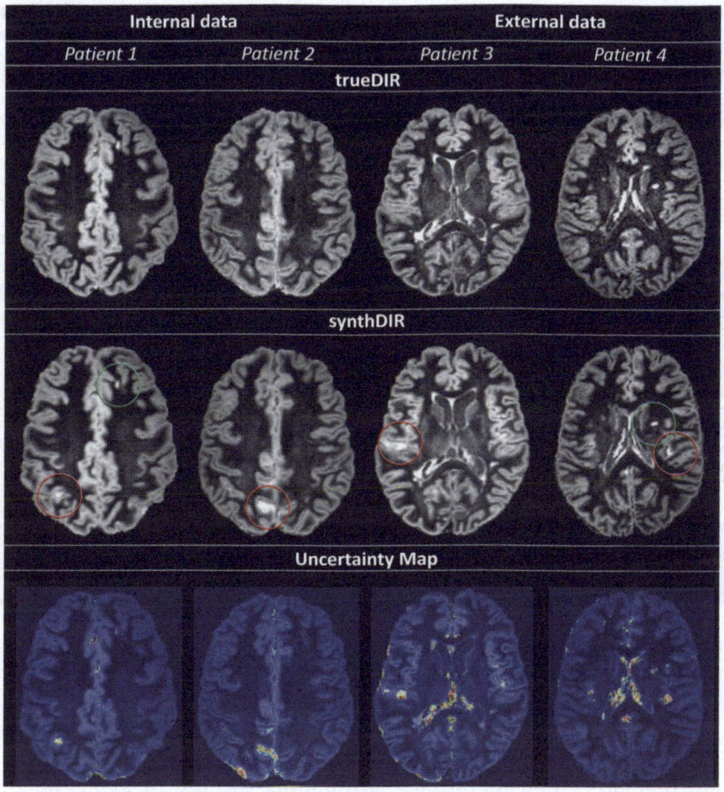

Fig. 9.5 Examples of synthetic images and the use of uncertainty map [3]. Uncertainty maps deliver critical insights into the accuracy of synthetic images. Highlighted in red (Patients 1–4), hyperintensities observed in synthDIR that do not match with trueDIR are distinctly marked as high-variance zones on the corresponding uncertainty maps. This feature aids in recognizing these discrepancies as artifacts generated during the synthesis process. Conversely, actual lesions are identified clearly as areas exhibiting minimal (Patient 1—green circle in synthDIR) or low (Patient 4—green circle in synthDIR) uncertainty values. Figure courtesy of [3]

9.6.2 Current Limitations and Ethical Considerations

Despite promising results, several challenges remain. The synthesis of contrast-enhanced images [16] and ensuring generalizability and adaptability [7] across various scanners and protocols are technical hurdles that need addressing. Although uncertainty map is one solution to remind clinicians about potential hallucinations, it complicates clinical flow. Task-specific, clinician-centric solutions might be needed considering the actual objectives of leveraging uncertainty quantification. For example, it might be clinically relevant to provide a hint about global confidence of the synthesis results and provide text to describe the issue in specific locations. This might connect interpretability and multi-modal learning. Additionally, the

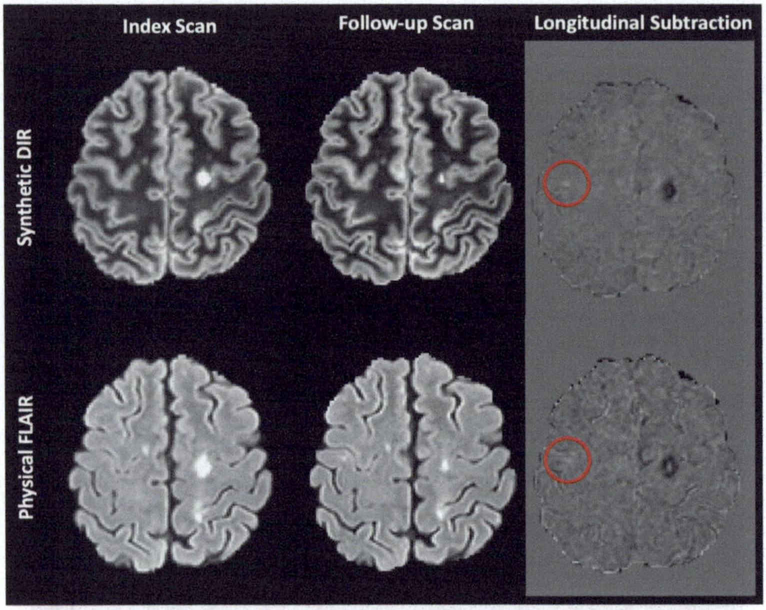

Fig. 9.6 Examples of synthetic images for longitudinal analysis [14]. In the longitudinal subtraction images, the juxtacortical lesion is more distinctly prominent and detectable in the synthetic DIR compared to those derived from physical FLAIR. Figure courtesy of [14]

ethical and regulatory considerations surrounding the use of synthetic images in clinical settings must be carefully managed to ensure patient safety and maintain trust in medical imaging technology.

9.6.3 Advancing Generative Models in Medical Imaging

Looking ahead, there are several exciting directions. Future work would focus on 3D/4D synthesis, enhancing model architectures to improve the fidelity and utility of synthetic images, particularly for capturing complex pathology details across diverse patient populations. One of the promising methods is diffusion models that operate on the latent space [12], making it applicable for 3D and even longitudinal synthesis.

Incorporating data from multiple imaging modalities or clinical data could enhance the diagnostic accuracy of synthetic images. Techniques like diffusion tensor imaging and perfusion imaging hold potential to add valuable dimensions to synthesized images.

The ability of generative models to produce consistent and high-quality images can significantly benefit longitudinal studies and personalized medicine. Developing models that account for temporal changes and individual patient data could revolutionize treatment planning and disease monitoring.

9.6.4 Broader Impact

The broader application of generative models could extend beyond MS to other medical fields where imaging is crucial, such as oncology or cardiology. This expansion could facilitate large-scale studies, enhance diagnostic efficiency, and enable more sensitive disease monitoring.

The journey of integrating generative models into medical imaging is only beginning. As methodology evolves, it holds the promise not only to enhance the quality of medical care but also to redefine the possibilities of medical treatment and research. Ongoing collaboration among clinicians, engineers, and computer scientists will be essential to navigate the challenges and realize the full potential of generative methods and clinician-centric, patient-centric AI.

Acknowledgments H.B.Li is supported by an SNF Postdoc Mobility grant.

Competing Interests The authors have no conflicts of interest to declare relevant to this chapter's content.

References

1. Filippi M, Brück W, Chard D, Fazekas F, Geurts JJ, Enzinger C, Hametner S, Kuhlmann T, Preziosa P, Rovira À et al (2019) Association between pathological and MRI findings in multiple sclerosis. Lancet Neurol 18(2):198–210
2. Finck T, Li H, Grundl L, Eichinger P, Bussas M, Mühlau M, Menze B, Wiestler B (2020) Deep-learning generated synthetic double inversion recovery images improve multiple sclerosis lesion detection. Investig Radiol 55(5):318–323
3. Finck T, Li H, Schlaeger S, Grundl L, Sollmann N, Bender B, Bürkle E, Zimmer C, Kirschke J, Menze B, et al (2022) Uncertainty-aware and lesion-specific image synthesis in multiple sclerosis magnetic resonance imaging: a multicentric validation study. Front Neurosci 16:889808
4. Gal Y, Ghahramani Z (2016) Dropout as a bayesian approximation: Representing model uncertainty in deep learning. In: International conference on machine learning, PMLR, pp 1050–1059
5. Goodfellow I, Pouget-Abadie J, Mirza M, Xu B, Warde-Farley D, Ozair S, Courville A, Bengio Y (2020) Generative adversarial networks. Commun ACM 63(11):139–144
6. Hernández-Lobato JM, Adams R (2015) Probabilistic backpropagation for scalable learning of bayesian neural networks. In: International conference on machine learning, PMLR, pp 1861–1869

7. Hu Q, Li H, Zhang J (2022) Domain-adaptive 3d medical image synthesis: An efficient unsupervised approach. In: International conference on medical image computing and computer-assisted intervention. Springer, pp 495–504
8. Isola P, Zhu JY, Zhou T, Efros AA (2017) Image-to-image translation with conditional adversarial networks. In: Proceedings of the IEEE conference on computer vision and pattern recognition, pp 1125–1134
9. Li H, Paetzold JC, Sekuboyina A, Kofler F, Zhang J, Kirschke JS, Wiestler B, Menze B (2019) Diamondgan: unified multi-modal generative adversarial networks for MRI sequences synthesis. In: Medical image computing and computer assisted intervention–MICCAI 2019: 22nd international conference, Shenzhen, China, October 13–17, 2019, Proceedings, Part IV 22. Springer, pp 795–803
10. Nichols TE, Das S, Eickhoff SB, Evans AC, Glatard T, Hanke M, Kriegeskorte N, Milham MP, Poldrack RA, Poline JB, et al (2017) Best practices in data analysis and sharing in neuroimaging using MRI. Nat Neurosci 20(3):299–303
11. Reid N (1996) Likelihood and bayesian approximation methods. Bayesian Stat 5:349–366
12. Rombach R, Blattmann A, Lorenz D, Esser P, Ommer B (2022) High-resolution image synthesis with latent diffusion models. In: Proceedings of the IEEE/CVF conference on computer vision and pattern recognition, pp 10684–10695
13. Ronneberger O, Fischer P, Brox T (2015) U-net: Convolutional networks for biomedical image segmentation. In: Medical image computing and computer-assisted intervention–MICCAI 2015: 18th international conference, Munich, Germany, October 5–9, 2015, Proceedings, part III 18. Springer, pp 234–241
14. Schlaeger S, Li HB, Baum T, Zimmer C, Moosbauer J, Byas S, Mühlau M, Wiestler B, Finck T (2023) Longitudinal assessment of multiple sclerosis lesion load with synthetic magnetic resonance imaging–a multicenter validation study. Investig Radiol 58(5):320–326
15. Song Y, Sohl-Dickstein J, Kingma DP, Kumar A, Ermon S, Poole B (2020) Score-based generative modeling through stochastic differential equations. In: International conference on learning representations
16. Thomas MF, Kofler F, Grundl L, Finck T, Li H, Zimmer C, Menze B, Wiestler B (2022) Improving automated glioma segmentation in routine clinical use through artificial intelligence-based replacement of missing sequences with synthetic magnetic resonance imaging scans. Investig Radiol 57(3):187–193
17. Upadhyay U, Chen Y, Hepp T, Gatidis S, Akata Z (2021) Uncertainty-guided progressive GANs for medical image translation. In: Medical image computing and computer assisted intervention–MICCAI 2021: 24th international conference, Strasbourg, France, September 27–October 1, 2021, Proceedings, Part III 24. Springer, pp 614–624
18. Wang Z, Bovik AC, Sheikh HR, Simoncelli EP (2004) Image quality assessment: from error visibility to structural similarity. IEEE Trans Image Process 13(4):600–612
19. Wang G, Li W, Aertsen M, Deprest J, Ourselin S, Vercauteren T (2019) Aleatoric uncertainty estimation with test-time augmentation for medical image segmentation with convolutional neural networks. Neurocomputing 338:34–45

Part III
Image Super-Resolution and Reconstruction

Chapter 10
Histopathological Synthetic Augmentation with Generative Models

Jiarong Ye, Peng Jin, Haomiao Ni, Sharon X. Huang, and Yuan Xue

Abstract In this chapter, we explore the application of generative models to enhance the fidelity and utility of artificially generated images for data augmentation in digital pathology. We employ *HistoGAN* for synthetic augmentation, filtering images based on label congruence and feature resemblance to real specimens. This ensures that only the most accurate synthetic images are used. Additionally, we utilize reinforcement learning for automated quality checks, optimizing synthetic sample selection, and improving image classification outcomes. However, GANs have limitations, such as instability during training and the need for large annotated datasets for conditional generation. To address these issues, we transition to *HistoDiffusion*, a model that utilizes diffusion processes, which are more stable to train and reduce the risk of mode collapse common in GANs. Furthermore, unconditional diffusion models can be guided with smaller annotated datasets to enable conditional synthesis. *HistoDiffusion* generates more complex and nuanced images, enhancing realism and diversity. Through this exploration of generative AI techniques for synthetic augmentation, each model addresses the limitations of its predecessor, advancing the effectiveness of data augmentation in digital pathology.

J. Ye · P. Jin · S. X. Huang
College of Information Sciences and Technology, The Pennsylvania State University, University Park, PA, USA
e-mail: jxy225@psu.edu; pqj5125@psu.edu; suh972@psu.edu

H. Ni
Department of Computer Science, The University of Memphis, Memphis, TN, USA
e-mail: hni@memphis.edu

Y. Xue (✉)
Department of Biomedical Informatics, The Ohio State University, Columbus, OH, USA
e-mail: yuan.xue@osumc.edu

L. Zhang et al. (eds.), *Generative Machine Learning Models in Medical Image Computing*, https://doi.org/10.1007/978-3-031-80965-1_10

10.1 Introduction

Image analysis of digitized histopathological slides is crucial for cancer diagnosis [20]. Machine learning, especially deep learning, has shown promise in classifying these images. Whole slide images (WSIs) are high-resolution, making direct analysis difficult. To address this, patch-level classification is used, where patches are analyzed individually and aggregated to determine the final label [19, 48, 52]. Accurate patch-level classification is essential for matching human diagnostic accuracy. Over the past decade, computer-assisted diagnosis (CAD) algorithms for histopathology images have been developed to enhance pathologists' accuracy in disease detection, diagnosis, and prognosis prediction [15]. These automatic histopathology image classification systems are particularly valuable in underdeveloped regions due to their low cost and accessibility. They help mitigate inter- and intra-pathologist variability, thereby supporting more consistent and accurate diagnoses (Fig. 10.1).

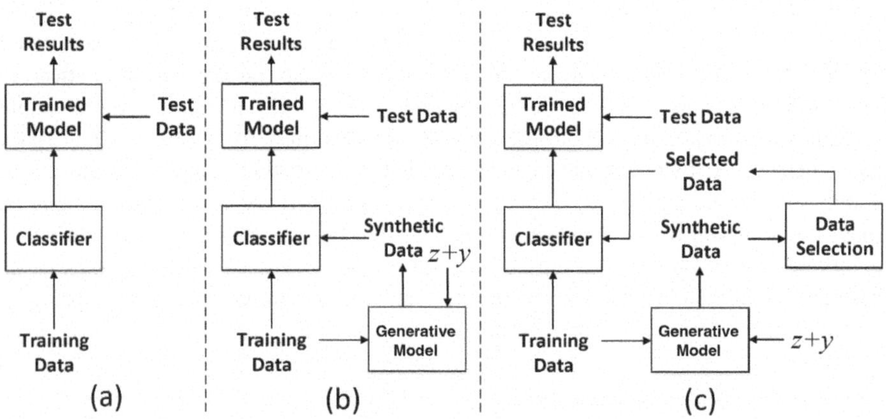

Fig. 10.1 Diagram of synthetic augmentation workflow. (**a**) Traditional training workflow using only real training data; (**b**) Augmenting the training dataset by incorporating synthetic data generated by a generative model; (**c**) Using synthetic augmentation, with filtered synthetic data to ensure only high-quality samples are added to the training set. (Note: The latent vector z is a random noise input fed into the generator part of a GAN. It is sampled from a predefined distribution, such as a Gaussian distribution; the conditional information y is used in conditional GANs (cGANs) to guide the generation process. It represents additional information like labels that the model uses to generate specific types of data.)

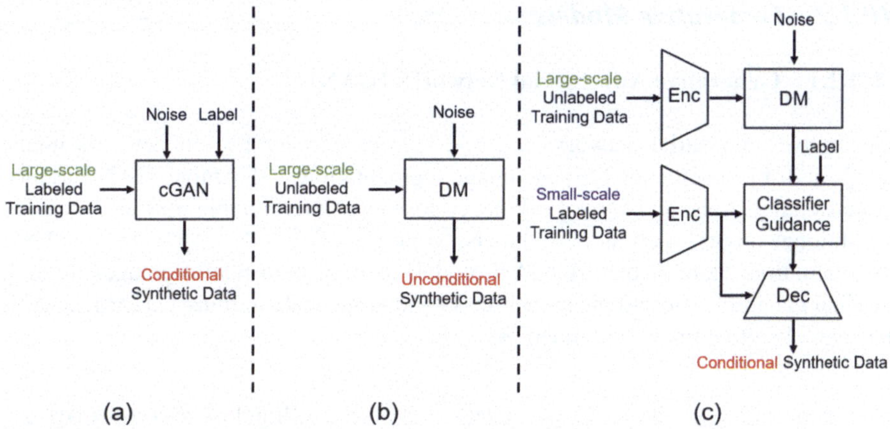

Fig. 10.2 Comparison between different deep generative models for synthetic augmentation. (**a**) Conditional Generative Adversarial Networks (cGANs) enhance the original GAN framework by integrating additional information, such as class labels, into both the generator and discriminator, guiding the data generation process to produce specific outputs based on the given conditions. However, cGAN-based method normally requires relatively large-scale annotated training data; (**b**) Unconditional diffusion model (DM) which cannot take conditional input; (**c**) Conditional diffusion model that can be pretrained on large-scale unannotated data and later applied to *unseen* small-scale annotated data for augmentation. The encoder (Enc) compresses the input data into a compact lower-dimensional latent representation. This process retains essential semantic information and enhances computational efficiency for subsequent processing within the latent space. After the diffusion model (DM) modifies the latent representation, the decoder (Dec) translates it back into the image space, reconstructing high-resolution images from the latent code while ensuring high visual fidelity to the real data

10.1.1 Synthetic Augmentation

Supervised training of image recognition systems requires large amounts of annotated data. However, histopathology image datasets are often small and imbalanced due to annotation costs and privacy concerns. Data augmentation is used to enhance training data and reduce overfitting. Effective augmentation generates new samples that follow the original data distribution, while poor augmentation can mislead training. Traditional data augmentation techniques [51], such as random transformations or distortions (e.g., cropping and flipping) and auto augmentations [5, 17] using hyper-parameter searching to automatically find the optimal augmentation policy, increase training data yet lack flexibility. To overcome data limitations in histopathology image recognition, we focus on expanding training sets with high-quality synthetic examples using GAN and diffusion models, termed as **Synthetic Augmentation**. In the following sections, we will discuss synthetic augmentation with images via generative models such as GANs and diffusion models, along with their pros and cons (Fig. 10.2).

10.1.2 Generative Models

10.1.2.1 Generative Adversarial Networks (GAN)

Generative adversarial networks (GANs) [13] enable applications such as image synthesis, object detection [25] and image segmentation [53]. Among GAN variants, conditional GANs (cGANs) [30] generate more interpretable results by using conditional inputs, such as class labels, to produce labeled samples for synthetic augmentation. State-of-the-art cGAN models achieve high-fidelity images through gradual generation or refinement sub-tasks and large-scale training [21, 56]. cGANs have an objective function defined as:

$$\min_{\theta_G} \max_{\theta_D} \mathcal{L}_{\text{cGAN}} = \mathbb{E}_{x \sim P_{\text{data}}}[\log D(x, y)] + \mathbb{E}_{z \sim \mathcal{N}}[\log(1 - D(G(z, y)))] \ . \tag{10.1}$$

In the equation above, x represents the real data from an unknown image distribution P_{data} and y is the conditional label. z is a random vector for the generator G, drawn from a standard normal distribution $\mathcal{N}(\mathbf{0}, \mathbf{I})$. During training, G and D are alternatively optimized to compete with each other.

To apply GANs for synthetic segmentation, Ratner et al. [37] learns data transformation with unlabeled data using GANs. GAGAN [1] and BAGAN [28] use cGANs [30] generated samples to augment the standard classifier in the low-data regime. Compared with works done in the natural image domain, issues related to insufficient and imbalanced data are more prominent in the medical image domain. To mitigate these problems, researchers have been working on synthetic augmentation for medical image recognition tasks. Frid-Adar et al. [10] proposes to use cGAN generated synthetic CT images to improve the performance of CNN in liver lesion classification. Gupta et al. [14] synthesizes lesion images from non-lesion ones using CycleGAN [61]. Bowles et al. [2] uses GAN derived synthetic images to augment medical image segmentation models. Zhao et al. [59] proposes a GAN model for synthesizing retinal images from small sized samples and uses the synthetic images to improve semantic segmentation performance. Mahapatra et al. [27] applies a Bayesian neural network (BNN) [26] to calculate the informativeness of the synthetic images for improved classification and segmentation results. Zhao et al. [60] uses transformations of labeled images for one-shot image segmentation. These approaches address insufficient and imbalanced data in medical imaging, enhancing recognition tasks.

10.1.2.2 Diffusion Models

More recently, diffusion models have become popular for natural image generation due to their impressive results and training stability [7, 18, 46]. A few studies have also demonstrated the potential of diffusion models for medical image synthesis [32,

36]. Diffusion models (DM) [18, 44, 45] are probabilistic models that are designed to learn a data distribution. Given a sample from the data distribution $z_0 \sim q(z_0)$, the DM *forward* process produces a Markov chain $z_1, \ldots, z_T$ by gradually adding Gaussian noise to z_0 based on a variance schedule $\beta_1, \ldots, \beta_T$, that is:

$$q(z_t|z_{t-1}) = \mathcal{N}(z_t; \sqrt{1-\beta_t} z_{t-1}, \beta_t \mathbf{I}) \ , \tag{10.2}$$

where variances β_t are constants. If β_t are small, the posterior $q(z_{t-1}|z_t)$ can be well approximated by diagonal Gaussian [35, 44]. Furthermore, when the T of the chain is large enough, z_T can be well approximated by standard Gaussian distribution $\mathcal{N}(\mathbf{0}, \mathbf{I})$. These suggest that the true posterior $q(z_{t-1}|z_t)$ can be estimated by $p_\theta(z_{t-1}|z_t)$ defined as [34]:

$$p_\theta(z_{t-1}|z_t) = \mathcal{N}(z_{t-1}; \mu_\theta(z_t), \Sigma_\theta(z_t)) \ . \tag{10.3}$$

The DM *reverse* process (also known as *sampling*) then generates samples $z_0 \sim p_\theta(z_0)$ by initiating a Markov chain with Gaussian noise $z_T \sim \mathcal{N}(\mathbf{0}, \mathbf{I})$ and progressively decreasing noise in the chain of $z_{T-1}, z_{T-2}, \ldots, z_0$ using the learnt $p_\theta(z_{t-1}|z_t)$. To learn $p_\theta(z_{t-1}|z_t)$, Gaussian noise ϵ is added to z_0 to generate samples $z_t \sim q(z_t|z_0)$, then a model ϵ_θ is trained to predict ϵ using the following mean-squared error loss:

$$L_{\text{DM}} = \mathbb{E}_{t\sim\mathcal{U}(1,T), z_0\sim q(z_0), \epsilon\sim\mathcal{N}(\mathbf{0},\mathbf{I})}[||\epsilon - \epsilon_\theta(z_t, t)||^2] \ , \tag{10.4}$$

where time step t is uniformly sampled from $\{1, \ldots, T\}$. Then $\mu_\theta(z_t)$ and $\Sigma_\theta(z_t)$ in Eq. 10.3 can be derived from $\epsilon_\theta(z_t, t)$ to model $p_\theta(z_{t-1}|z_t)$ [18, 34].

The denoising model ϵ_θ is typically implemented using a time-conditioned U-Net [39] with residual blocks [16] and self-attention layers [50]. Sinusoidal position embedding [50] is also usually used to specify the time step t to ϵ_θ.

10.1.3 Summary

To summarize, synthetic augmentation using generative models such as GANs and diffusion models addresses the challenges of small and imbalanced histopathology datasets. Conditional GANs generate high-fidelity images with class labels, enhancing interpretability. Diffusion models offer training stability and robust results. These techniques improve the quality of training data, enabling accurate patch-level classification in digital pathology. The following sections will delve into two specific synthetic augmentation techniques using HistoGAN and HistoDiffusion, respectively, and outline their applications and advantages in histopathology image recognition.

10.2 Synthetic Augmentation with HistoGAN

The motivation behind synthetic augmentation with HistoGAN addresses two critical needs in histopathology image analysis. First, we need a new HistoGAN framework to generate high-fidelity synthetic images that capture meaningful features, overcoming the limitations of existing GAN methods that produce visually appealing but not necessarily informative images. Second, a selective synthetic augmentation approach is essential to ensure that only high-quality synthetic images with high label confidence and accurate feature representation are incorporated into the training set. This selective process mitigates the risks of label ambiguity and feature misalignment, thereby enhancing the performance of histopathology image classification systems (Fig. 10.3).

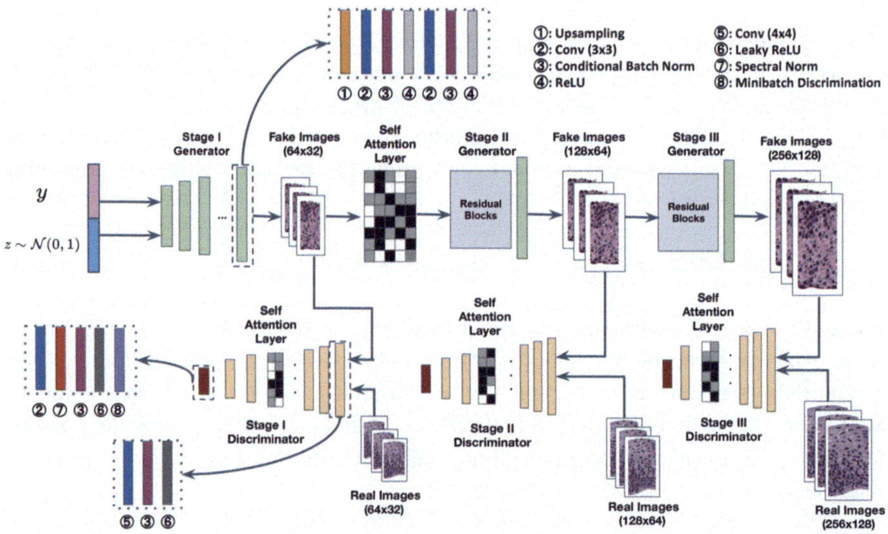

Fig. 10.3 Architecture of a 3-stage HistoGAN for histopathological patch synthesis. Inputs to GAN include y, a conditional input like class labels, to guide the generation process; and z, a latent vector sampled from a normal distribution to serve as a source of randomness and diversity. The number of stages can be adjusted based on the desired final image resolution. Features such as cytoplasm texture and nuclei shapes are progressively refined from stage I to III. Self-attention is applied after the stage I generator and in all stage discriminators to enhance local region consistency. Conditional batch normalization [6] follows convolutional layers for flexible feature map modulation

> **Highlights**

1. HistoGAN introduces an innovative conditional GAN model designed to synthesize realistic histopathology image patches;
2. The work explores a synthetic augmentation method based on handcrafted criteria;
3. Additionally, it examines a synthetic augmentation approach utilizing reinforcement learning.

10.2.1 Methodology

10.2.1.1 HistoGAN

We designed *HistoGAN*, a new model specifically for histopathology image synthesis, based on state-of-the-art conditional GAN techniques [3, 56, 58]. HistoGAN generates synthetic images in a coarse-to-fine manner through multiple stages, gradually refining details to ensure high fidelity. Following state-of-the-art conditional image synthesis techniques [3, 58], we use class-conditional batch normalization in both generators and discriminators to enhance learning effectiveness. Spectral normalization [31] is applied to all stages' discriminators to further improve model performance. To capture the distribution of nucleus density and color changes in histopathology images, we leverage self-attention [50, 58] at the early stages of generation and throughout all stages in the discrimination process. This mechanism allows the model to learn dependencies between spatial regions by examining the relationship between one pixel and all other positions in the same image. Similar to [58], the image features from the previous hidden layer x are first transformed into two feature spaces q, k as query and key in self attention [50] to calculate the attention map. Let $q(x) = W_q x$ and $k(x) = W_k x$, the attention map over the i-th location when synthesizing the j-th region is

$$\alpha_{j,i} = \frac{\exp\left(s_{ji}\right)}{\sum_{i=1}^{N} \exp\left(s_{ji}\right)}, \text{ where } s_{ji} = \boldsymbol{q}\left(\boldsymbol{x}_i\right)^T \boldsymbol{k}\left(\boldsymbol{x}_j\right) \ . \tag{10.5}$$

The output of the self-attention of the j-th region o_j is calculated by applying attention weight over the value v as

$$\boldsymbol{o}_j = \sum_{i=1}^{N} \alpha_{j,i} \boldsymbol{v}\left(\boldsymbol{x}_i\right), \text{ where } \boldsymbol{v}\left(\boldsymbol{x}_i\right) = \boldsymbol{W}_v \boldsymbol{x}_i \ . \tag{10.6}$$

In all transformation matrices W_q, W_k, and W_v, weight matrices are implemented as 1×1 convolutions. Compared with the StackGAN model implemented in our

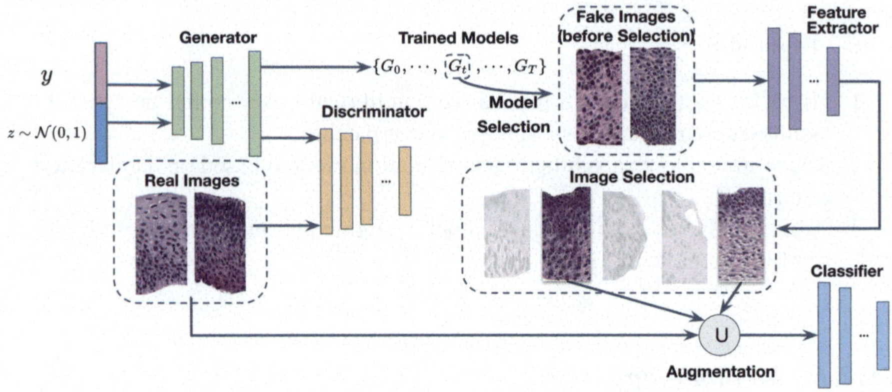

Fig. 10.4 The architecture of the proposed synthetic augmentation algorithm. The ∪ symbol indicates that the selected synthetic image set is unioned with the original training set to improve classification model training and test performance

previous work [54], our HistoGAN generates more realistic image patches which also benefits the following synthetic augmentation step (Fig. 10.4).

10.2.1.2 Synthetic Augmentation via Handcrafted Criteria

Given a trained cGAN model, one can sample infinite noise-vector inputs from a Gaussian distribution to generate infinite synthetic images. While a good cGAN model can generate realistic images, their usefulness for augmenting the original training set in visual recognition tasks is not guaranteed. Current GAN-based data augmentation methods vary the number of generated images based on the augmentation ratio, but effectiveness is affected by quality and diversity of synthetic images.

To reduce randomness and selectively add new images, we propose a two-step process: first, identify samples that can be confidently classified into certain classes; second, select samples whose features are within a certain neighborhood of class centroids in the feature space. This process uses a pre-trained feature extractor to calculate centroids for real samples and extract features for fake samples. To ensure robust feature extraction, we use a feature extractor with Monte Carlo dropout (MC-dropout) [11] and take the expectation value of multiple samplings. A depiction of our proposed synthetic augmentation algorithm is shown in Fig. 10.5 and a detailed description is given in Algorithm 10.1.

The first step of selection is based on label certainty. We evaluate the label certainty of a fake example by calculating the entropy score of its predicted class probabilities. If the feature extractor is certain about a sample's classification, the entropy score will be low. We rank the entropy scores of all generated images in ascending order and choose the first half with lower entropy.

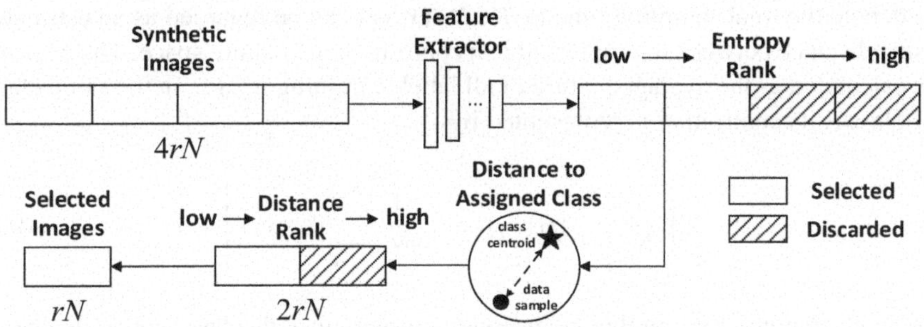

Fig. 10.5 Illustration of the image selection process. r and N represent the augmentation ratio and the number of original training data. The same feature extractor runs multiple times through MC-dropout for both entropy and class centroid distance calculations to increase robustness

Algorithm 10.1 Synthetic augmentation

Input: a set of trained HistoGAN models $\{G_t\}$, number of classes C, augmentation ratio r, number of original training samples $N = \sum_{i=1}^{C} N_i$.
Output: selected synthetic samples $\mathcal{X}$ with $|\mathcal{X}| = rN$.
Initialization: $\mathcal{X}_1 = \emptyset$, $\hat{t} = \arg\min(\hat{d}_t)$, $G_{\hat{t}}$ generated samples $\mathcal{X}_0 = \{x_j^i : i \leq C, j \leq 4rN_i\}$, entropy $\mathcal{E}^i = \{e_j^i : e_j^i = -\sum p_j^i \log p_j^i, i \leq C, j \leq 4rN_i\}$.
for $x_j^i \in \mathcal{X}_0$ **do**
  if $e_j^i < \text{Median}(\mathcal{E}^i)$ **then**
    $\mathcal{X}_1 = \mathcal{X}_1 \cup \{x_j^i\}$
  end if
end forclass centroid distance $\mathcal{D}^i = \{d_j^i : d_j^i = D_f(x_j^i, c_i)\}$.
for $x_j^i \in \mathcal{X}_1$ **do**
  $d_j^i = D_f\{x_j^i, c_i\}$
  if $d_j^i < \text{Median}(\mathcal{D}^i)$ **then**
    $\mathcal{X} = \mathcal{X} \cup \{x_j^i\}$
  end if
end for

The second step selects synthetic images based on their distance to class centroids in the feature space. We calculate the feature distances for the remaining samples and sort them in ascending order. The first half with smaller distances are kept. This ensures only samples that confidently match their assigned labels are selected. Similar to [54], the feature distance between image x and centroid c is defined as

$$D_f(x, c_i) = \frac{1}{K} \sum_k \sum_l \frac{1}{H_l W_l} \left\| \hat{\psi}_l^k(x) - \hat{\psi}_l^k(c_i) \right\|_2^2 , \qquad (10.7)$$

where $\hat{\psi}_l^k$ is the unit-normalized activation in the channel dimension A_l of the l-th layer of the k-th MC-sampling feature extraction network with shape $H_l \times W_l$.

We denote the total sampling time as K. $D_f(x, c_i)$ can be regarded as an estimated cosine distance between a sample and i-th centroid in the feature space. The centroid c is calculated as the average feature of all labeled training images in the same class. For class i, its centroid c_i is represented by

$$c_i = \left[\frac{1}{N_i} \sum_{j=1}^{N_i} \psi_1(x_j), \ldots, \frac{1}{N_i} \sum_{j=1}^{N_i} \psi_L(x_j) \right], \tag{10.8}$$

where N_i denotes the number of training samples in i-th class and x_j is the j-th training sample. Similar to Eq. 10.7, ψ_l is the activation extracted from the l-th layer of the feature extraction network. L is the total number of layers utilized in the feature distance selection. c_i is retained by one time MC-sampling and fixed during the distance calculation.

Given augmentation ratio r, we first generate $4rN_i$ images for each class i, then select rN_i images according to the two-step selection process described above. Regarding the choice of r, we provide an ablation study in Fig. 10.9, which indicates that the optimal augmentation ratio r for synthetic image pools generated by HistoGAN is $r = 0.5$, as it consistently provides the best performance across different pool sizes by balancing quality and diversity without introducing noise.

10.2.1.3 Synthetic Augmentation via Reinforcement Learning

While the traditional method using handcrafted metrics lacks generality and may not always capture the nuanced quality differences in synthetic images, its effectiveness in selective augmentation is somewhat limited. This limitation necessitates a more adaptive approach. Hence, we further employ a reinforcement learning (RL)-based approach to automate the selective augmentation process for synthetic medical images. By framing the selection mechanism as a model-free, policy-based RL process, we enable an agent to make decisions based on a comprehensive pool of learned features and classification performance gains. This approach ensures the selection of the most representative and high-quality synthetic samples, thereby enhancing the effectiveness of medical image recognition systems.

Background Theoretical Preliminaries About Proximal Policy Optimization (PPO) in RL

Proximal Policy Optimization (PPO) is a leading reinforcement learning algorithm known for its balance of simplicity and performance. It improves policy gradient methods by using a clipped objective function, which prevents large, unstable updates and ensures more stable learning. This makes PPO ideal for tasks like selective augmentation of synthetic medical images, where robust decision-making is crucial.

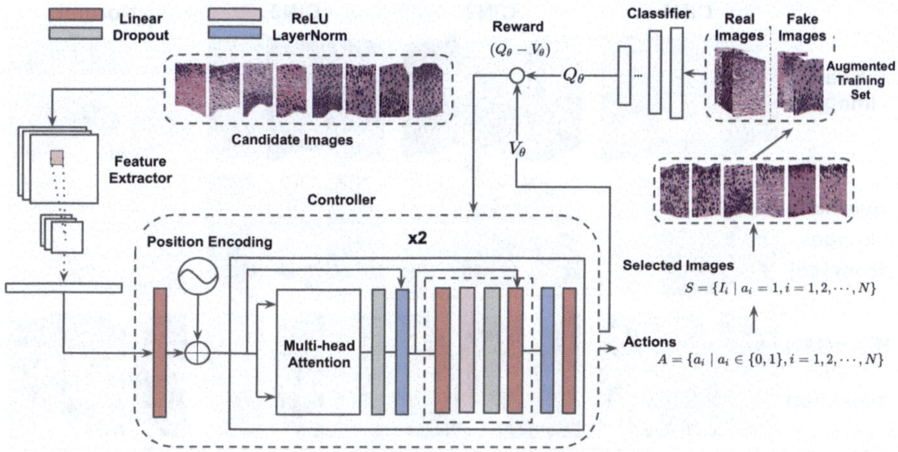

Fig. 10.6 The architecture of our proposed synthetic augmentation framework based on Reinforcement Learning

The detailed architecture of our proposed framework is shown in Fig. 10.6. We generate a candidate pool of synthetic images using HistoGAN. The controller, a transformer model [50], decides whether to select or discard each synthetic sample based on feature vectors from a ResNet34 model [16]. After selection, we train the classifier on the expanded dataset and use the maximum validation accuracy of the last five epochs [62] as the reward to update the policy. To ensure stable updates and avoid fluctuations, we use Proximal Policy Optimization (PPO) [41]. Next, we detail the design of the controller and policy gradient method, the two main components of our framework.

The controller leverages feature dependencies among candidate images, hypothesizing that augmentation order is not independent; later additions must differ from earlier ones to ensure diversity. To address this, we use the self-attention mechanism of the transformer model [50], which avoids recurrent structures by combining feature vectors with positional embeddings as input to the encoder. Skip connections combine features from different abstraction levels. The transformer's decoder, a linear layer, acts as the policy network, outputting binary actions for each input feature vector. Proximal Policy Optimization (PPO) [41] is used for efficient policy gradient optimization, stabilizing training with a clipped probability ratio. At time step t, let A_θ be the advantage function, the objective function is as follows:

$$\mathcal{L}(\theta) = \mathbb{E}\left[\min(\gamma_\theta(t)A_\theta(s_t, a_t), \text{clip}(\gamma_\theta(t), 1-\delta, 1+\delta)A_\theta(s_t, a_t))\right], \tag{10.9}$$

where $A_\theta(s_t, a_t) = Q_\theta(s_t, a_t) - V_\theta(s_t, a_t)$. As part of the transformer output, $V_\theta(s_t, a_t)$ is a learned state-value taken off as the baseline from the q-value to lower

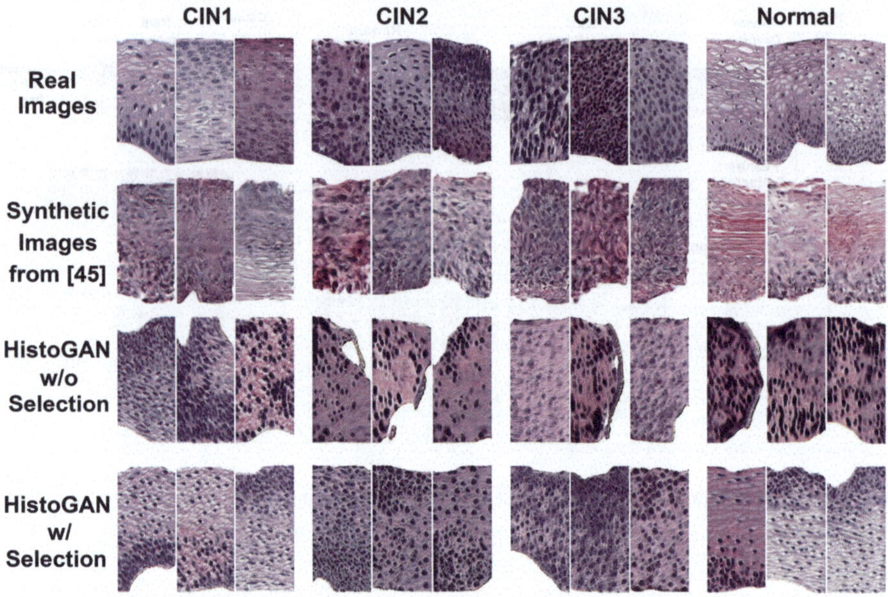

Fig. 10.7 Examples of real images, synthetic images generated from [54], and images generated by our HistoGAN model trained on cervical histopathology dataset before and after selection. Our HistoGAN generates realistic images with clearly better visual quality than those by [54]. Zoom in for a better view

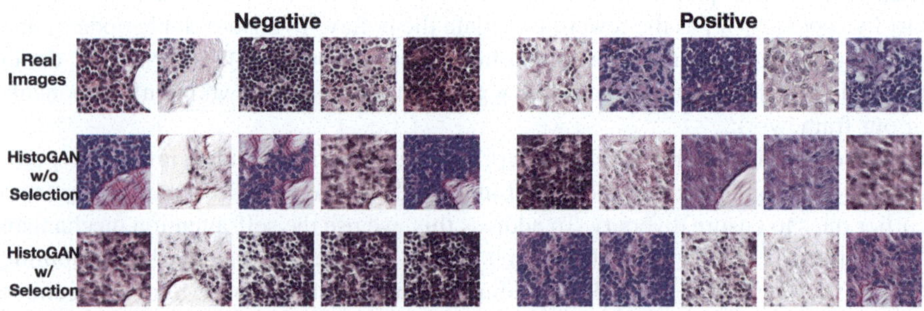

Fig. 10.8 Examples of real and synthetic images generated by HistoGAN trained on 10% of PCam dataset

the variation of the rewards along the training process. π refers to the probability of actions. $Q_\theta(s_t, a_t)$ is the q-value at time t defined as the smooth version of the max validation accuracy among the last 5 epochs in the classification task. The reward is smoothed using the Exponential Moving Average (EMA). The probability ratio $\gamma_\theta(t)$ between previous and current policies is: $\gamma_\theta(t) = \frac{\pi_\theta(a_t|s_t)}{\pi_\theta(a_{t-1}|s_{t-1})}$. If $a_i(t) = 0$, the candidate is discarded; otherwise, it is added to the training set (Figs. 10.7, 10.8, and 10.9).

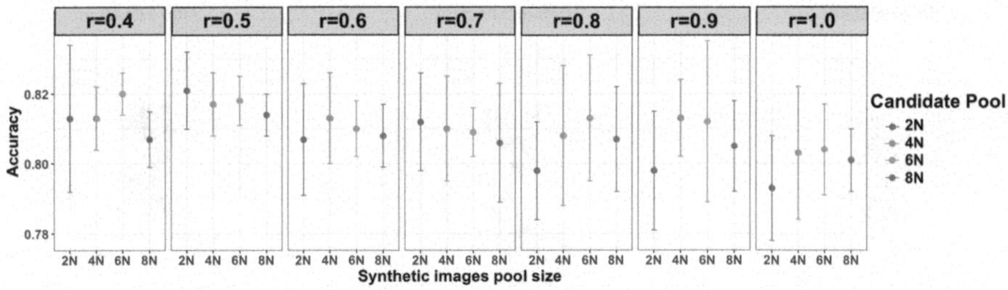

Fig. 10.9 Classification results of the proposed synthetic augmentation with different augmentation ratios on the cervical dataset. *N* in candidate pool sizes indicates the number of images in the original training dataset. For the same candidate pool size, selected images with different ratios are from the same pool. The error bar represents the standard deviation of classification accuracy from 5 multiple runs of each setting, the middle dot refers to the mean of 5 accuracy scores of the aforementioned multiple runs

10.2.2 Experiments and Results

To demonstrate the generality, experiments were conducted on two datasets. The first dataset contains labeled cervical histopathology images collected from a collaborating health sciences center, annotated by the same pathologist, resulting in 1284 Normal, 410 CIN1, 481 CIN2, and 472 CIN3 patches. The dataset is split by patients into training, validation, and testing sets (7:1:2 ratio), with image class ratios maintained across sets. The second dataset is the PatchCamelyon (PCam) benchmark, which includes 327,680 color patches of lymph node sections, each sized 96 × 96 pixels and annotated with binary labels for metastatic tissue. The dataset is split into 75% training, 12.5% validation, and 12.5% testing sets. Using only 10% of the training set (32,768 patches), we trained our HistoGAN model and a baseline classifier, then evaluated the models on the full test set.

To validate the quality of images generated by HistoGAN and the effectiveness of synthetic augmentation, two expert pathologists assessed 100 synthetic cervical histopathology images, split evenly between pre- and post-selection. Organized into 10 groups, the pathologists, blinded to the subgroup identities, consistently favored post-selection images in 7 out of 10 groups, with 2 ties and only 1 pre-selection preference, demonstrating the method's efficacy. They highlighted realistic features such as correct orientation and cell polarity, while noting areas for improvement like smudged chromatin. Despite some unrealistic aspects, most images were deemed diagnostically valuable, underscoring the potential of our selective augmentation approach (Figs. 10.10 and 10.11, Tables 10.1 and 10.2).

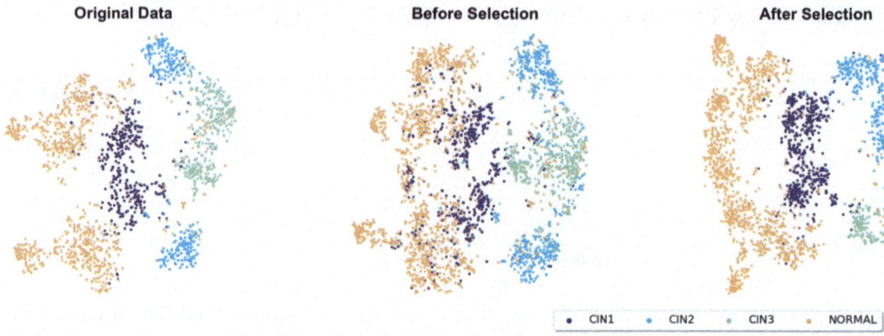

Fig. 10.10 t-SNE of the original and augmented cervical histopathology training set before and after image selection. The augmented training data after selection clearly have more distinguishable features than the ones without selection

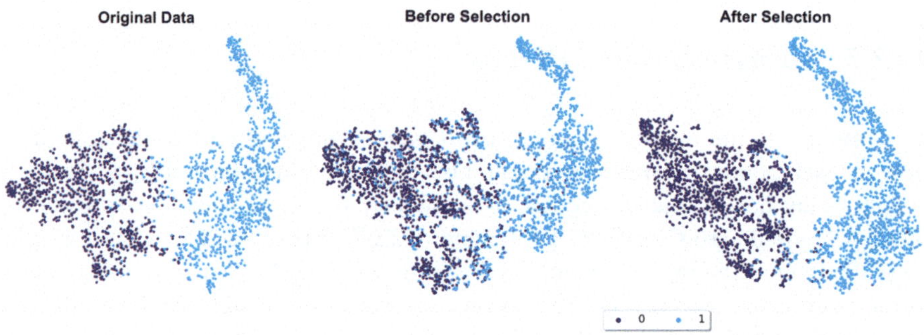

Fig. 10.11 t-SNE of the original and augmented PCam histopathology training set before and after image selection. While data augmentation without image selection increases the number of training samples, the original data distribution is distorted. After image selection, the original data distribution is recovered along with a greater number of data points

> **! Attention**
>
> While HistoGAN generates high-fidelity images, further improvements in realism and diversity are needed (smudged chromatin, missing nuclear details, and incorrect keratin texture).

10.2.3 Summary

This section introduces HistoGAN, a conditional GAN model for realistic histopathology image synthesis, and a synthetic augmentation method, using handcrafted criteria and reinforcement learning, which expands training datasets

Table 10.1 Classification results of baseline and augmentation models on the cervical dataset. We reimplemented [54] and a metric learning model with triplet loss [40] using the same pool of synthetic images generated by HistoGAN for fair comparison

	Accuracy ↑	AUC ↑	Sensitivity ↑	Specificity ↑
Baseline model	0.754 ± 0.012	0.836 ± 0.008	0.589 ± 0.017	0.892 ± 0.005
+ Traditional augmentation	0.766 ± 0.013	0.844 ± 0.009	0.623 ± 0.029	0.891 ± 0.006
+ GAN augmentation	0.787 ± 0.005	0.858 ± 0.003	0.690 ± 0.014	0.909 ± 0.003
+ Metric learning (Triplet loss)	0.798 ± 0.016	0.865 ± 0.010	0.678 ± 0.048	0.909 ± 0.013
+ Synthetic augmentation (Selective via centroid distance)*	0.808 ± 0.005	0.872 ± 0.004	0.639 ± 0.015	0.912 ± 0.006
+ Synthetic augmentation (Selective via transformer-PPO, Ours)	**0.835 ± 0.007**	**0.890 ± 0.005**	**0.747 ± 0.013**	**0.936 ± 0.003**

Table 10.2 Classification results of baseline and augmentation models on the PCam dataset

	Accuracy ↑	AUC ↑	Sensitivity ↑	Specificity ↑
Baseline model [16]	0.853 ± 0.003	0.902 ± 0.002	0.815 ± 0.008	0.877 ± 0.009
+ Traditional augmentation	0.860 ± 0.005	0.907 ± 0.003	0.823 ± 0.015	0.885 ± 0.017
+ GAN augmentation	0.859 ± 0.001	0.906 ± 0.001	0.822 ± 0.014	0.884 ± 0.011
+ Metric learning (Triplet loss) [40]	0.864 ± 0.004	0.910 ± 0.003	0.830 ± 0.012	0.887 ± 0.008
+ Synthetic augmentation (Selective via centroid distance) [54]*	0.868 ± 0.002	0.912 ± 0.002	0.835 ± 0.010	0.890 ± 0.006
+ Synthetic augmentation (Selective via Transformer-PPO, Ours)	**0.876 ± 0.001**	**0.917 ± 0.001**	**0.846 ± 0.010**	**0.895 ± 0.005**

without distorting the original distribution, significantly improving automated image recognition with minimal annotation. Our method complements existing data augmentation techniques and is applicable to other histopathology tasks with limited annotated data.

10.3 Synthetic Augmentation with HistoDiffusion

> **Highlights**
>
> **HistoDiffusion:** a synthetic augmentation method that pre-trains latent diffusion model on large unlabeled datasets and fine-tunes on small labeled datasets.

The transition from GANs to diffusion models in synthetic augmentation is motivated by the inherent limitations of GANs and the distinct advantages offered by diffusion models. GANs necessitate a substantial amount of labeled data to produce high-quality images and are prone to training instability. Conversely, diffusion models exhibit superior training stability and can be effectively pre-trained on extensive unlabeled datasets, enabling them to learn diverse image features without relying heavily on annotations. This capability significantly reduces the dependency on annotated data while still allowing for the generation of realistic, high-quality images. Therefore, diffusion models present a more practical and efficient approach for medical image synthesis and augmentation (Fig. 10.12).

> **Background Theoretical Preliminaries About Latent Diffusion Model (LDM)**
>
> Latent Diffusion Models (LDMs) enhance image synthesis by operating in a lower-dimensional latent space, thereby improving computational efficiency and training stability compared to pixel-space models. Utilizing an encoder-decoder architecture, it maps images into this latent space, where Gaussian noise is systematically added and reversed to generate high-quality images. Pre-training on extensive unlabeled datasets enables LDMs to capture a wide range of features, while subsequent fine-tuning on smaller labeled datasets minimizes the need for extensive annotations.

10.3.1 Methodology

10.3.1.1 HistoDiffusion Model Architecture

Our proposed HistoDiffusion is built on Latent Diffusion Models (LDM) [38], which requires fewer computational resources without degradation in performance, compared to prior works [7, 23, 42]. LDM first trains a latent autoencoder (LAE) [24] to encode images as lower-dimensional latent representations and then learns a diffusion model (DM) for image synthesis by modeling the latent space of the trained LAE. Particularly, the encoder $\mathcal{E}$ of the LAE encodes the input image

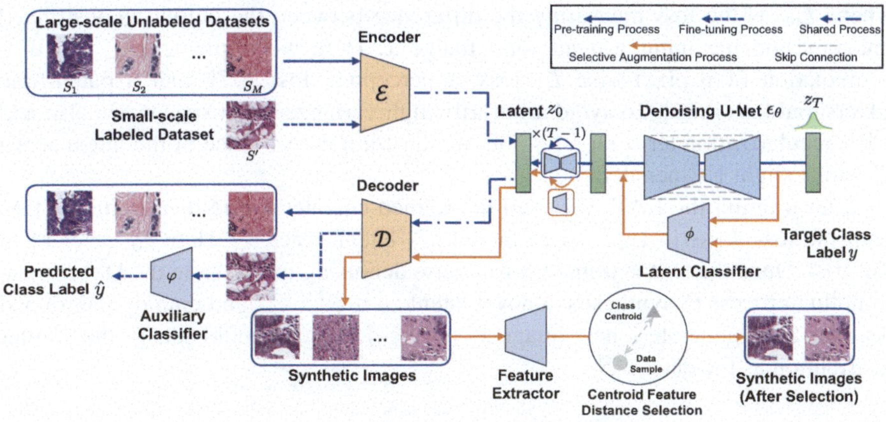

Fig. 10.12 The architecture of our proposed HistoDiffusion, which consists of a pre-training process (blue solid lines), a fine-tuning process (blue dashed lines), and a synthetic augmentation process (orange lines). During pre-training, a latent autoencoder (LAE) and a diffusion model (DM) are trained on large-scale unlabeled datasets for unconditional image synthesis. HistoDiffusion is then fine-tuned on a small-scale dataset for conditional image synthesis under the guidance of a trained latent classifier. During synthetic augmentation, given a target class label, the synthetic images generated by the fine-tuned model are selected and added to the training set based on their distances to the class centroids in the feature space

$x \in \mathbb{R}^{H\times W\times 3}$ into a latent representation $z = \mathcal{E}(x) \in \mathbb{R}^{h\times w\times c}$ in a lower-dimensional latent space $\mathcal{Z}$. Here H and W are the height and width of image x, and h, w, and c are the height, width, and channel of latent z, respectively. The latent z is then passed into the decoder $\mathcal{D}$ to reconstruct the image $\hat{x} = \mathcal{D}(z)$. Through this process, the compositional features from the image space $\mathcal{X}$ can be extracted to form the latent space $\mathcal{Z}$, and we then model the distribution of $\mathcal{Z}$ by learning a DM. For the DM in LDM, both the forward and reverse sampling processes are performed in the latent space $\mathcal{Z}$ instead of the original image space $\mathcal{X}$.

10.3.1.2 Unconditional Large-Scale Pre-training

To ensure the latent space $\mathcal{Z}$ can cover features of various data types, we first pre-train our proposed HistoDiffusion on large-scale unlabeled datasets. Specifically, we gather unlabeled images from M different sources to construct a large-scale set of datasets $\mathcal{S} = \{S_1, S_2, \ldots, S_M\}$. We then train an LAE using the data from $\mathcal{S}$ with the following self-reconstruction loss to learn a powerful latent space $\mathcal{Z}$ that can describe diverse features:

$$L_{\mathrm{LAE}} = \mathcal{L}_{\mathrm{rec}}(\hat{x}, x) + \lambda_{\mathrm{KL}} D_{\mathrm{KL}}(q(z)||\mathcal{N}(\mathbf{0}, \mathbf{I})) \ , \tag{10.10}$$

where $\mathcal{L}_{\text{rec}}$ is the loss measuring the difference between the output reconstructed image $\hat{x}$ and the input ground truth image x. Here we implement $\mathcal{L}_{\text{rec}}$ with a combination of a pixel-wise L_1 loss, a perceptual loss [57], and a patch-base adversarial loss [8, 9]. To avoid arbitrarily high-variance latent spaces, we also add a KL regularization term D_{KL} [24, 38] to constrain the variance of the latent space $\mathcal{Z}$ with a slight KL-penalty.

After training the LAE, we fixed the trained encoder $\mathcal{E}$ and then trained a DM with the loss L_{DM} in Eq. 10.4 to model $\mathcal{E}$'s latent space $\mathcal{Z}$. Here $z_0 = \mathcal{E}(x)$ in Eq. 10.4. Once the DM is trained, we can use denoising model ϵ_θ in the DM reverse sampling process to synthesize a novel latent $\tilde{z}_0 \in \mathbb{R}^{h \times w \times c}$ and employ the trained decoder $\mathcal{D}$ to generate a new image $\tilde{x} = \mathcal{D}(\tilde{z}_0)$, which should satisfy the similar distribution as the data in $\mathcal{S}$.

10.3.1.3 Conditional Small-Scale Fine-Tuning

Using the LAE and DM pretrained on $\mathcal{S}$, we can only generate the new image $\tilde{x}$ following the similar distribution in $\mathcal{S}$. To generalize our HistoDiffusion to the small-scale labeled dataset S' collected from a different source (i.e., $S' \not\subset \mathcal{S}$), we further fine-tune HistoDiffusion using the labeled data from S'. Let y be the label of image x in S'. To minimize the training cost, we fix both the trained encoder $\mathcal{E}$ and trained DM model ϵ_θ to keep latent space $\mathcal{Z}$ unchanged. Then we only fine-tune the decoder $\mathcal{D}$ using labeled data (x, y) from S' with the following loss function:

$$L_{\mathcal{D}} = \mathcal{L}_{\text{rec}}(\hat{x}, x) + \lambda_{\text{CE}} \mathcal{L}_{\text{CE}}(\varphi(\hat{x}), y) \ , \tag{10.11}$$

where $\mathcal{L}_{\text{rec}}(\hat{x}, x)$ is the self-reconstruction loss between the output reconstructed image $\hat{x} = \mathcal{D}(\mathcal{E}(x))$ and the input ground truth image x. To enhance the correlation between the decoder output $\hat{x}$ and label y, we also add an auxiliary image classifier φ trained with (x, y) on the top of $\mathcal{D}$ and impose the cross-entropy classification loss $\mathcal{L}_{\text{CE}}$ when fine-tuning $\mathcal{D}$. λ_{CE} is the balancing parameter. We annotate this fine-tuned decoder as $\mathcal{D}'$ for differentiation.

10.3.1.4 Classifier-Guided Conditional Synthesis

To enable conditional image generation with our HistoDiffusion, we further apply the classifier-guided diffusion sampling proposed in [7, 43, 44, 47] using the labeled data (x, y) from small-scale labeled dataset S'. We first utilize the trained encoder $\mathcal{E}$ to encode the data x from S' as latent z_0. Then we train a time-dependent latent classifier ϕ with paired (z_t, y) using the following loss function:

$$L_\phi = \mathcal{L}_{\text{CE}}(\phi(z_t), y) \ , \tag{10.12}$$

where $z_t \sim q(z_t|z_0)$ is the noisy version of z_0 at the time step t during the DM forward process, and $\mathcal{L}_{\mathrm{CE}}$ is the cross-entropy classification loss. Based on the trained unconditional diffusion model ϵ_θ, and a classifier ϕ trained on noisy input z_t, we enable conditional diffusion sampling by perturbing the reverse-process mean with the gradient of the log probability $p_\phi(y|z_t)$ of a target class y predicted by the classifier ϕ as follows:

$$\hat{\mu}_\theta(z_t|y) = \mu_\theta(z_t) + g \cdot \Sigma_\theta(z_t)\nabla_{z_t} \log p_\phi(y|z_t) \ , \tag{10.13}$$

where g is the guidance scale. Then the DM reverse process in HistoDiffusion can finally generate a novel latent $\tilde{z}_0$ satisfying the class condition y through a Markov chain starting with a standard Gaussian noise $z_T \sim \mathcal{N}(\mathbf{0}, \mathbf{I})$ using $p_{\theta,\phi}(z_{t-1}|z_t, y)$ defined as follows:

$$p_{\theta,\phi}(z_{t-1}|z_t, y) = \mathcal{N}(z_{t-1}; \hat{\mu}_\theta(z_t|y), \Sigma_\theta(z_t)) \ . \tag{10.14}$$

The final image $\tilde{x}$ of class y can be generated by applying the fine-tuned decoder $\mathcal{D}'$, i.e., $\tilde{x} = \mathcal{D}'(\tilde{z}_0)$.

10.3.1.5 Synthetic Augmentation

To further improve the efficacy of synthetic augmentation, we follow [55] to selectively add synthetic images to the original labeled training data based on centroid feature distance. The augmentation ratio is defined as the ratio between the selected synthetic images and the original training images. More results are demonstrated later in Table 10.3.

10.3.2 Experiments and Results

We employ three public datasets of histopathology images during the large-scale pre-training procedure. The first one is the H&E breast cancer dataset [4], containing 312,320 patches extracted from the hematoxylin & eosin (H&E) stained human breast cancer tissue micro-array (TMA) images [29]. Each patch has a resolution of 224 × 224. The second dataset is PanNuke [12], a pan-cancer histology dataset for nuclei instance segmentation and classification. The PanNuke dataset includes 7901 patches of 19 types of H&E stained tissues obtained from multiple data sources, and each patch has a unified size of 256 × 256 pixels. The third dataset is TCGA-BRCA-A2/E2 [49], a subset derived from the TCGA-BRCA breast cancer histology dataset [33]. The subset consists of 482,958 patches with a resolution of 256 × 256. Overall, there are 803,179 patches used for pre-training. As for fine-tuning and evaluation, we employ the NCT-CRC-HE-100K dataset that contains 100,000 patches from H&E stained histological images of human colorectal cancer (CRC)

Table 10.3 Quantitative comparison results of synthetic image quality and augmented classification. "Random" refers to directly augmenting the training dataset with synthesized images without any image selections while "selective" indicates applying selective module [55] to filter out low-quality images. The number ($X\%$) suggests that the number of the synthesized images is $X\%$ of the original training set

	FID ↓	Accuracy ↑	F1 Score ↑	Sensitivity ↑	Specificity ↑
Baseline (5% real images)	/	0.855	0.850	0.855	0.983
=—=—=—=—=—= StyleGAN2 [22]					
+ random 50%	5.714	0.860	0.856	0.860	0.980
+ selective [55] 50%	5.088	0.868	0.861	0.867	0.978
100%	5.927	0.879	0.876	0.879	0.982
200%	7.550	0.895	0.888	0.895	0.983
300%	10.643	0.898	0.896	0.898	0.987
=—=—=—=—=—= HistoDiffusion (Ours)					
+ random 50%	4.921	0.870	0.869	0.870	0.982
+ selective [55] 50%	4.544	0.891	0.888	0.891	0.983
100%	**3.874**	0.903	0.902	0.903	0.991
200%	4.583	**0.919**	**0.916**	**0.919**	**0.992**
300%	8.326	0.910	0.912	0.910	0.988

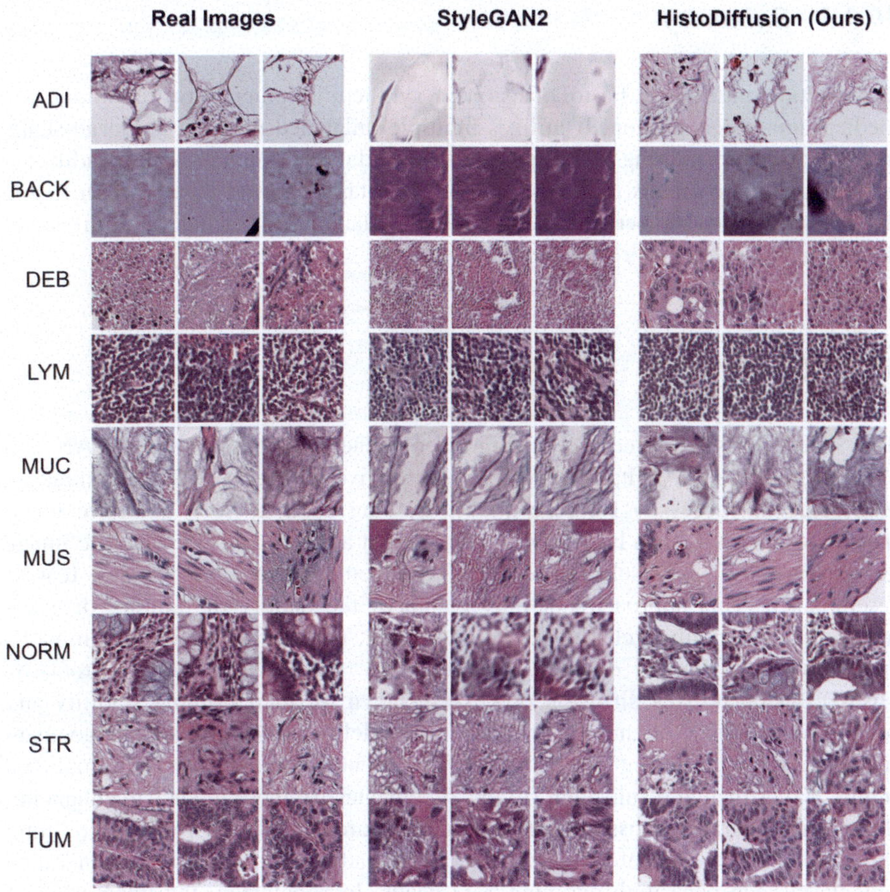

Fig. 10.13 Comparison of real images from training subset, synthesized images generated by StyleGAN2 [22] and our proposed HistoDiffusion (zoom in for clear observation). Qualitatively, our synthesized results contain more realistic and diagnosable patterns than results synthesized from StyleGAN2

and normal tissue. The patches have been divided into 9 classes: Adipose (ADI), background (BACK), debris (DEB), lymphocytes (LYM), mucus (MUC), smooth muscle (MUS), normal colon mucosa (NORM), cancer-associated stroma (STR), colorectal adenocarcinoma epithelium (TUM). The resolution of each patch is 224×224 (Fig. 10.13).

10.3.3 Summary

This section introduces HistoDiffusion, a synthetic augmentation technique for medical image recognition. It utilizes multiple unlabeled datasets for large-scale, unconditional pre-training and employs a labeled dataset for small-scale conditional fine-tuning. Experiments on a histopathology dataset showed that HistoDiffusion improves classification performance with limited labels and can handle future small datasets using the same pre-trained model.

10.4 Conclusion

This chapter has explored the integration of generative models, HistoGAN and HistoDiffusion, into digital pathology for effective synthetic data augmentation, addressing the necessity for high-quality training data. In Sect. 10.2, we introduced HistoGAN, which has marked a significant advancement in synthetic image generation, employing selective criteria based on label congruence and feature resemblance. This approach not only enhances the quality of training data but also mitigates common challenges of overfitting, thereby improving the model's performance on limited datasets. In Sect. 10.3, transitioning from HistoGAN, HistoDiffusion utilizes diffusion processes known for their training stability and reduced dependency on annotated data. This model is particularly advantageous in medical imaging, offering efficient synthesis of realistic images from minimal data inputs. Experimental results confirm the effectiveness of these models in enhancing diagnostic accuracy across various datasets. Future efforts will focus on refining these models with clinical insights and exploring advanced foundational generative models to keep pace with evolving data needs. In conclusion, the integration of HistoGAN and HistoDiffusion into the workflow of digital pathology represents a transformative shift toward more reliable, accessible, and efficient diagnostic practices. By harnessing the power of generative models, we can significantly expand the capabilities of pathological image analysis, ultimately leading to better patient outcomes and more streamlined medical processes.

References

1. Antoniou A, Storkey A, Edwards H (2017) Data augmentation generative adversarial networks. Preprint. arXiv:171104340
2. Bowles C, Chen L, Guerrero R, Bentley P, Gunn R, Hammers A, Dickie DA, Hernández MV, Wardlaw J, Rueckert D (2018) Gan augmentation: Augmenting training data using generative adversarial networks. Preprint. arXiv:181010863

3. Brock A, Donahue J, Simonyan K (2018) Large scale GAN training for high fidelity natural image synthesis. Preprint. arXiv:180911096
4. Claudio Quiros A, Murray-Smith R, Yuan K (2021) Pathologygan: Learning deep representations of cancer tissue. MELBA 2021(4):1–48
5. Cubuk ED, Zoph B, Mane D, Vasudevan V, Le QV (2019) Autoaugment: Learning augmentation strategies from data. In: Proceedings of the IEEE conference on computer vision and pattern recognition, pp 113–123
6. De Vries H, Strub F, Mary J, Larochelle H, Pietquin O, Courville AC (2017) Modulating early visual processing by language. In: Advances in neural information processing systems, pp 6594–6604
7. Dhariwal P, Nichol A (2021) Diffusion models beat GANs on image synthesis. In: NeurIPS 34, pp 8780–8794
8. Dosovitskiy A, Brox T (2016) Generating images with perceptual similarity metrics based on deep networks. In: NeurIPS 29
9. Esser P, Rombach R, Ommer B (2021) Taming transformers for high-resolution image synthesis. In: CVPR, pp 12873–12883
10. Frid-Adar M, Diamant I, Klang E, Amitai M, Goldberger J, Greenspan H (2018) GAN-based synthetic medical image augmentation for increased CNN performance in liver lesion classification. Neurocomputing 321:321–331
11. Gal Y, Ghahramani Z (2016) Dropout as a bayesian approximation: Representing model uncertainty in deep learning. In: International conference on machine learning, pp 1050–1059
12. Gamper J, Alemi Koohbanani N, Benet K, Khuram A, Rajpoot N (2019) Pannuke: an open pan-cancer histology dataset for nuclei instance segmentation and classification. In: ECDP. Springer, pp 11–19
13. Goodfellow I, Pouget-Abadie J, Mirza M, Xu B, Warde-Farley D, Ozair S, Courville A, Bengio Y (2014) Generative adversarial nets. In: NeurIPS, pp 2672–2680
14. Gupta A, Venkatesh S, Chopra S, Ledig C (2019) Generative image translation for data augmentation of bone lesion pathology. In: International conference on medical imaging with deep learning, pp 225–235
15. Gurcan MN, Boucheron LE, Can A, Madabhushi A, Rajpoot NM, Yener B (2009) Histopathological image analysis: A review. IEEE Rev Biomed Eng 2:147–171
16. He K, Zhang X, Ren S, Sun J (2016) Deep residual learning for image recognition. In: Proceedings of the IEEE conference on computer vision and pattern recognition, pp 770–778
17. Ho D, Liang E, Chen X, Stoica I, Abbeel P (2019) Population based augmentation: Efficient learning of augmentation policy schedules. In: International conference on machine learning, pp 2731–2741
18. Ho J, Jain A, Abbeel P (2020) Denoising diffusion probabilistic models. In: NeurIPS 33, pp 6840–6851
19. Hou L, Samaras D, Kurc TM, Gao Y, Davis JE, Saltz JH (2016) Patch-based convolutional neural network for whole slide tissue image classification. In: Proceedings of the IEEE conference on computer vision and pattern recognition, pp 2424–2433
20. Irshad H, Veillard A, Roux L, Racoceanu D (2013) Methods for nuclei detection, segmentation, and classification in digital histopathology: a review–current status and future potential. IEEE Rev Biomed Eng 7:97–114
21. Karras T, Aila T, Laine S, Lehtinen J (2017) Progressive growing of GANs for improved quality, stability, and variation. Preprint. arXiv:171010196
22. Karras T, Laine S, Aittala M, Hellsten J, Lehtinen J, Aila T (2020) Analyzing and improving the image quality of stylegan. In: CVPR, pp 8110–8119
23. Ker J, Wang L, Rao J, Lim T (2017) Deep learning applications in medical image analysis. IEEE Access 6:9375–9389
24. Kingma DP (2013) Auto-encoding variational bayes. arXiv preprint arXiv:1312.6114
25. Li J, Liang X, Wei Y, Xu T, Feng J, Yan S (2017) Perceptual generative adversarial networks for small object detection. In: Proceedings of the IEEE conference on computer vision and pattern recognition, pp 1222–1230

26. MacKay DJ (1992) A practical bayesian framework for backpropagation networks. Neural Comput 4(3):448–472
27. Mahapatra D, Bozorgtabar B, Thiran JP, Reyes M (2018) Efficient active learning for image classification and segmentation using a sample selection and conditional generative adversarial network. In: International conference on medical image computing and computer-assisted intervention. Springer, pp 580–588
28. Mariani G, Scheidegger F, Istrate R, Bekas C, Malossi C (2018) Bagan: Data augmentation with balancing GAN. Preprint. arXiv:180309655
29. Marinelli RJ, Montgomery K, Liu CL, Shah NH, Prapong W, Nitzberg M, Zachariah ZK, Sherlock GJ, Natkunam Y, West RB, et al (2007) The Stanford tissue microarray database. Nucleic Acids Res 36(suppl_1):D871–D877
30. Mirza M, Osindero S (2014) Conditional generative adversarial nets. Preprint. arXiv:14111784
31. Miyato T, Kataoka T, Koyama M, Yoshida Y (2018) Spectral normalization for generative adversarial networks. Preprint. arXiv:180205957
32. Moghadam PA, Van Dalen S, Martin KC, Lennerz J, Yip S, Farahani H, Bashashati A (2023) A morphology focused diffusion probabilistic model for synthesis of histopathology images. In: WACV, pp 2000–2009
33. Network TCGA (2012) Comprehensive molecular portraits of human breast tumours. Nature 490(7418):61–70
34. Nichol AQ, Dhariwal P (2022) GLIDE: Towards Photorealistic Image Generation and Editing with Text-Guided Diffusion Models. International Conference on Machine Learning. PMLR, pp 16784–16804
35. Nichol AQ, Dhariwal P, Ramesh A, Shyam P, Mishkin P, McGrew B, Sutskever I, Chen M (2022) Glide: Towards photorealistic image generation and editing with text-guided diffusion models. In: International conference on machine learning. PMLR, pp 16784–16804
36. Pinaya WH, Tudosiu PD, Dafflon J, Da Costa PF, Fernandez V, Nachev P, Ourselin S, Cardoso MJ (2022) Brain imaging generation with latent diffusion models. In: DGM4MICCAI. Springer, pp 117–126
37. Ratner AJ, Ehrenberg H, Hussain Z, Dunnmon J, Ré C (2017) Learning to compose domain-specific transformations for data augmentation. In: Advances in neural information processing systems, pp 3236–3246
38. Rombach R, Blattmann A, Lorenz D, Esser P, Ommer B (2022) High-resolution image synthesis with latent diffusion models. In: CVPR, pp 10684–10695
39. Ronneberger O, Fischer P, Brox T (2015) U-net: Convolutional networks for biomedical image segmentation. In: MICCAI. Springer, pp 234–241
40. Schroff F, Kalenichenko D, Philbin J (2015) Facenet: A unified embedding for face recognition and clustering. In: Proceedings of the IEEE conference on computer vision and pattern recognition, pp 815–823
41. Schulman J, Wolski F, Dhariwal P, Radford A, Klimov O (2017) Proximal policy optimization algorithms. Preprint. arXiv:170706347
42. Shen D, Wu G, Suk HI (2017) Deep learning in medical image analysis. Annu Rev Biomed Eng 19:221–248
43. Shi C, Ni H, Li K, Han S, Liang M, Min MR (2023) Exploring compositional visual generation with latent classifier guidance. In: CVPR, pp 853–862
44. Sohl-Dickstein J, Weiss E, Maheswaranathan N, Ganguli S (2015) Deep unsupervised learning using nonequilibrium thermodynamics. In: ICML, pp 2256–2265
45. Song Y, Ermon S (2019) Generative modeling by estimating gradients of the data distribution. In: NeurIPS 32
46. Song J, Meng C, Ermon S (2020) Denoising diffusion implicit models. ArXiv abs/2010.02502. https://api.semanticscholar.org/CorpusID:222140788
47. Song Y, Sohl-Dickstein J, Kingma DP, Kumar A, Ermon S, Poole B (2021) Score-based generative modeling through stochastic differential equations. In: International conference on learning representations. https://openreview.net/forum?id=PxTIG12RRHS

48. Tomita N, Abdollahi B, Wei J, Ren B, Suriawinata A, Hassanpour S (2019) Attention-based deep neural networks for detection of cancerous and precancerous esophagus tissue on histopathological slides. JAMA Netw Open 2(11):e1914645
49. van Treeck M, Cifci D, Laleh NG, Saldanha OL, Loeffler CM, Hewitt KJ, Muti HS, Echle A, Seibel T, Seraphin TP, et al (2021) DeepMed: a unified, modular pipeline for end-to-end deep learning in computational pathology. BioRxiv: 2021–12. Cold Spring Harbor Laboratory
50. Vaswani A, Shazeer N, Parmar N, Uszkoreit J, Jones L, Gomez AN, Kaiser Ł, Polosukhin I (2017) Attention is all you need. In: Advances in neural information processing systems, pp 5998–6008
51. Wang J, Perez L (2017) The effectiveness of data augmentation in image classification using deep learning. Convolutional Neural Netw Vis Recogn 11:1
52. Xu Y, Jia Z, Wang LB, Ai Y, Zhang F, Lai M, Eric I, Chang C (2017) Large scale tissue histopathology image classification, segmentation, and visualization via deep convolutional activation features. BMC Bioinf 18(1):281
53. Xue Y, Xu T, Zhang H, Long LR, Huang X (2018) Segan: Adversarial network with multi-scale L1 loss for medical image segmentation. Neuroinformatics 16(3–4):383–392
54. Xue Y, Zhou Q, Ye J, Long LR, Antani S, Cornwell C, Xue Z, Huang X (2019) Synthetic augmentation and feature-based filtering for improved cervical histopathology image classification. In: International conference on medical image computing and computer-assisted intervention. Springer, pp 387–396
55. Xue Y, Ye J, Zhou Q, Long LR, Antani S, Xue Z, Cornwell C, Zaino R, Cheng KC, Huang X (2021) Selective synthetic augmentation with histoGAN for improved histopathology image classification. Med Image Anal 67:101816
56. Zhang H, Xu T, Li H, Zhang S, Wang X, Huang X, Metaxas DN (2018) Stackgan++: Realistic image synthesis with stacked generative adversarial networks. IEEE Trans Pattern Anal Mach Intell 41(8):1947–1962
57. Zhang R, Isola P, Efros AA, Shechtman E, Wang O (2018) The unreasonable effectiveness of deep features as a perceptual metric. In: CVPR, pp 586–595
58. Zhang H, Goodfellow I, Metaxas D, Odena A (2019) Self-attention generative adversarial networks. In: International conference on machine learning, pp 7354–7363
59. Zhao H, Li H, Maurer-Stroh S, Cheng L (2018) Synthesizing retinal and neuronal images with generative adversarial nets. Med Image Anal 49:14–26
60. Zhao A, Balakrishnan G, Durand F, Guttag JV, Dalca AV (2019) Data augmentation using learned transformations for one-shot medical image segmentation. In: Proceedings of the IEEE conference on computer vision and pattern recognition, pp 8543–8553
61. Zhu JY, Park T, Isola P, Efros AA (2017) Unpaired image-to-image translation using cycle-consistent adversarial networks. In: Proceedings of the IEEE international conference on computer vision, pp 2223–2232
62. Zoph B, Le QV (2016) Neural architecture search with reinforcement learning. Preprint. arXiv:161101578

Chapter 11
Enhancing PET with Image Generation Techniques: Generating Standard-Dose PET from Low-Dose PET

Caiwen Jiang, Zixin Tang, Zhiming Cui, and Dinggang Shen

Abstract Positron Emission Tomography (PET) is an advanced imaging technique that vividly reflects human physiological activity and plays an indispensable role in diagnosing Alzheimer's disease (AD) and cancer. However, PET imaging involves injecting radionuclides into the body, inevitably leading to radiation exposure. Reducing the dose of radionuclide used during imaging is crucial for safer and more cost-effective PET imaging. However, reducing the dose in PET acquisition can degrade image quality, potentially failing to meet clinical requirements. To maintain high-quality PET imaging while reducing the radionuclide dose, besides developing imaging systems to improve sensitivity, another effective approach is to generate Standard-dose PET (SPET) from Low-dose PET (LPET) by generative technologies. In this work, we propose a novel and effective approach to estimate high-quality SPET images from LPET images. Specifically, We employ a semi-supervised training framework to fully utilize both the rare paired and the abundant unpaired LPET and SPET images. Additionally, using this framework as a foundation, we introduce a Region-adaptive Normalization (RN) and implement a structural consistency constraint to address task-specific challenges. RN customizes normalization procedures for distinct regions within each PET image, mitigating adverse effects stemming from significant intensity variations across different areas. Simultaneously, the structural consistency constraint ensures the preservation of structural details throughout the process of generating SPET images from LPET images. With extensive experimental validation, our approach can achieve superior

C. Jiang (✉) · Z. Tang · Z. Cui
School of Biomedical Engineering & State Key Laboratory of Advanced Medical Materials and Devices, ShanghaiTech University, Shanghai, China
e-mail: jiangcw@shanghaitech.edu.cn

D. Shen
School of Biomedical Engineering & State Key Laboratory of Advanced Medical Materials and Devices, ShanghaiTech University, Shanghai, China

Shanghai Clinical Research and Trial Center, Shanghai, China

Shanghai United Imaging Intelligence Co., Ltd., Shanghai, China
e-mail: dgshen@shanghaitech.edu.cn

L. Zhang et al. (eds.), *Generative Machine Learning Models in Medical Image Computing*, https://doi.org/10.1007/978-3-031-80965-1_11

performance over state-of-the-art methods, and shows stronger generalizability to the dose changes of PET imaging

11.1 Introduction

Positron Emission Tomography (PET) is an advanced nuclear imaging technology that has an essential role in early disease diagnosis and intervention in clinics [6, 24, 43]. By injecting radionuclides into the body and capturing signals from their decay, PET can visualize the metabolic and biochemical processes in the body by providing the radionuclides' distribution information [8, 26]. This unique feature allows PET to surpass other imaging methods, playing an indispensable role in the diagnosis and treatment of many diseases, particularly those affecting the body's physiological functions such as Alzheimer's Disease (AD) and cancer [10, 15, 31].

Nonetheless, given that those radionuclides are radioactive, which inevitably poses a risk of radiation exposure to patients [5, 28]. In addition, due to limitations in signal receiver sensitivity and noise interference, the dose of radionuclides must meet a certain threshold to produce PET images with sufficient quality for clinical diagnosis [1, 21]. Despite applying the As Low As Reasonably Achievable (ALARA) [32] principle in clinical imaging to minimize radiation exposure, PET imaging may still be deemed unacceptable for certain populations, such as pediatric subjects and pregnant women [4, 22]. To mitigate the radiation risks associated with PET imaging, designing advanced generation algorithms to enhance PET image quality (e.g., generating standard-dose PET (SPET) from low-dose PET (LPET)) is a promising alternative.

Generating SPET from LPET poses several challenges. Firstly, paired LPET and SPET data for training models are rare. In most clinical scenarios, paired PET data are not collected, and only a small amount of paired data is acquired in list mode by PET scanners [29] for research purposes. Secondly, There are dramatic variations in intensity distribution across different regions. As shown in Fig. 11.1, it is difficult to preserve intensity contrast among regions in generating SPET images from LPET images. Finally, PET is not a structural imaging technique and often lacks structural details, especially in LPET images with significant noise. This poses a challenge in accurately generating SPET images with sufficient structural details.

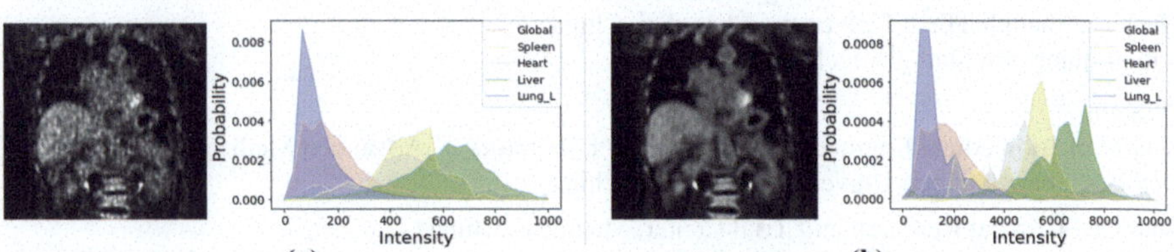

Fig. 11.1 (**a**) LPET and (**b**) SPET images, and their corresponding distributions of intensity across different regions

To address these challenges, we introduce a semi-supervised deep learning framework to accommodate training with those unpaired PET images. This framework incorporates a Region-adaptive Normalization (RN) technique and a structural consistency constraint, both aimed at enhancing the fidelity of generated SPET images by infusing them with more realistic intensity contrast and intricate structural details. Specifically, RN integrates semantic information into the normalization process, enabling tailored modulation of activations across different regions. Furthermore, the structural consistency constraint promotes alignment between predicted SPET features and real SPET images at various levels (e.g., vertex, line), ensuring the preservation of structural details during SPET generation. During training, unpaired LPET and SPET images are initially utilized to independently train corresponding network components in a self-supervised manner. Subsequently, a limited set of paired LPET and SPET images is employed to fine-tune the LPET-to-SPET mapping branch. With extensive experimental validation, we demonstrate that the SPET images generated by our approach are sufficiently realistic and have the potential for clinical application.

11.2 Previous Works on SPET Generation

From a technical standpoint, methods for generating SPET images can be broadly classified into two categories: (1) machine learning-based approaches and (2) deep learning-based approaches. In the former category, Kang et al. introduced a voxel-level prediction method for SPET images utilizing a random forest technique in 2015 [17]. Following this, Wang et al. proposed a sparse learning approach based on mapping to predict SPET images using both LPET images and corresponding MR images [35]. An et al. put forth a data-driven methodology employing multi-level correlation analysis to generate SPET images from LPET and MRI data [2], which were aligned using specific registration techniques [13, 14, 41]. However, due to the unavailability of corresponding MR images for most PET scans, Wang et al. devised a semi-supervised triple dictionary learning method to leverage a large number of unpaired training samples for SPET image generation [36]. Nonetheless, these methodologies are often semi-automated and time-intensive, posing challenges for clinical implementation.

In recent years, deep learning techniques have emerged as the predominant approach for generating SPET images, primarily owing to the unparalleled capabilities of Convolutional Neural Networks (CNNs) in image processing [18, 20]. In 2017, Xiang et al. introduced a deep auto-context CNN architecture, employing a series of CNN modules in an auto-context strategy to refine the initial SPET image estimations iteratively [42]. However, this approach involves slicing 3D images along the transverse plane to convert them into 2D images, leading to information loss in other directions and discontinuities in the final predicted 3D images across slices. To overcome this limitation, Kim et al. proposed an iterative generation framework based on 3D CNNs to predict complete SPET images [19]. Seeking more realistic results, Wang et al. devised a 3D conditional Generative Adversarial Network (GAN) for predicting SPET images from LPET images, replacing manual similarity loss definition with a discriminator [37]. They subsequently introduced a locally adaptive 3D GAN, incorporating MR images to provide anatomical information during SPET image generation [38]. Furthermore, Luo et al. introduced an Adaptive Rectification-based Generative Adversarial Network with Spectrum Constraint, referred to as AR-GAN, for SPET image generation [25]. However, the efficacy of deep learning methods relies on the availability of sufficient training data, which is often limited in practice due to the scarcity of paired LPET and SPET images.

11.3 Methodology

The proposed methodology is depicted in Fig. 11.2. Initially, we utilize a semi-supervised strategy to train the framework using unpaired data. Subsequently, we incorporate region-adaptive normalization and structural consistency constraint techniques to accurately maintain anatomical structure throughout the image generation process. Further elaboration on our approach is provided below.

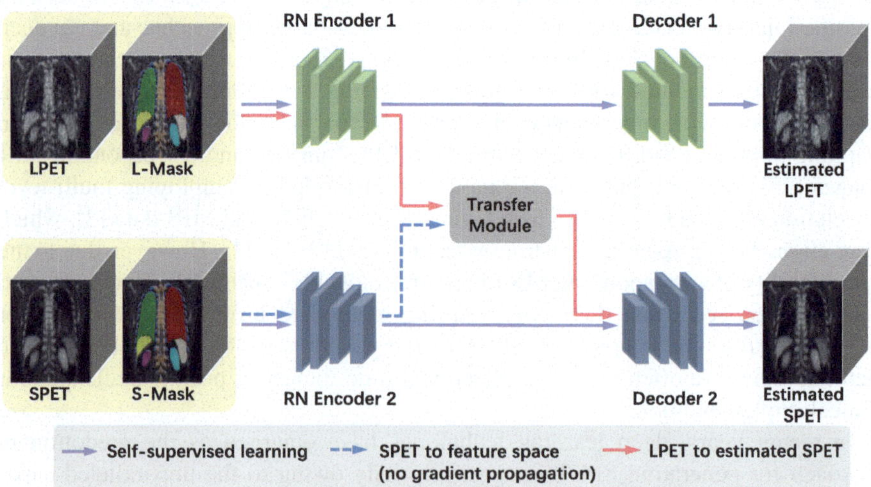

Fig. 11.2 Overview of our proposed semi-supervised framework, which involves training in two stages. The first stage employs unpaired data for self-supervised training, as indicated by the purple arrows. The second stage uses a small amount of unpaired data to fine-tune the trained network components, as indicated by the pink arrows

11.3.1 Utilization of Unpaired Data for Training

To tackle the challenge of insufficient paired data in SPET image generation, we propose a semi-supervised framework aimed at minimizing the dependency on paired images. The training process of this framework consists of two main stages: (1) self-supervised learning using unpaired data, and (2) supervised learning utilizing the limited set of paired data.

In the first stage of this semi-supervised learning process, depicted by the purple arrows in Fig. 11.2, LPET and SPET images are individually processed through a dose-specific auto-encoder network to acquire distinct embedding features. Here, RN Encoder E_1 and RN Encoder E_2 encode LPET and SPET images into the feature space, respectively, while Decoder D_1 and Decoder D_2 decode the features back into the corresponding PET images. Following this self-supervised training, the embedding features serve as representations of LPET or SPET images. However, minor discrepancies arising from dose variations may persist between the embedding features of LPET and SPET.

Subsequently, in the second stage, training is conducted using a subset of paired data to narrow the gap in the feature space via the Transfer Module T_{12}. This stage is represented by the flow of data indicated by the pink arrows in Fig. 11.2, traversing through RN Encoder E_1, Transfer Module T_{12}, and Decoder D_2.

Let X_L represent an LPET image and X_S a corresponding SPET image. In the first stage, $\{E_1, D_1\}$ and $\{E_2, D_2\}$ are individually trained under the loss functions $\mathcal{L}_{U1}$ and $\mathcal{L}_{U2}$, which are defined as

$$\mathcal{L}_{U1} = \mathcal{L}_{l2}(D_1(E_1(X_L)), X_L) + \lambda_1 \mathcal{L}_{d1}(D_1(E_1(X_L))), \tag{11.1}$$

$$\mathcal{L}_{U2} = \mathcal{L}_{l2}(D_2(E_2(X_S)), X_S) + \lambda_1 \mathcal{L}_{d2}(D_2(E_2(X_S))). \tag{11.2}$$

In the subsequent stage, $\{E_1, D_2\}$ undergo training using the following loss function $\mathcal{L}_S$,

$$\begin{aligned} \mathcal{L}_S = \; & \mathcal{L}_{l2}(D_2(E_1(X_L), X_S) \\ & + \lambda_2 \mathcal{L}_{d2}(D_2(T_{12}(E_1(X_L)), X_S) \\ & + \lambda_3 \mathcal{L}_{struc}(T_{12}(E_1(X_L)), E_2(X_S)). \end{aligned} \tag{11.3}$$

where λ_1, λ_2, and λ_3 represent hyperparameters that balance various loss terms. $\mathcal{L}l2$ and $\mathcal{L}struc$ denote the mean square error and structural consistency loss as outlined in Eq. (11.7), respectively. Additionally, $\mathcal{L}d1$ and $\mathcal{L}d2$ stand for the adversarial losses corresponding to LPET and SPET, respectively, each determined by a four-layer discriminator [11].

11.3.2 Implementation of Region-Specific Normalization in Different Regions

To enhance the network's generalization capabilities, various normalization techniques based on global statistics, such as Batch Normalization (BN) [12], Layer Normalization (LN) [3], Instance Normalization (IN) [34], and Group Normalization (GN) [40], have been proposed for tasks like classification, segmentation, and generation. However, these methods may not be optimal for generating PET images, which often exhibit significant intensity variations across different regions, as depicted in Fig. 11.1. Therefore, we introduce Region-adaptive Normalization (RN) in this study to adaptively learn distributions for different regions under segmentation guidance. Our goal is to generate SPET images that are noise-reduced yet exhibit clear organ boundaries.

To provide semantic guidance for RN operation, we utilize the TotalSegmentator [39], an openly available tool based on nnU-Net and trained with over one thousand samples, to segment multiple organs from the aligned CT images corresponding to their respective PET images in the spatial domain. For simplicity, we group these 104 anatomical structures into 8 independent tissues, comprising the heart, liver, spleen, lungs, stomach, kidneys, spine, and ribs. Additionally, we employ erosion operations to minimize small overlaps between different tissues. Given that the TotalSegmentator was trained on a diverse dataset of over a thousand samples, its segmentation performance is robust and sufficiently reliable for integration into our SPET generation algorithm. Selected segmentation results are presented in Fig. 11.4.

As depicted in Fig. 11.3, we integrate RN into the structure of encoder blocks, replacing BN. Following a methodology akin to [30, 44], the RN module utilizes two convolutional layers to learn region-specific affine transformation parameters β and γ from semantic segmentation m, with the first convolutional layer being shared to economize computational resources. Serving as adaptable functions applied to the input semantic map m, the modulation parameters γ and β are no longer C-dimensional vectors but tensors of identical dimensions as m, exhibiting varying values across different spatial locations.

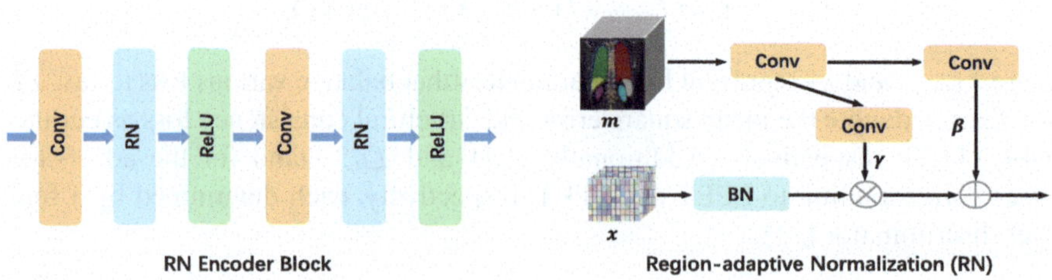

Fig. 11.3 Illustration of Region-adaptive Normalization (RN). The left side shows the differences between the RN encoder and traditional encoders, where BN is replaced with RN. The right side illustrates the specific operational details of RN

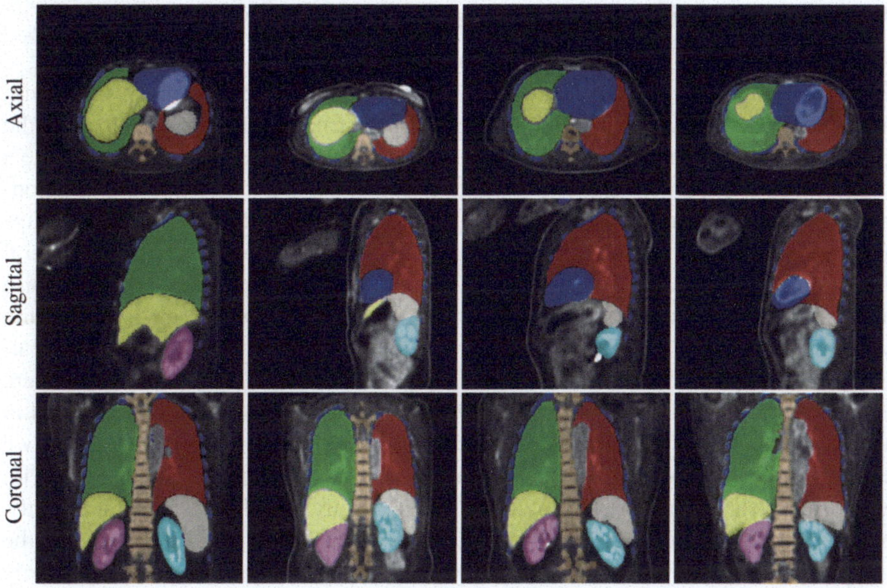

Fig. 11.4 Four typical cases of segmentation results, where the segmentation maps are overlayed on the PET images

Consider x as the input feature map of a batch comprising N samples, each having spatial dimensions of $H \times W \times Z$ and C channels. For the n-th sample in the c-th channel, $x_{n,c,i,j,k}$ represents the activation at spatial position (i, j, k) before normalization. Initially, we calculate the mean μ_c and standard deviation σ_c as follows:

$$\mu_c = \frac{1}{NHWZ} \sum_{n,i,j,k} x_{n,c,i,j,k}, \tag{11.4}$$

$$\sigma_c = \sqrt{\frac{1}{NHWZ} \sum_{n,i,j,k} ((x_{n,c,i,j,k})^2 - (\mu_c)^2) + \epsilon}, \tag{11.5}$$

where ϵ is a small constant for avoiding invalid denominators. Then, the normalized activation $h_{n,c,i,j,k}$ at spatial location (i, j, k) can be computed as:

$$h_{n,c,i,j,k} = \gamma_{c,i,j,k} \frac{x_{n,c,i,j,k} - \mu_c}{\sigma_c} + \beta_{c,i,j,k}. \tag{11.6}$$

11.3.3 Constraint of Multi-Level Structural Consistency

Because of artifacts and noise present in LPET images, certain small tissues with fuzzy boundaries (such as pulmonary bronchial structures) may vanish after the generation of SPET images from LPET data. To address this issue, we introduce a structural consistency loss. This loss initially establishes specific structural relationships among input image patches and subsequently ensures that these relationships are maintained in the resulting SPET images. It's important to note that the structural consistency loss is computed exclusively in the feature space to mitigate noise interference and computational burden. Specifically, the process involves feeding seven pairs of LPET and SPET patches into the network simultaneously. One pair is initially cropped from the entire PET image, while the remaining six pairs are taken from its surrounding areas. Theoretically, these six pairs can be selected at any distance and direction around the central patch. However, for simplicity, we choose patches in six directions along the positive and negative axes (x, y, z) with equal Euclidean distances. During training, the central patch is selected randomly, but sequentially during testing. In cases where the central patch is located at the image's edge, the number of surrounding patches may be fewer than six, with only three in extreme scenarios (such as corners).

LPET patches are processed through RN Encoder E_1 and Transfer Module T_{12} (i.e., two $1 \times 1 \times 1$ convolutional layers) to yield the estimated standard-dose features $f^{ES} = \{f_i^{ES}\}_{i=1}^{7}$. Similarly, SPET patches obtained from the same spatial locations traverse RN Encoder E_2 to produce the standard-dose features $f^S = \{f_i^S\}_{i=1}^{7}$. The subsequent step involves calculating the structural consistency loss between f^S and f^{ES} across hierarchical levels, specifically, the *vertex level* and *line level*. Here, each cropped patch fed into the network is regarded as a *vertex*. The vertex-level loss $\mathcal{L}vertex$ quantifies the error in patch generation, while the line-level loss $\mathcal{L}line$ measures the patch-to-patch distance computed from f^S and f^{ES}. Thus, the structural consistency loss is formulated as follows:

$$\mathcal{L}_{struc}(f^{ES}, f^S) = \sum_{i=1}^{7} \mathcal{L}_{vertex}(f_i^S, f_i^{ES}) + \alpha \sum_{i=1}^{7} \sum_{j=1}^{7} \mathcal{L}_{line}(f_i^S - f_i^{ES}, f_j^S - f_j^{ES}), \tag{11.7}$$

where the hyperparameter α is employed to weigh the loss terms in $\mathcal{L}struc$. $\mathcal{L}vertex$ and $\mathcal{L}_{line}$ represent the functions utilized to gauge similarity at the vertex and line levels, respectively, employing MSE and cosine similarity, respectively.

11.4 Experiments

11.4.1 Materials

To assess our proposed SPET image generation framework, PET images are sourced from the (total-body) uEXPLORER PET/CT scanner [45]. Paired LPET and SPET images are obtained through list mode scanning with an injection of 256 MBq of [^{18}F]-FDG. Specifically, SPET images are reconstructed using 1200 s data acquired between 60 and 80 min post-injection via the ordered-subsets expectation maximization (OSEM) algorithm [27]. Simultaneously, corresponding 1/10th LPET images are reconstructed using 120 s data sampled uniformly from the 1200 s data. Additionally, unpaired SPET images are collected from other research efforts conducted on the uEXPLORER scanner. Ultimately, the PET dataset we compile comprises 50 unpaired SPET images and 20 paired LPET and SPET images.

In the first stage, 10 LPET images (from 10 randomly-selected sets of paired LPET and SPET images) are used for training the RN Encoder E_1 and Decoder D_1, while 60 SPET images (including those 10 SPET images from 10 selected sets of paired LPET and SPET images) are used for training the RN Encoder E_2 and Decoder D_2. In the second stage, those 10 selected sets of paired LPET and SPET images in the first stage are used for training the E_1, Transfer Module T_{12}, and D_2, while the rest 10 paired LPET and SPET images are used for testing.

11.4.2 Experiment Setup

During the data preprocessing, all images are resampled to a voxel spacing of $2 \times 2 \times 2$ mm^3 with dimensions of $256 \times 256 \times 160$. Intensity normalization is applied to bring the intensity range within [0, 1] using min-max normalization. To expand the training dataset and mitigate GPU memory dependency, we extract overlapping patches sized $96 \times 96 \times 96$ from the whole PET image. Specifically, for calculating the structural consistency loss, we randomly select the first patch and then crop six additional pairs from its neighboring areas, each located 98 voxels away from the centroid of the first patch. Additionally, to ensure result stability and minimize randomness, we conduct two-fold cross-validation during evaluation. The experiment is repeated five times with varying dataset splits, and the average and standard deviation of the results are reported.

We employ the Adam optimizer with an initial learning rate of 0.001 for network training. All experiments are conducted on the PyTorch platform using an NVIDIA Tesla V100 GPU. Empirically, we set λ_1, λ_2, and λ_3 in Eqs. (11.1), (11.2), and (11.3) to 1, 1, and 0.5, respectively, and α in Eq. (11.7) is set to 0.2. Quantitative assessment adopts three metrics: Normalized Root Mean Squared Error (NMSE), Peak Signal to Noise Ratio (PSNR), and Structural Similarity Index (SSIM).

Table 11.1 Quantitative comparison with state-of-the-art SPET image generation methods, in terms of PSNR, SSIM, and NMSE

Method	PSNR (dB) ↑	SSIM ↑	NMSE ↓
LPET	17.735 ± 2.145	0.974 ± 0.014	0.028 ± 0.004
Cycle-GAN	21.531 ± 1.872	0.980 ± 0.011	0.025 ± 0.003
3D-cGAN	23.266 ± 1.339	0.982 ± 0.009	0.024 ± 0.003
CT-assisted	22.947 ± 1.531	0.984 ± 0.007	0.024 ± 0.003
LA-GAN	24.258 ± 1.276	0.985 ± 0.006	0.023 ± 0.002
AR-GAN	24.845 ± 1.037	0.987 ± 0.006	0.022 ± 0.001
Our proposed	**25.154 ± 0.933**	**0.989 ± 0.005**	**0.021 ± 0.001**

The optimal results are highlighted in bold

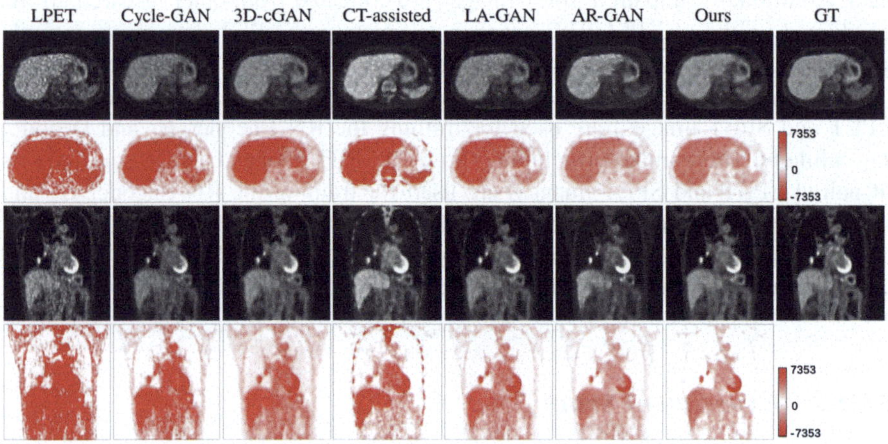

Fig. 11.5 Visual comparison of SPET images produced by six different methods. From left to right are the LPET images, results of five other comparison methods (2nd–6th columns) and our approach (7th column), and the GT (SPET image). The corresponding difference maps between the generated results and GT are shown in the 2nd (axial view) and 4th (coronal view) rows

11.4.3 Comparison with State-of-the-Art Methods

We conducted a comprehensive comparison between our proposed approach and several state-of-the-art SPET generation methods, namely Cycle-GAN [46], 3D-cGAN [37], CT-assisted [23], LA-GAN [38], and AR-GAN [25]. The results, both quantitative and qualitative, are presented in Table 11.1 and Fig. 11.5, respectively.

Quantitative results obtained by various methods, including PSNR, SSIM, and NMSE, are presented in Table 11.1, highlighting the superior performance of our proposed approach. Notably, compared to Cycle-GAN, which demonstrates the worst results, our method showcases significant enhancements in PSNR, SSIM, and NMSE by 3.623 dB, 0.009, and 0.004, respectively. This demonstrates that, even if the same additional unpaired SPET can be used, reasonable network architecture and utilization are still needed to help SPET generation. Even though both our approach and Cycle-GAN can use additional unpaired SPET data, our method achieves better SPET generation performance due to a more rational design of framework and utilization strategy. Additionally, paired t-test analysis reveals that the p-value between our approach and each of the other methods is less than 0.05, indicating a statistically significant improvement achieved by our proposed approach.

The visual comparisons among different methods are depicted in Fig. 11.5. Our approach showcases the generation of SPET images with enhanced clarity in boundaries and reduced noise. Notably, our method excels in producing superior results, particularly in regions prone to ambiguity, such as the bronchial region illustrated in the third row of Fig. 11.5. Furthermore, when comparing our approach with CT-assisted and LA-GAN, both of which utilize additional CT images either directly or indirectly, it is evident that SPET images generated by CT-assisted exhibit noticeable oversaturation, retaining excess content from CT images. This underscores the limitations of simply integrating additional CT images in enhancing SPET generation. Moreover, the difference maps highlight that our approach generates SPET images with minimal difference from the ground truth, further confirming its superiority over existing state-of-the-art methods, a conclusion supported by visual inspection of the results.

11.4.4 The Roles of Different Components

In our proposed method, we incorporate three primary strategies, i.e., semi-supervised strategy, region-adaptive normalization, and structural consistency constraint. To assess the effectiveness of each strategy in SPET image generation, we conduct comprehensive experiments in this section. We establish a baseline approach, referred to as blNet, comprising an encoder, two convolutional layers, a decoder, and a discriminator arranged sequentially. Subsequently, we enhance blNet by integrating the self-supervised strategy, region-adaptive normalization, and structural consistency loss, resulting in blNet-SS, blNet-SS-RN, and blNet-SS-RN-SC, respectively. All models undergo training under identical settings, and their performance is evaluated based on results presented in Fig. 11.6 and Table 11.2.

Semi-supervised Strategy When training the end-to-end SPET generation network with paired PET images, different components are tasked with learning various functionalities. For instance, an encoder extracts features from LPET images, while a decoder reconstructs SPET images from these extracted features. This versatility can also be achieved through training with unpaired PET images. Hence, we introduce the semi-supervised strategy to enable the utilization of additional unpaired data for network training.

A comparison between the performance of blNet and blNet-SS, as presented in the first and second rows of Table 11.2, reveals the benefits of the semi-supervised

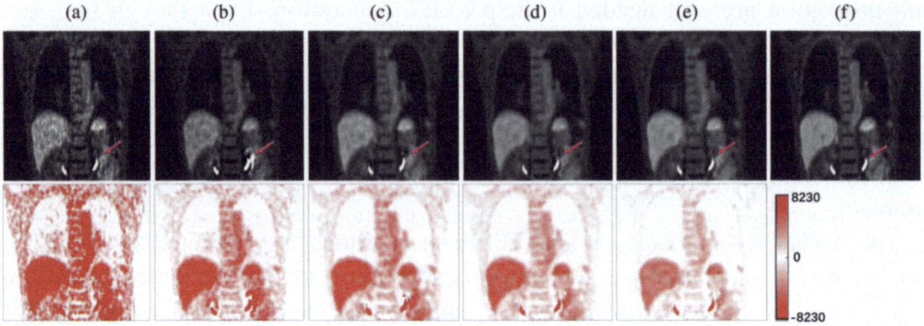

Fig. 11.6 Visual comparison of SPET images generated by different network components and loss functions. From left to right are the LPET image, results by four different methods (2nd–5th columns), and the ground truth (GT) (last column). The corresponding difference maps are shown in the second row. (**a**) LPET. (**b**) blNet. (**c**) blNet-SS. (**d**) blNet-SS-RN. (**e**) blNet-SS-RN-SC. (**f**) GT

Table 11.2 Performance comparison of SPET images generated by different network components and loss functions, in terms of PSNR, SSIM, and NMSE

Method	PSNR (dB) ↑	SSIM ↑	NMSE ↓
blNet	21.176 ± 1.932	0.979 ± 0.012	0.026 ± 0.003
blNet-SS	22.532 ± 1.617	0.981 ± 0.010	0.024 ± 0.003
blNet-SS-RN	24.463 ± 1.112	0.986 ± 0.007	0.022 ± 0.002
blNet-SS-RN-SC	**25.154 ± 0.933**	**0.989 ± 0.005**	**0.021 ± 0.001**

The optimal results are highlighted in bold

strategy in SPET image generation. Notably, there is a consistent enhancement across all three metrics (PSNR, SSIM, and NMSE) with the adoption of the semi-supervised approach. Moreover, visual samples in Fig. 11.6b and c showcase that SPET images generated by blNet-SS exhibit reduced noise and clearer boundaries compared to blNet. This observation underscores the efficacy of our proposed semi-supervised strategy, which leverages both paired and unpaired PET images for training, rather than relying solely on paired PET images.

Region-Adaptive Normalization Batch Normalization (BN) is a widely used technique in deep learning networks, known for its ability to significantly enhance training efficiency. However, as a method relying on global-wise (batch-wise) statistics, BN may not be the optimal choice for the SPET image generation task. This is because PET images exhibit wide intensity variations across different regions, and applying the same normalization operation to all regions can potentially diminish the contrast differences between them, leading to blurred boundaries in the resulting SPET images.

This observation is supported by the typical sample depicted in Fig. 11.6c and d, where blNet-SS utilizes BN and blNet-SS-RN replaces BN with RN within the same network framework. Comparing the results, the SPET image generated by blNet-SS-

RN exhibits notably stronger regional variance. Particularly, the boundaries of the spine and ribs are clearer in the results of blNet-SS-RN, as highlighted by the red boxes and arrows. This validates our hypothesis that RN can better preserve regional variance compared to BN for the SPET image generation task. Moreover, the quantitative results presented in Table 11.2 demonstrate that blNet-SS-RN improves the PSNR, SSIM, and NMSE by 1.931 dB, 0.005, and 0.002 respectively, compared to blNet-SS. This further confirms the superiority of RN over BN for SPET image generation.

Structural Consistency Constraint PET images originate from real human tissues, implying that neighboring patches in PET images exhibit certain associations. Consequently, we devised the structural consistency loss to uphold such associations during the generation process, thereby aiding in the generation of unclear regions (e.g., pulmonary bronchial) by leveraging information from neighboring regions (e.g., heart). We conducted specific experiments to confirm the efficacy of our proposed structural consistency loss, presenting the results in Table 11.2 and Fig. 11.6e.

From the visual outcomes depicted in Fig. 11.6d and e, it is evident that blNet-SS-RN-SC significantly enhances the clarity of previously unclear regions (i.e., the bronchi highlighted by the red box) compared to blNet-SS-RN. Additionally, the corresponding difference maps exhibit smaller discrepancies (indicated by lighter colors) with the ground truth. The quantitative results in Table 11.2 further support this observation, demonstrating that blNet-SS-RN-SC achieves improvements in PSNR, SSIM, and NMSE by 0.691 dB, 0.003, and 0.001, respectively, compared to blNet-SS-RN without the structural consistency loss. These findings serve as evidence of the efficacy of our devised structural consistency loss in enhancing the generation of SPET images.

11.5 Discussion

11.5.1 The Effect of Region-Adaptive Normalization

As illustrated in Fig. 11.1, PET images exhibit noticeable intensity variations across different regions, which is the important image information. In our endeavor to capture these variances during SPET image generation, we integrate the Region-adaptive Normalization (RN) module into our proposed framework. To underscore the benefits of RN, we conduct a comparative analysis with Batch Normalization (BN) [12] and Instance Normalization (IN) [34], commonly employed in generation tasks. Specifically, employing a 3D-UNet as the baseline, we replace the normalization technique with BN, IN, and RN, respectively, while maintaining other conditions constant. The results of these experiments are presented in Fig. 11.7.

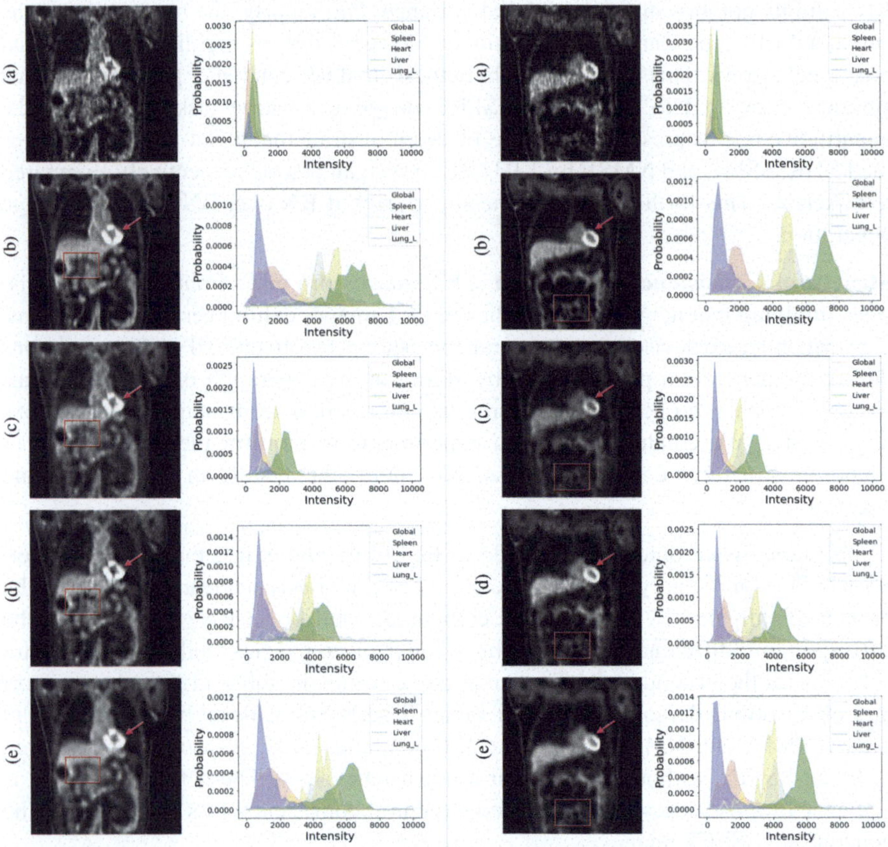

Fig. 11.7 Visual comparison of two SPET images of two subjects, produced by three different normalization methods. The first column shows the coronal views of the PET image, and the second column shows the corresponding region-wise intensity distributions. From top to bottom are the (**a**) LPET image, (**b**) GT (SPET image), and three results using (**c**) BN, (**d**) IN, and (**e**) RN (the 3rd–5th rows), respectively. Red boxes and red arrows show detailed results for comparison

In Fig. 11.7, SPET images generated with RN exhibit clearer inter-region boundaries and fewer artifacts in hypermetabolic regions compared to other normalization methods. Additionally, focusing on intensity distribution, the region-wise intensity variation of RN is more distinct and closely resembles the ground truth (GT). This highlights the superior normalization performance of RN in the context of SPET generation, surpassing both BN and IN.

The segmentation of multiple organs derived from CT images inevitably contains some errors, primarily stemming from two sources. Firstly, spatial misalignment between PET and CT images due to physiological motion introduces errors. Secondly, errors in the prediction of CT segmentation masks contribute to inaccuracies. Concerning the former, PET attenuation correction relies on corresponding CT

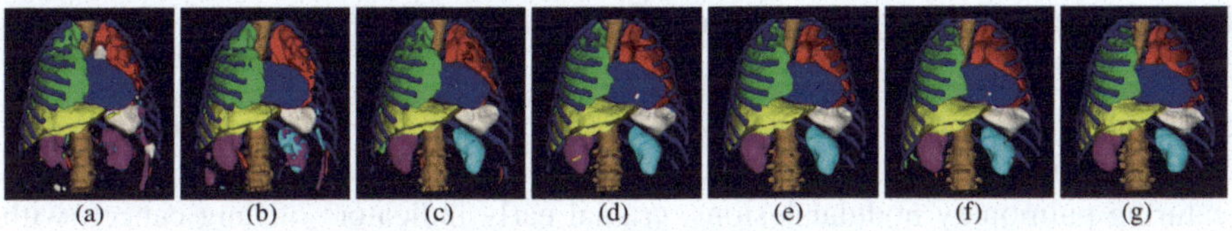

Fig. 11.8 Multi-organ segmentation achieved by TotalSegmentator with different accuracy. **(a)** m_1. **(b)** m_2. **(c)** m_3. **(d)** m_4. **(e)** m_5. **(f)** m_6. **(g)** "GT"

Table 11.3 Quantitative results of SPET generation with different segmentation accuracy

	Multi-organ segmentation		SPET generation		
	Dice (%)	IoU	PSNR (dB) ↑	SSIM ↑	NMSE ↓
m_1	80.72 ± 2.53	67.67 ± 7.33	20.543 ± 1.987	0.978 ± 0.013	0.026 ± 0.004
m_2	83.62 ± 2.14	71.85 ± 5.28	21.457 ± 1.447	0.980 ± 0.009	0.025 ± 0.003
m_3	87.41 ± 1.86	77.64 ± 4.86	23.654 ± 1.245	0.982 ± 0.008	0.024 ± 0.003
m_4	92.27 ± 1.73	85.65 ± 3.15	24.813 ± 0.987	0.987 ± 0.007	0.023 ± 0.002
m_5	94.11 ± 1.58	88.87 ± 2.52	24.875 ± 0.965	0.988 ± 0.007	0.023 ± 0.002
m_6	97.03 ± 1.19	94.23 ± 1.27	25.087 ± 0.942	0.989 ± 0.005	0.021 ± 0.001
"GT"	100.00	100.00	25.154 ± 0.933	0.989 ± 0.005	0.021 ± 0.001

images to compute attenuation coefficients, thereby inheriting spatial misalignment errors (e.g., induced by breathing) during the attenuation correction process. Hence, such errors are inherent in the attenuated PET images themselves and cannot be mitigated by our SPET generation algorithm. Regarding the latter, we conducted additional experiments to assess the impact of segmentation accuracy on our SPET generation approach.

Specifically, we retrained the TotalSegmentator [39] and applied it to our dataset, producing seven sets of multi-organ segmentations by controlling the number of training epochs. Since ground truth segmentation data for our dataset are unavailable, we approximate the last group, exhibiting the most favorable visualization, as pseudo "GT" and then compute the Dice and IoU metrics for the remaining six groups relative to this pseudo "GT". Figure 11.8 provides a visual illustration of the seven groups of multi-organ segmentations, while Table 11.3 presents the corresponding SPET generation results under varying segmentation accuracy.

Observing Table 11.3, we note the robustness of our approach to segmentation accuracy when segmentation results are satisfactory (e.g., m_4, m_5, and m_6). However, in cases of notably poor segmentation outcomes (e.g., m_1, m_2, and m_3), our approach exhibits sensitivity to segmentation accuracy, with SPET generation performance deteriorating. Notably, the performance of SPET generation is even inferior to that without utilizing multi-organ segmentation maps (i.e., the generated results with m_1 and m_2 are inferior to those by the blNet-SS in Table 11.2).

11.5.2 The Diagnostic Value of Generated PET Images

To evaluate the impact of different network components and loss functions on the detectability of lesion areas, we manually curated and annotated six samples featuring pulmonary nodular lesions, crucial early indicators of lung cancer, with guidance from radiologists possessing over five years of diagnostic expertise. Standard uptake value (SUV) serves as a prevalent reference indicator in PET tumor diagnosis. Following the methodology outlined in [7, 23], we leveraged the biases of SUV_{mean} and SUV_{max} to quantitatively appraise the detectability of lesion areas. Here, SUV_{mean} corresponds to the average value computed across all voxels within the nodule's ROI, while SUV_{max} represents the highest uptake observed among the individual nodule voxels. The calculation is delineated below:

$$Bias = \frac{SUV^{ES}_{mean/max} - SUV^{S}_{mean/max}}{SUV^{S}_{mean/max}} \times 100\%, \tag{11.8}$$

which indicates difference in nodule quantification between estimated SPET and true SPET. The smaller bias means that the nodule area of the estimated SPET is more similar to that of true SPET, i.e., the nodule is more easily to be detected.

We designed four groups of experiments to investigate the influence of different components of our approach on nodule detection, denoted as blNet, blNet-SS, blNet-SS-RN, and blNet-SS-RN-SC, where blNet is composed of encoder, two convolutional layers, decoder, and discriminator in sequence, and blNet-SS, blNet-SS-RN, and blNet-SS-RN-SC are adopted semi-supervised strategy, region-adaptive normalization, and structural consistency constraint sequentially based on blNet.

The biases of SUV_{mean} and SUV_{max} for these six samples are illustrated in Fig. 11.9. It is evident from the figure that the biases of SUV_{mean} and SUV_{max} progressively decrease from blNet to blNet-SS-RN-SC. This trend indicates a gradual reduction in the differences in nodule area between the estimated SPET and the ground truth SPET, thereby suggesting an enhancement in the detectability of

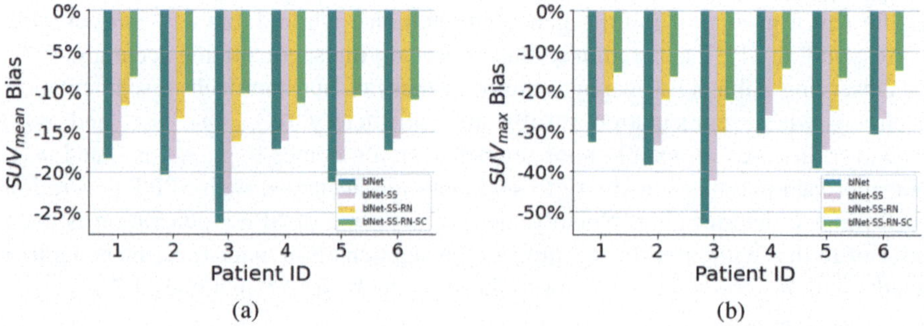

Fig. 11.9 (**a**) SUV_{mean} and (**b**) SUV_{max} biases of generated SPET under different network components and loss functions

pulmonary nodular lesion areas. Thus, the semi-supervised strategy, region-adaptive normalization, and structural consistency constraint are all useful in enhancing the detection of pulmonary nodular lesion areas.

11.5.3 The Impact of Variations in Radionuclide Dosage

To assess the robustness of our semi-supervised approach to changes in radionuclide dosage, we acquired a separate external dataset using the methodology outlined in Sect. 11.4.1. This dataset comprises 40 samples, each containing six PET images acquired at different doses. Specifically, the SPET images were reconstructed using 1200 s data collected between 60 and 80 min post-injection, while the remaining five LPET images were reconstructed using 600, 300, 200, 120, and 90 s data, uniformly sampled from the 1200 s data, respectively. Additionally, to ensure the robustness of our models, this external dataset was sourced from new PET scans distinct from those used in Sect. 11.4.1. Consequently, the 120 and 1200 s data from the external dataset were not part of the original dataset. The reconstructed SPET and LPET images are depicted in Fig. 11.10, where shorter durations correspond to lower doses. Subsequently, we compared our approach with a conventional fully-supervised SPET generation method, 3D-cGAN [37], across various doses and provided quantitative results in Fig. 11.11. It is noteworthy that both our approach and 3D-cGAN are trained in Sect. 11.4.3 and tested on the new external dataset only.

From the findings, our approach consistently outperforms 3D-cGAN across all doses. Additionally, the reduction rates in PSNR and SSIM are notably gentler compared to those of 3D-cGAN as the dose diminishes (i.e., time duration decreases), suggesting that our approach exhibits greater resilience to dose variations. This resilience can be attributed to the incorporation of a semi-supervised strategy, enabling the utilization of a larger dataset (i.e., 50 unpaired SPET images) for network training, in contrast to the fully-supervised 3D-cGAN. Generally, semi-supervised methodologies tend to demonstrate greater robustness than fully-supervised approaches when confronted with a certain volume of unpaired training data, a phenomenon corroborated by numerous studies [9, 16, 33].

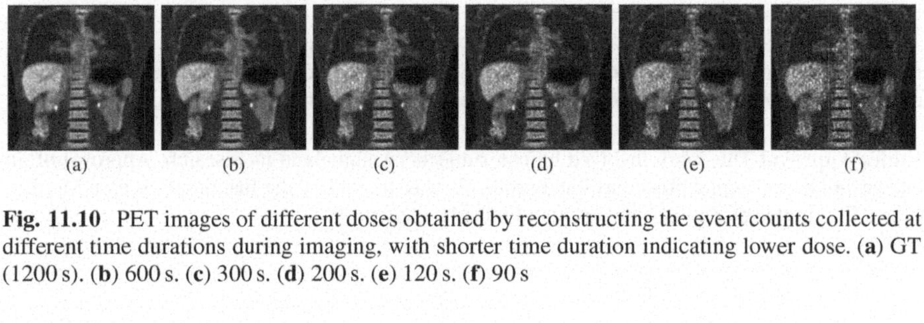

Fig. 11.10 PET images of different doses obtained by reconstructing the event counts collected at different time durations during imaging, with shorter time duration indicating lower dose. (**a**) GT (1200 s). (**b**) 600 s. (**c**) 300 s. (**d**) 200 s. (**e**) 120 s. (**f**) 90 s

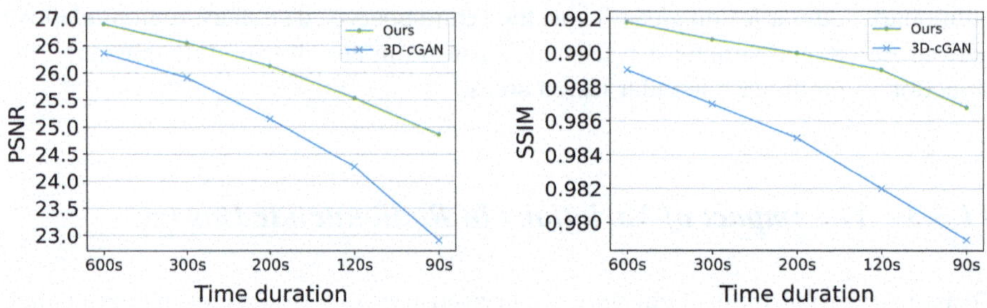

Fig. 11.11 Influence of dose change to fully-supervised method (3D-cGAN) and semi-supervised method (Ours), respectively

11.6 Conclusion

In this study, we present a novel and efficient approach for tackling three primary challenges encountered in SPET generation: (1) the scarcity of paired training data, (2) the presence of blurred boundaries in generated SPET images, and (3) the difficulty in accurately reproducing unclear regions. Specifically, we introduce a semi-supervised methodology that integrates both supervised and unsupervised techniques, allowing for the utilization of both paired and unpaired PET images during network training. Additionally, we incorporate region-adaptive normalization (RN) and a structural consistency constraint into our framework to leverage semantic information from CT scans. This integration helps prevent the generated SPET images from retaining extraneous content and enhances structural details, particularly in regions with blurred boundaries, by leveraging information from clearer regions. We validate the efficacy of each proposed strategy through comprehensive ablation experiments conducted on real human chest-abdomen PET images. Furthermore, extensive experimentation demonstrates that our approach outperforms existing state-of-the-art methods both quantitatively and qualitatively.

Acknowledgments This work was supported in part by the National Natural Science Foundation of China (grant numbers U23A20295, 62131015, 82441023, 82394432, 62250710165, 82402394), Shanghai Municipal Central Guided Local Science and Technology Development Fund (grant number YDZX20233100001001), Shanghai Pujiang Program (no. 23PJ1430200), and HPC Platform of ShanghaiTech University.

Competing Interests The authors declare that they have no competing interests or personal relationships that could have appeared to influence the work reported in this paper.

Ethics Approval This work involved human subjects or animals in its research. Approval of all ethical and experimental procedures and protocols was granted by the Institute Research Medical Ethics Committee of Zhongshan Hospital, Fudan University.

References

1. Amirrashedi M, Sarkar S, Ghadiri H, Ghafarian P, Ay M (2021) Standard-dose PET reconstruction from low-dose preclinical images using an adopted all convolutional U-Net. Biomed Appl Mol Struct Funct Imaging 11600:834–848
2. An L, Zhang P, Adeli E, Wang Y, Ma G, Shi F, Lalush DS, Lin W, Shen D (2016) Multi-level canonical correlation analysis for standard-dose PET image estimation. IEEE Trans Image Process 25(7):3303–3315
3. Ba JL, Kiros JR, Hinton GE (2016) Layer normalization. arXiv preprint arXiv:160706450
4. Barbosa F, Queiroz MA, Nunes RF, Costa LB, Zaniboni EC, Marin JG, Cerri GG, Buchpiguel CA (2020) Nonprostatic diseases on PSMA PET imaging: a spectrum of benign and malignant findings. Cancer Imaging 20(1):1–23
5. Buchbender C, Heusner TA, Lauenstein TC, Bockisch A, Antoch G (2012) Oncologic PET/MRI, part 1: tumors of the brain, head and neck, chest, abdomen, and pelvis. J Nucl Med 53(6):928–938
6. Chen W (2007) Clinical applications of PET in brain tumors. J Nucl Med 48(9):1468–1481
7. Cui J, Gong K, Guo N, Wu C, Meng X, Kim K, Zheng K, Wu Z, Fu L, Xu B, et al. (2019) PET image denoising using unsupervised deep learning. Eur J Nucl Med Mol Imaging 46(13):2780–2789
8. Decazes P, Hinault P, Veresezan O, Thureau S, Gouel P, Vera P (2021) Trimodality PET/CT/MRI and radiotherapy: a mini-review. Front Oncol 10:3392
9. Diaz-Pinto A, Colomer A, Morales S, Xu Y, Frangi A (2019) Retinal image synthesis and semi-supervised learning for glaucoma assessment. IEEE Trans Med Imaging 38(9):2211–2218
10. Dimitrakopoulou-Strauss A, Pan L, Sachpekidis C (2021) Kinetic modeling and parametric imaging with dynamic PET for oncological applications: general considerations, current clinical applications, and future perspectives. Eur J Nucl Med Mol Imaging 48:21–39
11. Goodfellow I, Pouget-Abadie J, Mirza M, Xu B, Warde-Farley D, Ozair S, Courville A, Bengio Y (2014) Generative adversarial nets. Adv Neural Inf Process Syst 27(11):100–109
12. Ioffe S, Szegedy C (2015) Batch normalization: accelerating deep network training by reducing internal covariate shift. In: International conference on machine learning, pp 448–456
13. Jia H, Wu G, Wang Q, Shen D (2010) ABSORB: atlas building by self-organized registration and bundling. NeuroImage 51(3):1057–1070
14. Jia H, Yap P, Shen D (2012) Iterative multi-atlas-based multi-image segmentation with tree-based registration. NeuroImage 59(1):422–430
15. Jiang C, Pan Y, Cui Z, Shen D (2022) Reconstruction of standard-dose PET from low-dose PET via dual-frequency supervision and global aggregation module. In: 2022 IEEE 19th International Symposium on Biomedical Imaging (ISBI), pp 1–5
16. Kamran S, Hossain K, Tavakkoli A, Zuckerbrod S, Baker S (2021) VtGAN: semi-supervised retinal image synthesis and disease prediction using vision transformers. In: Proceedings of the IEEE/CVF International Conference on Computer Vision, pp 3235–3245
17. Kang J, Gao Y, Shi F, Lalush DS, Lin W, Shen D (2015) Prediction of standard-dose brain PET image by using MRI and low-dose brain [18F]FDG PET images. Med Phys 42(9):5301–5309
18. Kawahara J, Brown CJ, Miller SP, Booth BG, Hamarneh G (2017) BrainNetCNN: convolutional neural networks for brain networks; towards predicting neurodevelopment. NeuroImage 146:1038–1049
19. Kim K, Wu D, Gong K, Dutta J, Kim JH, Son YD, Hang KK, Fakhri GE, Li Q (2018) Penalized PET reconstruction using deep learning prior and local linear fitting. IEEE Trans Med Imaging 37(6):1478–1487
20. Kleesiek J, Urban G, Hubert A, Schwarz D, Maier-Hein K, Bendszus M, Biller A (2016) Deep MRI brain extraction: a 3D convolutional neural network for skull stripping. NeuroImage 129:460–469
21. Kreisl WC, Kim M, Coughlin JM, Henter ID, Owen DR, Innis RB (2020) PET imaging of neuroinflammation in neurological disorders. Lancet Neurol 19(11):940–950

22. Lei Y, Dong X, Wang T, Higgins K, Yang X (2020) Estimating standard-dose PET from low-dose PET with deep learning. Image Process 113:73–82
23. Lu W, Onofrey J, Lu Y, Shi L, Ma T, Liu Y, Liu C (2019) An investigation of quantitative accuracy for deep learning based denoising in oncological PET. Phys Med Biol 64(16):165019
24. Luo Y, Wang Y, Zu C, Zhan B, Wu X, Zhou J, Shen D, Zhou L (2021) 3D transformer-GAN for high-quality PET reconstruction. In: International conference on medical image computing and computer-assisted intervention, pp 276–285
25. Luo Y, Zhou L, Zhan B, Fei Y, Zhou J, Wang Y, Shen D (2022) Adaptive rectification based adversarial network with spectrum constraint for high-quality PET image synthesis. Med Image Anal 77:102335
26. Maurer L, Wang J (2005) Positron Emission Tomography: applications in drug discovery and drug development. Curr Top Med Chem 5(11):1053–1075
27. Mehranian A, Reader A (2020) Model-based deep learning PET image reconstruction using forward–backward splitting expectation–maximization. IEEE Trans Radiat Plasma Med Sci 5(1):54–64
28. Meyer JH, Cervenka S, Kim M, Kreisl WC, Henter ID, Innis RB (2020) Neuroinflammation in psychiatric disorders: PET imaging and promising new targets. Lancet Psychiatry 7(12):1064–1074
29. Nichols T, Qi J, Asma E, Leahy R (2002) Spatiotemporal reconstruction of list-mode pet data. IEEE Trans Med Imaging 21(4):396–404
30. Park T, Liu M, Wang T, Zhu J (2019) Semantic image synthesis with spatially-adaptive normalization. In: Proceedings of the IEEE/CVF conference on computer vision and pattern recognition, pp 2337–2346
31. Sakthivel P, Thakar A, Prashanth A, Angamuthu M, Sharma SC, Kumar R (2020) Clinical applications of 68 ga-psma PET/CT on residual disease assessment of juvenile nasopharyngeal angiofibroma (JNA). Nucl Med Mol Imaging 54(1):63–64
32. Slovis TL (2002) The ALARA concept in pediatric CT: myth or reality? Radiology 223(1):5–6
33. Spurr A, Aksan E, Hilliges O (2017) Guiding infoGAN with semi-supervision. In: Joint European conference on machine learning and knowledge discovery in databases, pp 119–134
34. Ulyanov D, Vedaldi A, Lempitsky V (2016) Instance normalization: the missing ingredient for fast stylization. arXiv preprint arXiv:160708022
35. Wang Y, Zhang P, An L, Ma G, Kang J, Shi F, Wu X, Zhou J, Lalush DS, Lin W (2015) Predicting standard-dose PET image from low-dose PET and multimodal MR images using mapping-based sparse representation. Phys Med Biol 61(2):791–801
36. Wang Y, Ma G, An L, Shi F, Zhang P, Wu X, Zhou J, Shen D (2016) Semi-supervised tripled dictionary learning for standard-dose PET image prediction using low-dose PET and multimodal MRI. IEEE Trans Biomed Eng 64(3):569–579
37. Wang Y, Yu B, Wang L, Zu C, Lalush DS, Lin W, Wu X, Zhou J, Shen D, Zhou L (2018) 3D conditional generative adversarial networks for high-quality PET image estimation at low dose. NeuroImage 174:550–562
38. Wang Y, Zhou L, Yu B, Wang L, Zu C, Lalush DS, Lin W, Wu X, Zhou J, Shen D (2019) 3D auto-context-based locality adaptive multi-modality GANs for PET synthesis. IEEE Trans Med Imaging 38(6):1328–1339
39. Wasserthal J, Meyer M, Breit H, Cyriac J, Yang S, Segeroth M (2022) Totalsegmentator: robust segmentation of 104 anatomical structures in CT images. arXiv preprint arXiv:220805868
40. Wu Y, He K (2018) Group normalization. In: Proceedings of the European conference on computer vision (ECCV), pp 3–19
41. Wu G, Jia H, Wang Q, Shen D (2011) SharpMean: groupwise registration guided by sharp mean image and tree-based registration. NeuroImage 56(4):1968–1981
42. Xiang L, Qiao Y, Nie D, An L, Lin W, Wang Q, Shen D (2017) Deep auto-context convolutional neural networks for standard-dose PET image estimation from low-dose PET/MRI. Neurocomputing 267(6):406–416

43. Xiang L, Wang L, Gong E, Zaharchuk G, Zhang T (2020) Noise-aware standard-dose PET reconstruction using general and adaptive robust loss. In: International workshop on machine learning in medical imaging, pp 654–662
44. Xiao J, Yu L, Xing L, Yuille A, Zhou Y (2021) DualNorm-UNet: incorporating global and local statistics for robust medical image segmentation. arXiv preprint arXiv:210315858
45. Zhang X, Xie Z, Berg E, Judenhofer MS, Liu W, Xu T, Ding Y, Lv Y, Dong Y, Deng Z (2020) Total-body dynamic reconstruction and parametric imaging on the uEXPLORER. J Nucl Med 61(2):285–291
46. Zhu JY, Park T, Isola P, Efros AA (2017) Unpaired image-to-image translation using cycle-consistent adversarial networks. In: Proceedings of the IEEE international conference on computer vision, pp 2223–2232

Chapter 12
EyesGAN: Synthesize Human Face from Human Eyes

Xiaodong Luo and Xiang Chen

Abstract Face recognition has achieved notable success across various domains, including mobile payment, authentication, criminal investigation, and urban management. Despite these advances, face occlusion remains a critical challenge in person identification, particularly in anti-terrorism efforts, criminal cases, and public security contexts. To address this issue, we introduce an enhanced deep generative adversarial network (EyesGAN) designed to synthesize human faces from eye images, offering a promising approach for masked face recognition. BicycleGAN is chosen as the baseline and effective improvements have been achieved. First, the self-attentional mechanism is introduced so that the improved model can more effectively learn about the internal mapping between human eyes and face. Second, the perceptual loss is applied to guide the model cyclic training and help with updating the network parameters so that the synthesized face can be of higher-similarity to the ground truth face. Third, EyesGAN has been designed by getting the utmost out of the performance of the perceptual loss and the self-attentional mechanism in GANs. To train and evaluate EyesGAN, we have reconstructed a dataset for eyes-to-face synthesis, leveraging public face datasets. The synthesized faces generated by EyesGAN have been rigorously compared with existing methods, both quantitatively and qualitatively. Extensive experiments demonstrate that our method outperforms state-of-the-art techniques across multiple metrics including Average Euclidean Distance, Average Cosine Similarity, Synthesis Accuracy Percentage, Fréchet Inception Distance. Notably, we achieved a Baidu face recognition rate of 96.1% on 615 test samples from the CelebA database. This study explores the feasibility of facial synthesis from eye images, with the attention map indicating that our network can accurately predict other facial regions based on the eyes alone. Furthermore, we extend our investigation to assess the performance of our

X. Luo (✉)
School of Information and Engineering, Sichuan Tourism University, Chengdu, China
e-mail: luoxd@sctu.edu.cn

X. Chen
College of Electrical and Information Engineering, Hunan University, Changsha, China
e-mail: xiangc@hnu.edu.cn

L. Zhang et al. (eds.), *Generative Machine Learning Models in Medical Image Computing*, https://doi.org/10.1007/978-3-031-80965-1_12

proposed method in the recovery of noisy X-ray images. Our approach successfully synthesizes high-quality images that demonstrate a high degree of consistency with the corresponding ground truth images, underscoring its potential for enhancing image quality in medical imaging applications.

12.1 Introduction

Over the past decades, face recognition technology has experienced a remarkable surge, permeating various sectors to address a multitude of practical challenges, such as mobile payments, authentication, and public security. Despite these advancements, the recognition of occluded faces remains a significant hurdle in the field. In real-world applications, particularly in counter-terrorism, criminal investigations, and public safety, the need to identify individuals wearing facial coverings is paramount. However, recognizing occluded faces is exceedingly challenging due to the limited visible information, typically restricted to the eyes and adjacent areas. To tackle this issue, researchers have integrated computer vision techniques into surveillance systems, offering tangible assistance for face recognition in occluded conditions. The typical approach to masked face recognition involves two stages: synthesizing a face from the visible information, followed by applying recognition algorithms to the synthesized image. Consequently, the efficacy of the face synthesis methodology is directly linked to the accuracy of masked face recognition. Like the majority of face synthesis techniques, our approach is fundamentally grounded in generative adversarial networks (GANs) [15]. To synthesize human faces from masked faces, extensive, high-quality datasets are essential. However, constructing a robust dataset of real masked faces is a formidable task, and no public database is available. In this paper, we propose a novel three-step process for masked face recognition. The initial phase involves extracting the human eyes from the masked face image. This is succeeded by the synthesis of the human face from the extracted eyes, and the final phase encompasses face recognition. The operational principle is depicted in Fig. 12.1.

The main work of this paper is to study the second step, and the datasets of eyes-to-face synthesis can be constructed based on the general face datasets. The human eye is one of the most distinctive features of the face, encapsulating a

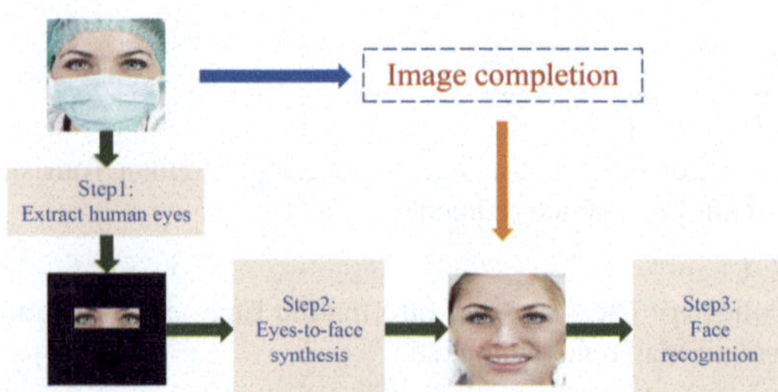

Fig. 12.1 A potential scheme for masked face recognition

wealth of unique characteristics. Zhou et al. [45] identified a comprehensive set of 68 facial landmarks, including detailed inner points for the eyes, eyebrows, mouth, and nose, totaling 51, and 17 contour points along the face's periphery. Notably, the eyes and eyebrows alone account for over 20 of these feature points. Because of the internal relational mapping between human eyes and the face, it is possible that a photorealistic face can be constructed based on the information of human eyes. The objective of eyes-to-face synthesis is to generate a facial image that aligns with the original at both the pixel level and within the semantic space—a challenging yet promising task. This process falls within the realms of face synthesis, image generation, and image translation. The GANs have garnered significant acclaim since their inception, particularly in the domains of image generation and translation. The majority of synthetic face research has concentrated on generating faces of varying ages, expressions, and hairstyles, and translating photos into face sketches.

In recent years, there has been a growing interest in the field of completing incomplete face images. The synthesis of faces from eye images represents an emerging research direction, fraught with technical hurdles that require innovative solutions. Chen et al. [6] were the pioneers in this space, developing a method to synthesize human faces from eye images, building upon the conditional GAN pix2pix framework proposed by Isola et al. [22]. However, there is still a discernible discrepancy between the synthesized faces and the ground truth, particularly in aspects such as age, expression, resolution, and semantic similarity. To surmount these obstacles, this study introduces a novel methodology designed to narrow the gap between synthetic and ground truth faces, advancing the state-of-the-art. This work provides a robust technical foundation for masked face recognition applications.

In this study, we have undertaken several innovative steps to achieve eyes-to-face synthesis. We have constructed a novel dataset tailored for this task, leveraging two publicly available face datasets, CelebA [25] and LFW [21], to facilitate model training and testing. Building upon the BicycleGAN framework [46] as our baseline network, we introduce several key enhancements. A pre-trained face feature extraction model, Resnet [18], is employed to extract feature vectors from both the synthetic face and the ground truth. The Euclidean Distance between these feature vectors is computed and incorporated into the total loss function as a perceptual loss. Drawing from recent successes in the application of self-attention mechanisms in GANs [29, 36, 41], which have significantly bolstered performance in image generation, we have designed a new end-to-end network, EyesGAN. This network fully exploits the self-attention mechanism to learn the internal connections between human eyes and the face, enabling the synthesis of high-quality faces in both pixel level and semantic space. To substantiate the superiority of our proposed network, the synthetic faces generated have been rigorously evaluated across three dimensions: pixel level, semantic space, and validity. Our results, benchmarked against existing methods, demonstrate that EyesGAN consistently produces high-quality images, achieving optimal scores across all four metrics. Furthermore, we have utilized the Baidu face recognition API (https://ai.baidu.com/tech/face/

compare) to evaluate the synthesized faces, providing additional evidence that our method generates faces with the highest similarity to the ground truth.

Overall, the main contributions of this paper are four aspects.

- In this work, an effective solution for face occlusion recognition has been explored, including three steps: eye extraction, eyes-to-face synthesis and face recognition.
- A new end-to-end deep generative adversarial network EyesGAN has been designed to synthesize the human face from human eyes, which takes advantage of the perceptual loss function and the self-attentional mechanism in GANs.
- Our evaluation demonstrates that EyesGAN outperforms existing methods across all metrics. Furthermore, we employ a real-world face recognition algorithm, the Baidu face recognition API, to assess the synthesized faces. Notably, EyesGAN achieves an accuracy of 96.10% on a test set of 615 images from the CelebA database, surpassing the performance of current methods and indicating its potential as a solution for face occlusion recognition.
- This work delves into the feasibility of human face synthesis from eye images. By analyzing the attention maps generated by our model, we reveal that EyesGAN can predict the remainder of the face, including features such as the nose, mouth, chin, age, and skin colour, based solely on the input of the eyes.

12.2 Related Work

The purpose of synthesizing human faces from human eyes is to explore a scheme of masked face recognition, which belongs to image inpainting, image translation or image generation. This work has benefited from these technological breakthroughs.

12.2.1 GAN-Based Image Generation

With the continuous development of the deep neural network, GANs are widely applied in the field of computer vision, which are usually composed of a generator and discriminator for training in an adversarial way, and can generate high-definition images [27, 28]. Although these algorithms can generate high-resolution images in pixel level, the synthesized images were random in semantic space. The purpose of image-to-image translation is to convert an image into another one or more with a particular target. Recently, significant achievements were made in the image-to-image translation [12, 42]. Because of the lack of datasets, most studies focused on unsupervised methods [9, 28]. Typically, the StarGAN proposed by Choi et al. [9] is a multi-domain unsupervised image transformation model, which can complete facial expression translation, face gender change, and hair colour change. Recently, a novel unsupervised Groupwise-Deep Whitening-and-Coloring

Transformation (GDWCT) [8] network was allowed end-to-end training in image translation for delivering esoteric style semantics. Besides, conditional GANs are also widely explored, and researchers have made significant achievements in the field of image translation. For instance, pix2pix proposed by Isola et al. [22] utilised the conditional GANs to construct the mapping equation between input and output images of multi-domain. BicycleGAN [46] was a hybrid model based on the conditional GANs, which combined advantages of cVAE-GAN [23, 24] and cLR-GAN [13, 14] to learn a multi-modal mapping between two image domains.

12.2.2 Face Recognition

Recently, face recognition technology has been rapidly developed and applied to solve many practical problems. For example, Wang et al. [37] proposed a feature augmentation method termed Large Margin Feature Augmentation (LMFA) to improve the face recognition rate effectively. Deng et al. [11] designed Additive Angular Margin Loss (ArcFace) to obtain highly discriminative features for face recognition, which required negligible computational overhead. Abudarham et al. [1] found the critical features for which humans had high perceptual sensitivity to detect differences between different identities. Goswami et al. [16] studied three aspects related to the robustness of DNNs for face recognition. Other researchers have also made major breakthroughs in face recognition and graphic recognition [44]. Till now, these research mainly focused on unshaded face recognition, and the authors promoted the improvement of face recognition accuracy from different angles. In practical applications, face occlusion recognition is a challenging task for us. Cao et al. [5] proposed a new face recognition method based on RPCA and facial symmetry to provide a solution for face occlusion recognition. Chen et al. [7] proposed the nuclear norm-based matrix regression method to recover low-rank error images in the presence of severe occlusion and illumination changes. Song et al. [35] designed a mask learning strategy to find and discard corrupted feature elements from recognition, which can effectively solve the partial occlusion of face recognition. These schemes are effective at partial face occlusion recognition, but not for masked face recognition. Therefore, synthesizing photorealistic human faces from human eyes can provide more effective technical support for masked face recognition than existing methods.

12.2.3 Face Synthesis

In recent years, significant breakthroughs have been made in the field of computer vision, drawing increasing numbers of researchers to the area of face synthesis. Generally, the research community has concentrated on three principal areas. The first of these is face completion. The methods realized the recovery of local face occlusion, and the quality of synthetic face was also improved [17, 33]. For example, Wang et al. [38] proposed a deep generative adversarial network with a Laplacian pyramid mechanism, that recover the spatial information of missing face regions in a coarse-to-fine manner. The second is facial style transfer, such as expression changes, posture changes, hair colour changes and face sketch image generation [26, 40]. Zhao et al. [43] designed a Dual-Agent Generative Adversarial Network (DA-GAN) model to synthesize the realistic profile face from the front face. Bao et al. [3] proposed a new GAN to recombine different identities and attributes for identity-preserving face synthesis in open domains. The third is face attribute editing. For example, TraVeLGAN [2] based on preserving intra-domain vector transformations in a potential space learned with a siamese network, which can successfully realize the wearing and removing of hats, glasses and other ornaments. There is no doubt that recent studies have addressed key challenges in the realm of face synthesis. However, existing models typically operate on full-pixel-sized input and output face images, focusing primarily on partial face occlusion scenarios. Furthermore, they fall short when it comes to the task of facial recovery using only the eye region. Consequently, these methods cannot effectively synthesize a human face that closely resembles the ground truth based solely on the information available from the eyes.

12.3 Method

This section provides a comprehensive overview of our proposed methodology. Synthesizing a face from eye images is to generate a photorealistic facial representation that closely resembles the ground truth. To achieve this, we introduce an end-to-end architectural framework designed to synthesize a human face image Y^i base on eyes image X_A^i, by forming a mapping function $G(x)$, which can synthesize the corresponding faces from given human eye images, formulated as Eq. 12.1:

$$Y^i = G\left(X_A^i\right). \tag{12.1}$$

In this work, an improved GANs has been proposed to realize such a mapping function $G(x)$. To train such a network, the pairs of human eyes and corresponding ground truth face image $\left\{X_A^i, X_B^i\right\}$ are set as input, Y^i is set as output, X_B^i is set as ground truth face. Both the input X_A^i and output Y^i come from pixel level and semantic space. The network's parameters θ_G have been optimized by minimizing a specifically designed synthesis loss L_{gn}. For the training datasets with N training pairs of $\left\{X_A^i, X_B^i\right\}$, the optimization problem can be formulated as Eq. 12.2:

$$\hat{\theta}_G = \arg\min_{\theta_G} \sum_{n=1}^{N} L_{gn}\left(G_{\theta_G}\left(X_A^n\right), X_B^n\right), \tag{12.2}$$

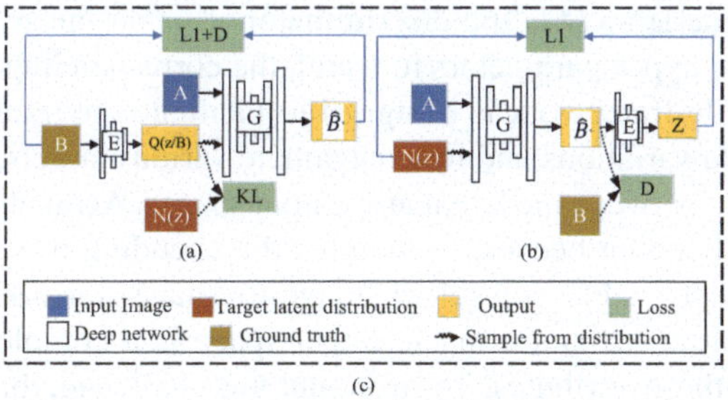

Fig. 12.2 BicycleGAN architecture, (**a**) cVAE-GAN started from a ground truth image B and encoded it into the latent space. The generator then attempted to map the input image A along with a sampled z back into the ground truth image B. (**b**) cLR-GAN randomly sampled a latent code from a known distribution, used it to map A into the output $\hat{B}$, and then tried to reconstruct the latent code from the output. (**c**) The BicycleGAN method combined constraints in both directions

where L_{gn} is defined as a weighted sum of several losses that jointly constrain an image to reside in the desired manifold. In the following parts, we describe these loss functions and the proposed model in detail.

12.3.1 Baseline: BicycleGAN ($B \rightarrow z \rightarrow \hat{B}$ and $z \rightarrow \hat{B} \rightarrow \hat{z}$)

BicycleGAN initially proposed by Zhu et al. [46] shows high-quality results in the image-to-image translation setting, learning a multi-modal mapping between two image domains. BicycleGAN combined with Conditional Variational Autoencoder GAN (cVAE-GAN) and Conditional Latent Regressor GAN (cLR-GAN) [22, 24] objectives in a hybrid model, the formulation was illustrated in Fig. 12.2. (a) cVAE-GAN forced the latent code z to directly map the ground truth B to it which used an encoding function E. The generator G then used both the latent code z and the input image A to synthesize the desired output $\hat{B}$. The distribution $Q(z/B)$ of latent code z used by the encoder E was a Gaussian assumption. (b) cLR-GAN started from a randomly drawn latent code z and recovered it with $\hat{z} = E(G(A, z))$, which enforced the generator G to utilize the latent code embedding z, while stayed close to the actual test time distribution $p(z)$. The encoder E here produced a point estimate for $\hat{z}$ not a Gaussian distribution. (c) BicycleGAN combined constraints in both directions.

BicycleGAN was proposed to train with constraints in both directions, aiming to take advantage of both cycles $B \rightarrow z \rightarrow \hat{B}$ and $z \rightarrow \hat{B} \rightarrow \hat{z}$. The total loss function is described as Eq. 12.3:

$$\begin{aligned} G^*, E^* = \arg\min_{G,E}\max_{D} \mathcal{L}_{GAN}^{VAE}(G, D, E) + \lambda_1 \mathcal{L}_1^{VAE}(G, E) \\ + \mathcal{L}_{GAN}(G, D) + \lambda_{\text{latent}} \mathcal{L}_1^{\text{latent}}(G, E) + \lambda_{KL} \mathcal{L}_{KL}(E) \end{aligned}, \tag{12.3}$$

where G is the generator, D is the discriminator, E is an image encoder, $\mathcal{L}$ is the loss function, λ are hyper-parameters to weigh the corresponding losses.

The BicycleGAN framework is designed to facilitate the translation of a single image into multiple variations and to amalgamate various targets, thereby fostering a bijective mapping between the latent and output spaces. Achieving such a mapping is particularly challenging because it requires the encoding of semantically meaningful attributes that enable controlled image-to-image transformations. Directly enforcing a specific distribution in the latent space is a complex task due to the intricate nature of these attributes. To surmount this challenge, this study introduces a novel approach that harnesses the self-attention mechanism to encode the latent information, thereby driving the synthesis of a single object image.

12.3.2 Proposed Framework

The framework of our proposed approach is shown in Fig. 12.3. To synthesize a photorealistic human face from eyes, a new GAN is proposed, containing two generators which share the training parameters.

G_1 **Model** The G_1 generator based on cLR-GAN. The latent code embedding z is utilized by the generator network to stay close to the actual test time distribution p(z). The noise vector $N(z)$ starts from a randomly drawn underlying code z and attempts to recover it with $\hat{z} = E(G(A, z))$. Note that $\hat{z}$ produced by the encoder E is an estimate function rather than a distribution. Particularly, the residual network

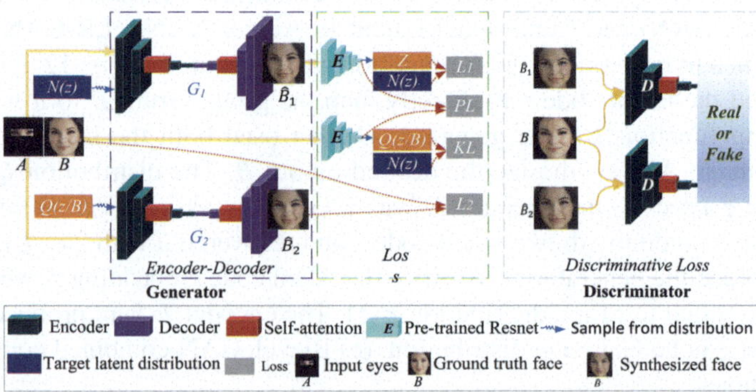

Fig. 12.3 Overview of proposed model. (1) Eye image A is simultaneously input into two generators for encoding and decoding, both G_1 and G_2 models have shared training parameters. (2) In encoder-decoder network, the self-attention mechanism is added to extract attention feature map. (3) G_2 starts from a ground truth image B and encode it into the latent space. The generator then attempts to map the input image A along with a sampled z back into the original image B. G_1 randomly samples a latent code from a known distribution $N(z)$, uses it to map A into the output $\hat{B}$, and then tries to reconstruct the latent code from the output. (4) Proposed model combines the constraints in perceptual loss and attention map

proposed by He et al. [18] is used as the encoder E to translate the image into the feature vectors effectively. The discriminator loss $L_{1GAN}(G, D)$ on $\hat{B}$ is used to facilitate the network to synthesize photorealistic faces. The loss functions are expressed as Eq. 12.4 and Eq. 12.5, respectively,

$$L_1(G, E) = \mathbb{E}_{A \sim P(A), Z \sim P(Z)} \|z - E(G(A, z))\|_1, \tag{12.4}$$

$$G^*, E^* = \arg\min_{G,E} \max_{D} L_{1GAN}(G, D) + \lambda_1 L_1(G, E). \tag{12.5}$$

G_2 Model The G_2 generator based on cVAE-GAN, which has used both the distribution $Q(z/B)$ of latent code z by the encoder E and the input eyes A to synthesize the desired output face $\hat{B}$. This model can be easily understood as the reconstruction of ground truth faces B, the latent encode $Q(z/B)$ is encoded with B as a prior condition and the A combine to guide the mode training in pairs, and expect the output face $\hat{B}$ close to ground truth face B. This scheme is similar to an autoencoder [20]. As a conditional scenario, the distribution $Q(z/B)$ of latent code z is no longer an estimate but a Gaussian assumption [46], $Q(z/B) \triangleq E(B)$. During model hyper-parametric training, sampling $z \sim E(B)$ is allowed to be directly back-propagation [23]. The G_2 GAN loss can be shown as Eq. 12.6:

$$\begin{aligned} L_{2GAN} =& \mathbb{E}_{A,B \sim P(A,B)}[\log(D(A, B))]+ \\ & \mathbb{E}_{A,B \sim P(A,B), z \sim E(B)}[\log(1 - D(A, G(A, z)))] \end{aligned}, \tag{12.6}$$

$L_2(G)$ loss is also added to make the reconstructed face image $\hat{B}$ close to ground truth face image B on the pixel level, the value is given as Eq. 12.7:

$$L_2(G) = \mathbb{E}_{A,B \sim P(A,B), z \sim E(B)} \|B - G(A, z)\|_1, \tag{12.7}$$

further, the distribution $Q(z/B)$ of latent code z by $E(B)$ is encouraged to approach a random Gaussian distribution $N(z)$ to enable sampling at inference time. The KL loss function is given as Eq. 12.8:

$$L_{KL}(E) = \mathbb{E}_{B \sim p(B)} [\mathcal{D}_{KL}(E(B) \| \mathcal{N}(0, I))], \tag{12.8}$$

where $\mathcal{D}_{KL}(p\|q) = -\int p(z) \log \frac{p(\mathcal{Z})}{q(\mathcal{Z})} d\mathcal{Z}$. L_{2GAN}, L_2, L_{KL} are weighted together formed the synthesis loss function, a conditional version of the VAE-GAN [24, 46] is given as Eq. 12.9:

$$G^*, E^* = \arg\min_{G,E} \max_{D} L_{2GAN}(G, D, E) + \lambda_2 L_2(G, E) + \lambda_{KL} L_{KL}(E) \quad . \tag{12.9}$$

Proposed Generator Model A growing body of research has demonstrated the effectiveness of integrating self-attention mechanisms into GANs to enhance their performance. The self-attention mechanism is particularly adept at assessing the relevance of different positions within a sequence by considering the entire sequence, as illustrated in [29]. Parmar et al. [30] incorporated self-attention into an image transformer for image generation, setting new benchmarks for the state-of-the-art. In a similar vein, Zhang et al. [41] introduced the SAGAN, which integrates self-attention between convolutional layers within the generator. Self-attention mechanism GANs excel at identifying both global and long-term dependencies within the internal representations of images, providing a more nuanced and comprehensive approach to image generation and synthesis.

BicycleGAN [46] and pix2pix [22] models shown high-quality results in image-to-image translation. Chen et al. [6] proposed a GAN model which made a breakthrough in the task of synthesizing the human face from the eyes. These methods all used the traditional convolutional U-net [31] as the generator. Traditional convolutional GANs generate high-resolution details by relying solely on spatially local points within lower-resolution feature maps. This approach, while effective, can be limited in capturing long-range dependencies within the data. In contrast, the self-attention mechanism offers a superior balance for modelling these long-range dependencies. It maintains computational efficiency and statistical effectiveness, generating a response at a given position as a weighted sum of features across all positions. The weights, or attention vectors, are determined with minimal computational overhead. In this study, we have integrated the self-attention mechanism [41] into our encoder-decoder framework, specifically calculating the self-attention map between two convolutional layers of the U-net architecture. The enhanced generator framework is depicted in Fig. 12.4. The self-attention module is a supplement to convolutions, helping to establish long-term, multi-level dependencies between adjacent regions of the image. By introducing this mechanism, our network can effectively find global and long-term dependence in the internal representation of the face, which can facilitate generators to synthesize more a photorealistic face.

In the proposed generator architecture, the self-attention mechanism is shown in Fig. 12.5.

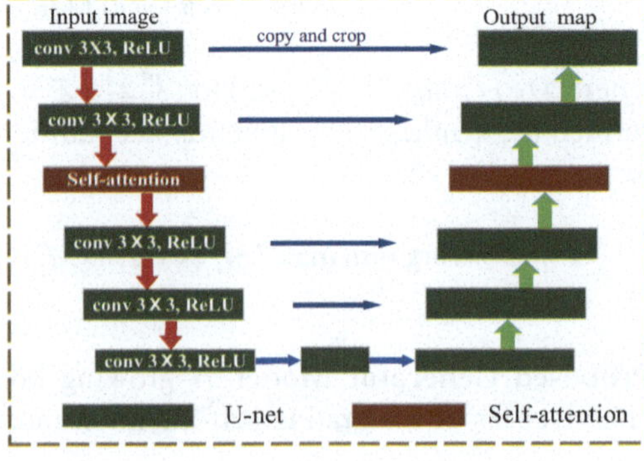

Fig. 12.4 The proposed generator architecture

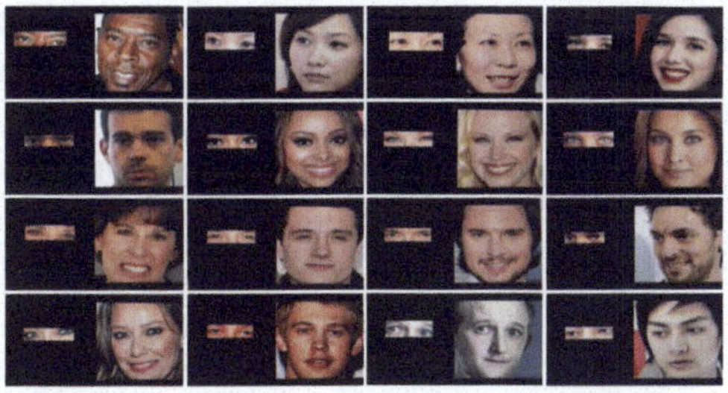

Fig. 12.5 Samples of eyes-to-face datasets. The size of each data pair image is 512 × 256 pixels, the left of each image is eyes A and the right is the corresponding ground truth human face B

The feature vectors of the image from the previous hidden layer $x \in \mathbb{R}^{c\times N}$ are transformed into three feature spaces f, g, h to calculate the attention map, where $f(x) = W_f x, g(x) = W_g x, h(x) = W_h x$. First, $f(x), g(x)$ matrix multiplication are made to calculate a feature map $\beta_{j,i}$ as in Eq. 12.10:

$$\beta_{j,i} = \frac{\exp\left(s_{ij}\right)}{\sum_{i=1}^{N} \exp\left(s_{ij}\right)}, s_{ij} = f\left(x_i\right)^T g\left(x_j\right), \tag{12.10}$$

where $\beta_{j,i}$ indicates the extent to which the model attends to the ith location when synthesizing the jth region. Then the output of the attention layer is $o = \left(o_1, o_2, o_3, \ldots, o_j, \ldots, o_N\right) \in \mathbb{R}^{C\times N}$ as Eq. 12.11:

$$o_j = \sum_{i=1}^{N} \beta_{j,i} h_{(x_i)}, \tag{12.11}$$

in the above formulation, $W_f \in \mathbb{R}^{\bar{C}\times C}$, $W_g \in \mathbb{R}^{\bar{C}\times C}$, $W_h \in \mathbb{R}^{C\times C}$ are the learned weight matrices, they are implemented as 1×1 convolutions. To match the convolution layer, $\bar{C} = C/8$ is used in this experiment.

Besides, the output of the attention layer o multiplies by a scale parameter β and adds the feature vectors x of the previous convolutional layer to form the output y, and y is as an input of the following convolution layer. y is given as Eq. 12.12:

$$y = \beta o + x, \tag{12.12}$$

where β is initialized as 0. Experimental results show that this scheme is effective in the task of human face synthesis.

Proposed Perceptual Loss Function Unlike style transfer [8] and multi-domain image translation [9, 46], the eyes-to-face synthesis is more concerned about the consistency and similarity between the synthesized face and the ground truth. Chen et al. [6] used a pre-trained VGG19 model [34] to extract the feature of the synthesized face and ground truth, and then calculated the loss of every feature maps between them. The VGG19 model is adept at linearizing the manifold of the original image into a subspace within the global Euclidean depth feature space [4].

In this work, a pre-trained Resnet model [18] has been used to extract feature vectors pertaining to the synthesized and ground truth human faces. We then calculate the Euclidean Distance between these vectors, with the resulting value being fed back to the generator as the perceptual loss. Our experimental results indicate that the pre-trained Resnet model outperforms the pre-trained VGG19 in the extraction of facial features, such as eyes, eyebrows, nose, mouth, age, and contour. This superiority can be attributed to the fact that the pre-trained Resnet has been specifically trained on the large-scale face recognition dataset CASIA-WebFace [39], which is specialized for face recognition tasks. In contrast, the pre-trained VGG19 model has been trained to extract general image features and is commonly used for image classification tasks. The perceptual loss function of feature maps between synthesis face and ground truth is shown as Eq. 12.13:

$$PL\left(E_{PR}\right) = \mathbb{E}_{\widehat{B},B\sim P(\widehat{B},B)} \left\| E_{PR}(\widehat{B}) - E_{PR}(B) \right\|_2 , \tag{12.13}$$

where $E_{PR}(\widehat{B})$ and $E_{PR}(B)$ represent the feature maps of the synthesized face and the ground truth face outputs by the pre-trained Resnet model, respectively.

Proposed Total Loss Function As mentioned above, the final loss function proposed in this paper can be expressed as Eq. 12.14:

$$\begin{aligned} L_{gn} = \arg \min_{G,E} \max_{D} & L_{1GAN}(G, D) + L_{2GAN}(G, D, E) \\ & + \lambda_1 L_1(G, E) + \lambda_2 L_2(G, E) \\ & + \lambda_{KL} L_{KL}(E) + \lambda_{PL} PL\left(E_{PR}\right), \end{aligned} \tag{12.14}$$

where the hyper-parameters λ_1, λ_2, λ_{KL} and λ_{PL} are the weights of each part, which is to be decided in the experiments. They can be dynamically adapted to different mission objectives. The values of these hyper-parameters require abundant experiments to excavate.

12.4 Experiments and Discussion

12.4.1 Datasets

To accomplish the task of synthesizing photorealistic human faces from eye images, our proposed EyesGAN model necessitates appropriate dataset training. In this study, we have constructed an eyes-to-face synthesis dataset leveraging two well-known face datasets: CelebA [25] and LFW [21]. The construction process is outlined as follows: First, the size of the original face image should be reshaped as 256×256, and the normalized face images are taken as the ground truth face B. Second, the human eyes in the face is detected, and replace the RGB information of the face except for the eyes with black, then the image of only eyes A can be obtained. Third, the eyes image A and ground truth image B combine in left-to-right order to form a size of 512×256 data image, the examples of the database are shown in Fig. 12.5. These paired datasets form a novel collection for eyes-to-face synthesis. In total, 20,150 eyes-to-face image pairs have been assembled, comprising 6730 pairs from the LFW dataset, 13,220 pairs from the CelebA dataset, and an additional 200 pairs sourced from publicly available online resources. In the experimental design of this work, 12,605 image pairs from CelebA have been designated as the training dataset, with the remaining 615 CelebA pairs and all 6730 LFW pairs selected as the test datasets. The faces in this new dataset exhibit a diverse range of characteristics, including various skin colours, genders, facial expressions, ages, poses, and resolutions.

12.4.2 Experimental Design

Prior to training the proposed model, it is essential to establish the hyper-parameters for the total loss function with fixed values. Extensive experimental validation has indicated that setting the hyper-parameters to $\lambda_1 = 1.0$, $\lambda_2 = 0.5$, $\lambda_{KL} = 1.0$ and $\lambda_{PL} = 0.2$, yields superior performance for our model. The initial learning rate for both the generator and discriminator is configured at 0.0002. Furthermore, the computational requirements for our model necessitate a GPU setup that is at least on par with a GTX1080Ti. The model presented in this paper was trained utilizing a batch size of 16 over 300 epochs, employing the PyTorch framework.

12.4.3 Qualitative Evaluation

The objective of eyes-to-face synthesis is to generate synthetic human faces that closely approximate the ground truth across multiple dimensions, including pixel accuracy, gender, age, skin colour, and facial features. In accordance with the experimental procedures outlined previously, the results of our study have been compared with those of state-of-the-art methods. A qualitative comparative analysis of the results is presented in Fig. 12.6, offering a visual representation of the performance of different algorithms in the context of eyes-to-face synthesis.

The experimental outcomes demonstrate that the BicycleGAN's performance in the task of eyes-to-face synthesis is suboptimal. The generated faces exhibit a lower degree of similarity to the ground truth, with some images displaying blurring and a lack of clarity in defining facial features, such as the nose and mouth. BicycleGAN, originally designed for one-to-many image translation tasks, excels in generating multiple target outputs. However, it shows limited capability in capturing the intricate internal mapping between human eyes and the overall facial structure when tasked with generating a human face from eye images alone.

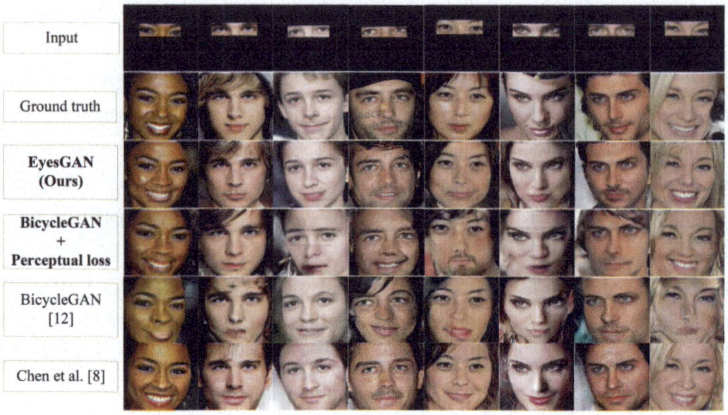

Fig. 12.6 Comparison of different algorithms to synthesize the human faces from the human eyes

When the perceptual loss function $PL\,(E_{PR})$ is added into BicycleGAN to guide the training, the quality of the generated images is improved. Obviously, they are almost the same as that of Chen et al. [6]. This consequence shows that it is useful to add the perceptual loss function to the primary network.

The results indicate that EyesGAN outperforms other algorithms in synthesizing high-quality human faces, particularly in the rendering of fine details. EyesGAN demonstrates its capability to generate more realistic faces that closely resemble the ground truth across various attributes, including image resolution, age, facial expression, and head posture. The comparative analysis of the experimental outcomes suggests that EyesGAN effectively captures the mapping relationship between human eyes and facial features.

Synthetic Face Analysis on CelebA

The proposed method underwent rigorous verification on the test set from CelebA. To comprehensively demonstrate the performance of EyesGAN, this study selected human eye images varying in age, skin colour, and gender as inputs to evaluate the synthesized facial outputs. The experimental results are illustrated in Fig. 12.7. While the synthesized faces do not precisely replicate the ground truth faces, they exhibit a high degree of resemblance, encompassing facial expressions, gender characteristics, skin colouration, head orientation, and features such as the nose and mouth. The synthesized faces are remarkably photorealistic, closely mirroring the original images in both pixel-level detail and semantic attributes.

Extensive experimental results have demonstrated that the quality of synthesized faces on both the LFW and CelebA datasets is predominantly influenced by the quality of the input human eye images and the richness of the information they contain. In general, the synthesis of a high-definition face is contingent upon the use of high-resolution eye images. The integrity and completeness of the eye information are instrumental in producing a generated face that closely resembles

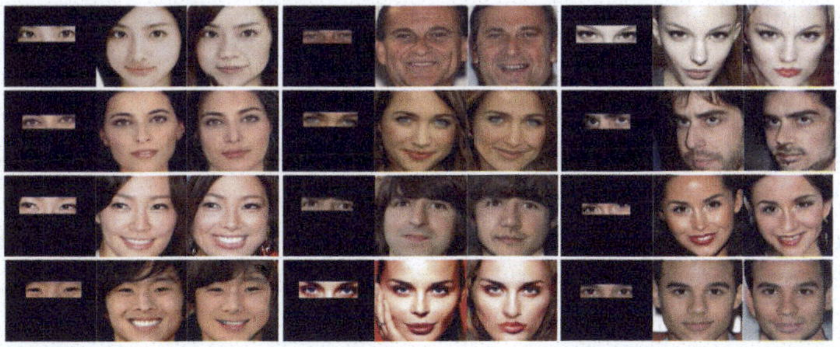

Fig. 12.7 Samples of synthesized faces on CelebA. For each set of samples, the left column is input eyes, the middle column is ground truth, and the right column is synthetic face. The faces are of different genders, ages, skin tones, facial expressions, postures

the ground truth. Our EyesGAN model, when trained on one dataset, such as CelebA, exhibits the capacity to perform effectively on other datasets, including LFW. This capability underscores the generalization and robustness of EyesGAN, highlighting its ability to adapt and provide reliable performance across varied datasets.

12.4.4 Quantitative Evaluation

To underscore the advanced nature of EyesGAN, we have conducted comparative analyses with state-of-the-art methods [6, 46]. Building upon the evaluation criteria proposed by Chen et al. [6], this study introduces three additional metrics to assess the quality of synthesized faces: the FID, verification through the Baidu face recognition API, and the computational time required for face synthesis. The quality of the synthesized faces is quantitatively evaluated from the following four aspects.

Euclidean Distance (ED) For facial images, even small pose variations from the same person would lead to significant differences in the pixels. Consequently, directly calculating the ED between the pixels of synthesized and ground truth faces to assess their consistency is not a valid approach. In this work, we have utilized a pre-trained face recognition model, ResNet, to extract 128-byte feature vectors from both the synthesized and original faces. The ED of these vectors is then computed to provide a quantitative evaluation of the synthesized faces.

Cosine Similarity (CS) Cosine Similarity (CS) measures the cosine of the angle between two vectors, providing a metric to assess the similarity between them. The value of CS ranges from 0 to 1, where a higher cosine value indicates greater similarity, reflecting a smaller angular difference between the vectors. Inspired by the concepts presented in previous works [6], we employ a pre-trained face recognition model, ResNet, to extract 128-byte feature vectors from both the synthesized and original faces.

Synthesis Accuracy Percentage (SAP) Drawing upon the principles established by FaceNet [32], the ED is utilized as a foundational measure for face recognition, with a threshold set at 1.1.

Fréchet Inception Distance (FID) The Fréchet Inception Distance (FID), introduced by Heusel et al. [19], is a metric designed to assess the similarity between generated images and their original counterparts.

Consequently, the four proposed criteria—Average Euclidean Distance (AED), Average Cosine Similarity (ACS), Synthesis Accuracy Percentage (SAP), and Fréchet Inception Distance (FID)—are subjected to a final averaging calculation. The experiments were conducted using test datasets derived from CelebA, comprising 615 test samples, and LFW, comprising 6730 test samples.

To substantiate the stability and generalization capabilities of EyesGAN, we conducted comparative experiments with other state-of-the-art algorithms on the LFW test set, which comprises 6730 test samples. The outcomes of these experiments for each algorithm are detailed in Table 12.1. The analysis of the results leads to the conclusion that our proposed EyesGAN method outperforms other algorithms across all four evaluation metrics.

Baidu Face Recognition API Furthermore, we conducted an evaluation using a contemporary face recognition technology, the Baidu face recognition API. This assessment was applied to 615 test faces based on the CelebA dataset. We compared the recognition scores, recognition rates, average scores, as well as the lowest and highest scores against existing methods. The comparative results are presented in Table 12.2.

Table 12.1 The comparison results of different algorithms on CelebA (615 test data) and LFW (6730 test data)

Evaluation indicators	AED ↓	ACS ↑	SAP ↑	FID ↓
CelebA				
BicycleGAN [46]	0.9094	78.55%	85.53%	24.55
BicycleGAN+Perceptual loss (PL)	0.8300	82.01%	93.33%	25.32
Chen et al. [6]	0.8002	83.26%	95.29%	22.04
EyesGAN(ours)	**0.7547**	**85.14%**	**98.04%**	**20.51**
LFW				
BicycleGAN [46]	0.9954	74.57%	60.86%	34.93
BicycleGAN+Perceptual loss (PL)	0.9300	77.00%	83.36%	27.37
Chen et al. [6]	0.8686	80.51%	91.87%	26.67
EyesGAN(ours)	**0.8493**	**81.38%**	**94.19%**	**26.53**

The bold values denote the best performance over the rest results

Table 12.2 Authentication results comparison by Baidu face recognition algorithm (API) on the CelebA (615 test data)

Evaluation indicators	Lowest score	Highest score	Average score	Face recognition rate
BicycleGAN [46]	4.54	95.38	73.88	20.30%
BicycleGAN+Perceptual loss (PL)	7.55	97.97	90.57	85.40%
Chen et al. [6]	32.43	96.51	84.40	64.07%
EyesGAN(ours)	**65.32**	**98.73**	**94.21**	**96.10%**

The bold values denote the best performance over the rest results

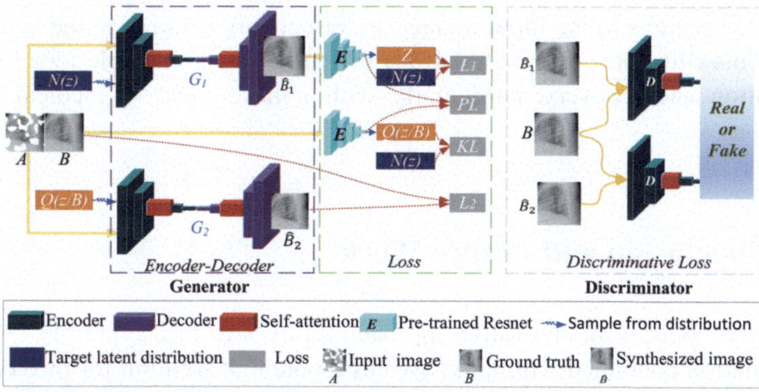

Fig. 12.8 Extension of the proposed method to X-ray images

Both qualitative and quantitative evaluation results show that EyesGAN can synthesize high-quality faces from human eyes, which exceeds the currently optimal results, and provide a potentially effective solution for face occlusion recognition.

12.4.5 Extension of Our Approach on Medical Images

The methodologies developed for image completion from limited regions are equally applicable to medical imaging scenarios. To further assess the efficacy of our proposed method, we selected X-ray images from the Open-i dataset [10] for the task of image completion. To address potential issues with corrupted images, we introduced random occlusions in certain regions of the original images. These noisy images were then utilized as inputs for the image completion process, with corresponding adjustments made to the network as depicted in Fig. 12.8. The outcomes of the X-ray image completion task are detailed in Fig. 12.9. The results demonstrate that our proposed method is capable of predicting high-quality images that exhibit a high degree of consistency with the ground truth images. Notably,

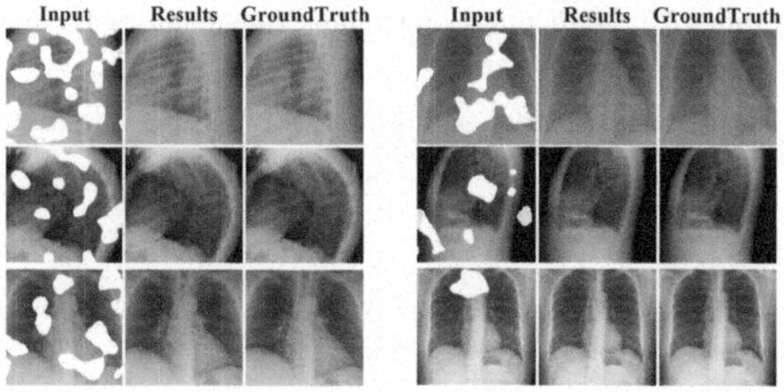

Fig. 12.9 Synthesised images from noisy X-ray images, using our proposed method

the occluded regions in the input images are effectively restored in the synthesized outputs. This illustrates the potential of our method as a valuable tool for image augmentation and recovery, particularly within the context of medical imaging applications.

12.5 Conclusion and Future Work

This study introduces an innovative approach for eyes-to-face synthesis, leveraging the information contained within the eyes as a potential solution for face occlusion recognition. To address this challenge, we have designed EyesGAN, an end-to-end deep neural network that incorporates an enhanced perceptual loss function and a self-attention mechanism to guide the training of the generator. Our experimental results indicate that our proposed method surpasses existing optimal methods across four key evaluation metrics. The faces synthesized by EyesGAN exhibit greater realism compared to those generated by existing methods. Furthermore, we employed the Baidu face recognition API, a real-world face recognition algorithm, to assess the synthesized faces. Our model achieved a higher recognition accuracy, demonstrating its effectiveness. Additionally, the experimental results of our model performance analysis confirm that the proposed network possesses high stability. We have also explored the application of our method in medical imaging scenarios, yielding promising results that highlight the method's efficiency and potential as an image augmentation tool and for image recovery.

While EyesGAN has exhibited remarkable capabilities in part-to-whole synthesis, there are specific scenarios where the quality of the generated images does not meet the highest standards, especially when the input region's information is of low clarity. These challenges underscore the need for future enhancements, particularly in improving the resolution and fidelity of the generated images. Addressing these aspects is crucial for ensuring that the technology can be seamlessly integrated into practical applications and deliver reliable results across various conditions.

References

1. Abudarham N, Shkiller L, Yovel G (2019) Critical features for face recognition. Cognition 182:73–83
2. Amodio M, Krishnaswamy S (2019) TraVeLGAN: image-to-image translation by transformation vector learning. In: Proceedings of the IEEE conference on computer vision and pattern recognition, pp 8983–8992
3. Bao J, Chen D, Wen F, Li H, Hua G (2018) Towards open-set identity preserving face synthesis. In: Proceedings of the IEEE conference on computer vision and pattern recognition, pp 6713–6722
4. Bengio Y, Mesnil G, Dauphin Y, Rifai S (2013) Better mixing via deep representations. In: International conference on machine learning, pp 552–560
5. Cao L, Li H, Guo H, Wang B (2019) Robust pca for face recognition with occlusion using symmetry information. In: 2019 IEEE 16th international conference on networking, sensing and control (ICNSC). IEEE, pp 323–328
6. Chen X, Qing L, He X, Su J, Peng Y (2018) From eyes to face synthesis: a new approach for human-centered smart surveillance. IEEE Access 6:14567–14575
7. Chen Z, Wu XJ, Kittler J (2019) A sparse regularized nuclear norm based matrix regression for face recognition with contiguous occlusion. Pattern Recognit Lett 125:494–499
8. Cho W, Choi S, Park DK, Shin I, Choo J (2019) Image-to-image translation via group-wise deep whitening-and-coloring transformation. In: Proceedings of the IEEE conference on computer vision and pattern recognition, pp 10639–10647
9. Choi Y, Choi M, Kim M, Ha JW, Kim S, Choo J (2018) Stargan: unified generative adversarial networks for multi-domain image-to-image translation. In: Proceedings of the IEEE conference on computer vision and pattern recognition, pp 8789–8797
10. Demner-Fushman D, Kohli MD, Rosenman MB, Shooshan SE, Rodriguez L, Antani S, Thoma GR, McDonald CJ (2016) Preparing a collection of radiology examinations for distribution and retrieval. J Am Med Inform Assoc 23(2):304–310
11. Deng J, Guo J, Xue N, Zafeiriou S (2019) Arcface: additive angular margin loss for deep face recognition. In: Proceedings of the IEEE conference on computer vision and pattern recognition, pp 4690–4699
12. Deshpande A, Lu J, Yeh MC, Jin Chong M, Forsyth D (2017) Learning diverse image colorization. In: Proceedings of the IEEE conference on computer vision and pattern recognition, pp 6837–6845
13. Donahue J, Krähenbühl P, Darrell T (2016) Adversarial feature learning. arXiv preprint arXiv:160509782
14. Dumoulin V, Belghazi I, Poole B, Mastropietro O, Lamb A, Arjovsky M, Courville A (2016) Adversarially learned inference. arXiv preprint arXiv:160600704
15. Goodfellow I, Pouget-Abadie J, Mirza M, Xu B, Warde-Farley D, Ozair S, Courville A, Bengio Y (2014) Generative adversarial nets. In: Advances in neural information processing systems, pp 2672–2680
16. Goswami G, Agarwal A, Ratha N, Singh R, Vatsa M (2019) Detecting and mitigating adversarial perturbations for robust face recognition. Int J Comput Vis 127(6–7):719–742
17. Han X, Liu Y, Yang H, Xing G, Zhang Y (2020) Normalization of face illumination with photorealistic texture via deep image prior synthesis. Neurocomputing 386:305–316
18. He K, Zhang X, Ren S, Sun J (2016) Deep residual learning for image recognition. In: Proceedings of the IEEE conference on computer vision and pattern recognition, pp 770–778
19. Heusel M, Ramsauer H, Unterthiner T, Nessler B, Hochreiter S (2017) GANs trained by a two time-scale update rule converge to a local Nash equilibrium. In: Advances in neural information processing systems, pp 6626–6637
20. Hinton GE, Salakhutdinov RR (2006) Reducing the dimensionality of data with neural networks. Science 313(5786):504–507

21. Huang GB, Mattar M, Berg T, Learned-Miller E (2008) Labeled faces in the wild: a database forstudying face recognition in unconstrained environments. Workshop on faces in'Real-Life'Images: detection, alignment, and recognition
22. Isola P, Zhu JY, Zhou T, Efros AA (2017) Image-to-image translation with conditional adversarial networks. In: Proceedings of the IEEE conference on computer vision and pattern recognition, pp 1125–1134
23. Kingma DP, Welling M (2013) Auto-encoding variational bayes. arXiv preprint arXiv:13126114
24. Larsen ABL, Sønderby SK, Larochelle H, Winther O (2015) Autoencoding beyond pixels using a learned similarity metric. arXiv preprint arXiv:151209300
25. Liu Z, Luo P, Wang X, Tang X (2018) Large-scale celebfaces attributes (celeba) dataset. Retrieved 15 Aug 2018
26. Ma D, Liu B, Kang Z, Zhou J, Zhu J, Xu Z (2019) Two birds with one stone: transforming and generating facial images with iterative GAN. Neurocomputing 396:278–290
27. Ma L, Jia X, Georgoulis S, Tuytelaars T, Van Gool L (2018) Exemplar guided unsupervised image-to-image translation with semantic consistency. arXiv preprint arXiv:180511145
28. Mirza M, Osindero S (2014) Conditional generative adversarial nets. arXiv preprint arXiv:14111784
29. Parikh AP, Täckström O, Das D, Uszkoreit J (2016) A decomposable attention model for natural language inference. arXiv preprint arXiv:160601933
30. Parmar N, Vaswani A, Uszkoreit J, Kaiser Ł, Shazeer N, Ku A, Tran D (2018) Image transformer. arXiv preprint arXiv:180205751
31. Ronneberger O, Fischer P, Brox T (2015) U-net: convolutional networks for biomedical image segmentation. In: International conference on medical image computing and computer-assisted intervention. Springer, Berlin, pp 234–241
32. Schroff F, Kalenichenko D, Philbin J (2015) Facenet: a unified embedding for face recognition and clustering. In: Proceedings of the IEEE conference on computer vision and pattern recognition, pp 815–823
33. Shen W, Liu R (2017) Learning residual images for face attribute manipulation. In: Proceedings of the IEEE conference on computer vision and pattern recognition, pp 4030–4038
34. Simonyan K, Zisserman A (2014) Very deep convolutional networks for large-scale image recognition. arXiv preprint arXiv:14091556
35. Song L, Gong D, Li Z, Liu C, Liu W (2019) Occlusion robust face recognition based on mask learning with pairwise differential siamese network. In: Proceedings of the IEEE international conference on computer vision, pp 773–782
36. Vaswani A, Shazeer N, Parmar N, Uszkoreit J, Jones L, Gomez AN, Kaiser Ł, Polosukhin I (2017) Attention is all you need. In: Advances in neural information processing systems, pp 5998–6008
37. Wang P, Su F, Zhao Z, Guo Y, Zhao Y, Zhuang B (2019) Deep class-skewed learning for face recognition. Neurocomputing 363:35–45
38. Wang Q, Fan H, Sun G, Cong Y, Tang Y (2019) Laplacian pyramid adversarial network for face completion. Pattern Recognit 88:493–505
39. Yi D, Lei Z, Liao S, Li SZ (2014) Learning face representation from scratch. arXiv preprint arXiv:14117923
40. Zhang Z, Song Y, Qi H (2017) Age progression/regression by conditional adversarial autoencoder. In: Proceedings of the IEEE conference on computer vision and pattern recognition, pp 5810–5818
41. Zhang H, Goodfellow I, Metaxas D, Odena A (2018) Self-attention generative adversarial networks. arXiv preprint arXiv:180508318
42. Zhang H, Sun Y, Liu L, Xu X (2019) CascadeGAN: a category-supervised cascading generative adversarial network for clothes translation from the human body to tiled images. Neurocomputing 382:148–161

43. Zhao J, Xiong L, Jayashree PK, Li J, Zhao F, Wang Z, Pranata PS, Shen PS, Yan S, Feng J (2017) Dual-agent GANs for photorealistic and identity preserving profile face synthesis. In: Advances in neural information processing systems, pp 66–76
44. Zhi H, Liu S (2019) Face recognition based on genetic algorithm. J Vis Commun Image Represent 58:495–502
45. Zhou E, Fan H, Cao Z, Jiang Y, Yin Q (2013) Extensive facial landmark localization with coarse-to-fine convolutional network cascade. In: Proceedings of the IEEE international conference on computer vision workshops, pp 386–391
46. Zhu JY, Zhang R, Pathak D, Darrell T, Efros AA, Wang O, Shechtman E (2017) Toward multimodal image-to-image translation. In: Advances in neural information processing systems, pp 465–476

Part IV
Various Applications

Chapter 13
Deep Generative Models for 3D Medical Image Synthesis

Paul Friedrich, Yannik Frisch, and Philippe C. Cattin

Abstract Deep generative modeling has emerged as a powerful tool for synthesizing realistic medical images, driving advances in medical image analysis, disease diagnosis, and treatment planning. This chapter explores various deep generative models for 3D medical image synthesis, with a focus on Variational Autoencoders (VAEs), Generative Adversarial Networks (GANs), and Denoising Diffusion Models (DDMs). We discuss the fundamental principles, recent advances, as well as strengths and weaknesses of these models and examine their applications in clinically relevant problems, including unconditional and conditional generation tasks like image-to-image translation and image reconstruction. We additionally review commonly used evaluation metrics for assessing image fidelity, diversity, utility, and privacy and provide an overview of current challenges in the field.

13.1 Introduction

Medical imaging plays a critical role in diagnosing, monitoring, and treating disease by providing unique structural, functional, and metabolic information about the human body. While natural images usually capture data in two dimensions, medical practice often requires the acquisition of three-dimensional volumes like Magnetic Resonance Imaging (MRI), Computed Tomography (CT), or Positron Emission Tomography (PET) scans. Acquiring these volumetric scans can be time-consuming, costly, limited by scanner availability, and in the case of CT and PET scans, expose patients to harmful radiation. In addition, privacy and ethical concerns make it difficult to share medical data. Together, these factors limit the availability of large-scale medical image datasets for scientific studies, deep learning

P. Friedrich (✉) · P. C. Cattin
Department of Biomedical Engineering, University of Basel, Allschwil, Switzerland
e-mail: paul.friedrich@unibas.ch; philippe.cattin@unibas.ch

Y. Frisch
Graphical-Interactive Systems, Technical University Darmstadt, Darmstadt, Germany
e-mail: yannik.frisch@gris.tu-darmstadt.de

L. Zhang et al. (eds.), *Generative Machine Learning Models in Medical Image Computing*, https://doi.org/10.1007/978-3-031-80965-1_13

in medical image analysis, or physician training. Driven by advances in generating synthetic natural images, the application of deep generative models to medical images has emerged as a promising solution to address data scarcity and enable various medical image analysis tasks [25, 26]. However, the three-dimensionality and distinct distribution characteristics of medical images present unique challenges for image synthesis, requiring a careful adaptation of standard methods [100]. This chapter explores the basics of popular image generation models such as Variational Autoencoders (VAEs), Generative Adversarial Networks (GANs), and Denoising Diffusion Models (DDMs), discusses the advantages and disadvantages of each model type, reviews their applications in various medical image analysis tasks, and takes a look at common evaluation metrics for assessing model performance.

13.2 Background on Deep Generative Models

13.2.1 Deep Generative Models

Generative models are a class of machine learning models that aim to learn the underlying distribution p_{data} of some input data x to (1) generate new samples from that same distribution or (2) assign probability values to existing samples, allowing for certain downstream tasks. In Deep Generative Models (DGMs), this probability density estimation task is solved using deep neural networks that either explicitly model the distribution p_{model} or parameterize a model that can sample from p_{model} without explicitly estimating it. This general principle of finding a model that accurately represents the underlying data distribution of some input data x is shown in Fig. 13.1. In recent years, deep generative modeling has been applied to various data modalities, including text, audio, shapes, and images, using models such as Restricted Boltzmann Machines [23], Normalizing Flows [79], Variational Autoencoders [51], Generative Adversarial Networks [29], and Denoising Diffusion Models [37, 85].

13.2.2 Variational Autoencoders

The basic principle of VAEs [51] builds on that of standard autoencoders. Both encode an input x into a low-dimensional latent representation $z = E(x)$ using an encoder network E. The original image $x' = D(z)$ is then reconstructed from this representation z using a decoder network D. VAEs, however, differ in the way they parameterize this latent representation. Instead of directly encoding the image x into a single vector z, they encode it into the parameters of a normal distribution by designing the encoder in a way to predict the mean $\mu = E_\mu(x)$ and variance $\sigma^2 = E_\sigma(x)$ of that distribution. The latent representation z can then be drawn from

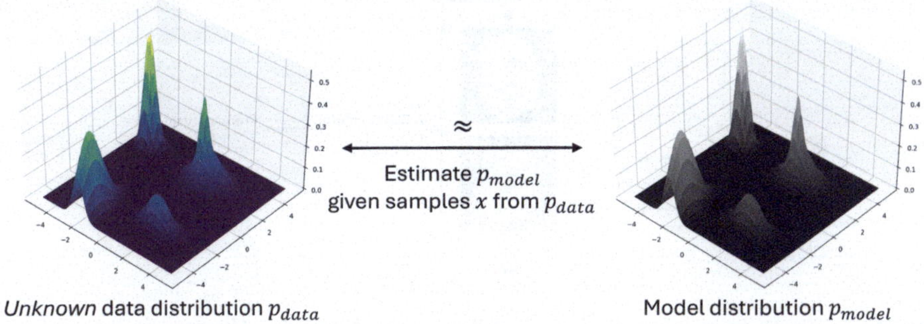

Fig. 13.1 The basic principle of generative modeling. Using data from the data distribution p_{data}, we try to find a model p_{model} that closely follows this distribution. We can then use this model to generate new samples that resemble the original data distribution

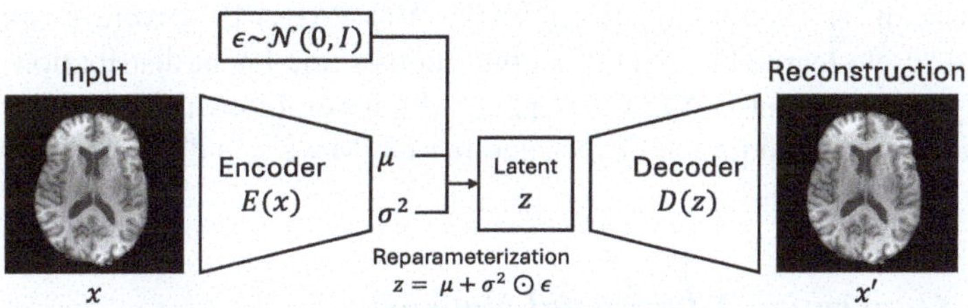

Fig. 13.2 The basic principle of Variational Autoencoders. An input image x is encoded into a KL regularized latent representation $z = E(x)$ and is subsequently reconstructed as $x' = D(z)$. By minimizing the reconstruction error, as well as the KL-divergence between the latent and a standard normal distribution, the model learns to generate new data and encode data in a meaningful way

$\mathcal{N}(\mu, \sigma^2)$. As backpropagating through this stochastic part would be impossible, VAEs apply a reparameterization trick and instead sample an auxiliary variable $\epsilon \sim \mathcal{N}(0, I)$ to define $z = \mu + \sigma^2 \odot \epsilon$. In addition, VAEs apply a KL-divergence regularization term to this latent distribution to make it close to a standard normal distribution. This allows generating new samples by drawing $z \sim \mathcal{N}(0, I)$ and passing it through the trained decoder network. This general setup is shown in Fig. 13.2. Combining these two principles, VAEs can be trained by minimizing the reconstruction error between input and reconstructed image, as well as by applying the KL-divergence regularization, which results in the following training objective:

$$\mathcal{L}_{VAE} = \|x - D(E(x))\|_2^2 + D_{KL}(\mathcal{N}(E_\mu(x), E_\sigma(x))\|\mathcal{N}(0, I)). \qquad (13.1)$$

This objective maximizes the evidence lower bound (ELBO) on the log-likelihood of the data. The model, therefore, learns to generate new data and compress data into a meaningful latent representation. While VAEs have a relatively short inference time and are known for their ability to produce diverse images, they suffer from poor sample quality and often produce blurry images [104]. To overcome this problem,

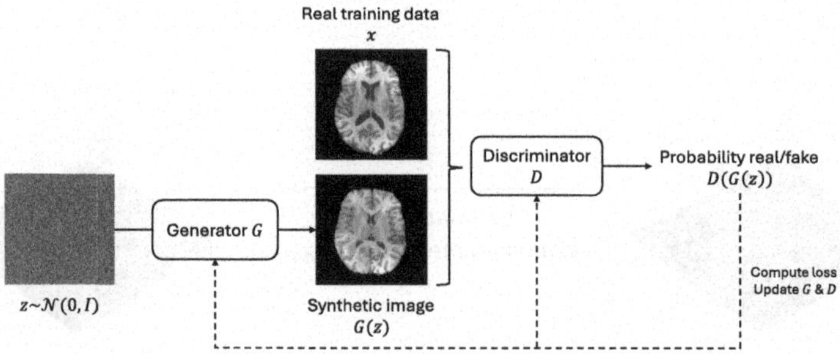

Fig. 13.3 The basic principle of Generative Adversarial Networks. The generator G and the discriminator D play an adversarial game against each other, where the generator tries to synthesize realistic images that the discriminator cannot distinguish from the real training data

variations such as Vector Quantized VAEs (VQ-VAEs) [93] were proposed that map to a discrete learned instead of a continuous static latent distribution. Another commonly used variant is VQ-GAN [21], which combines the VQ-VAE concept with the adversarial training of GANs, another DGM we will discuss in next section.

13.2.3 Generative Adversarial Networks

In recent years, GANs [29] have successfully been used to generate medical images, and form the basis of many applications in the medical field. Unlike most other generative models, GANs don't explicitly model the underlying data distribution in terms of a probability density function but take a different approach by implicitly modeling the distribution through a process of adversarial training. GANs are trained following a two-player min-max game shown in Fig. 13.3, and generally consist of two networks: the Generator $G(z)$ that aims to generate realistic fake samples from random noise $z \sim N(0, I)$ and the Discriminator $D(x)$ that tries to distinguish real and fake samples by solving a classification task. Both networks are iteratively optimized using the following training objective:

$$\min_G \max_D \mathcal{L}_{GAN}(D, G) = \mathbb{E}_{x \sim p_{data}}[\log D(x)] + \mathbb{E}_{z \sim N(0,I)}[\log(1 - D(G(z)))] \tag{13.2}$$

Intuitively, the generator aims to produce increasingly realistic fake data to fool the discriminator, while the discriminator tries to get better at distinguishing real data from fake data. While GANs have demonstrated impressive image generation capabilities [46], they often suffer from problems such as training instabilities and convergence problems. These issues can be caused by a mismatch between the capacity of the generator and the discriminator or an overconfident discriminator that makes it difficult for the generator to learn and optimize its parameters.

Another common problem is mode collapse, where the generator learns to output limited variations of samples by ignoring certain modes of the data distribution. To overcome these problems, various GAN modifications that apply improved training techniques, regularization strategies, or loss modifications have been introduced. Those include Wasserstein GAN (WGAN) [2], WGAN with Gradient Penalty (WGAN-GP) [32], Spectral Normalization GAN (SNGAN) [70], or Least Squares GAN (LSGAN) [66]. These adaptations have successfully reduced GAN-related problems but do not completely eliminate them.

13.2.4 Denoising Diffusion Models

Denoising Diffusion Models [37, 85] are latent variable models that sample from a distribution by reversing a defined diffusion process. This *diffusion* or *forward process* progressively perturbs the input data with Gaussian noise and maps the data distribution to a simple prior, namely a standard normal distribution. To generate new samples, we aim to learn the *reverse process*, which maps from this prior to the data distribution. New samples are generated by drawing random noise from the prior and passing it through the reverse process. This general principle is shown in Fig. 13.4. The diffusion process consists of T timesteps and can be described as a Markov chain, with each transition being a Gaussian that follows a predefined variance schedule $\beta_1, \ldots, \beta_T$:

$$q(x_{1:T}|x_0) := \prod_{t=1}^{T} q(x_t|x_{t-1}), \quad \text{with} \quad q(x_t|x_{t-1}) := \mathcal{N}(\sqrt{1-\beta_t}x_{t-1}, \beta_t I). \tag{13.3}$$

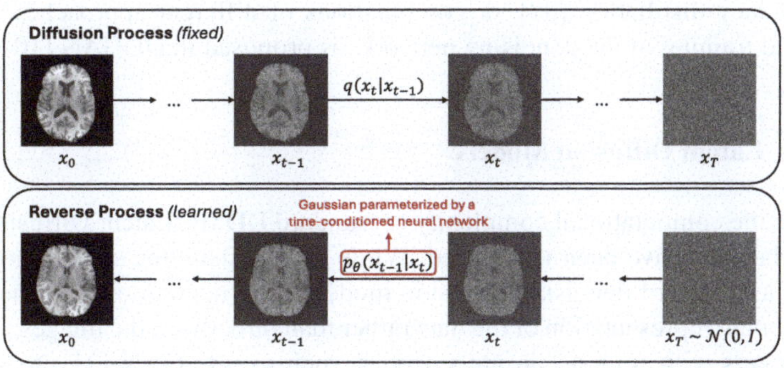

Fig. 13.4 The basic principle of Denoising Diffusion Models. The diffusion model consists of two main components: a fixed *diffusion process* that gradually perturbs input data with Gaussian noise and maps the data distribution to a simple prior, and a learned *reverse process* with each transition being a Gaussian parameterized by a time-conditioned neural network

The reverse process can also be described as a Markov chain with learned Gaussian transition kernels, starting at a simple prior distribution $p(x_T) = \mathcal{N}(0, I)$:

$$p_\theta(x_{0:T}) := \prod_{t=1}^{T} p_\theta(x_{t-1}|x_t), \quad \text{with} \quad p_\theta(x_{t-1}|x_t) := \mathcal{N}(\mu_\theta(x_t, t), \Sigma_\theta(x_t, t)). \tag{13.4}$$

While $\Sigma_\theta(x_t, t)$ is often fixed to the forward process variances β_t, $\mu_\theta(x_t, t)$ is usually estimated by a time-conditioned neural network. This network is trained by minimizing the variational lower bound of the negative log-likelihood. Following a reparameterization trick [37], we can configure the network to predict the noise $\epsilon_\theta(x_t, t)$ to be removed from a corrupted sample x_t and simplify the training objective to an MSE loss, with $\alpha_t = 1 - \beta_t$, $\bar{\alpha}_t = \prod_{s=1}^{t} \alpha_s$, and $\epsilon \sim \mathcal{N}(0, \boldsymbol{I})$:

$$\mathcal{L}_{simple} = \|\epsilon - \epsilon_\theta(x_t, t)\|_2^2, \quad \text{where} \quad x_t = \sqrt{\bar{\alpha}_t} x_0 + \sqrt{1 - \bar{\alpha}_t}\epsilon. \tag{13.5}$$

Given a trained network $\epsilon_\theta(x_t, t)$ and a randomly drawn starting point $x_T \sim \mathcal{N}(0, I)$, we can iteratively produce a new sample by applying the following equation T times:

$$x_{t-1} = \frac{1}{\sqrt{\alpha_t}} \left(x_t - \frac{1 - \alpha_t}{\sqrt{1 - \bar{\alpha}_t}} \epsilon_\theta(x_t, t) \right) + \sigma_t \epsilon \tag{13.6}$$

While diffusion models have demonstrated impressive image generation capabilities [16], their iterative nature requires multiple network evaluations for generating a single sample, making them slow and resource-intensive. To speed up this sampling process, several adaptations have been introduced, such as the Denoising Diffusion Implicit Model (DDIM) [86], which formulates a deterministic non-Markovian process to sample with fewer steps, different knowledge distillation methods, such as consistency distillation [87], or combinations of different approaches, such as adversarial training of the denoising network, as proposed in DDGAN [104].

13.2.4.1 Latent Diffusion Models

To reduce the computational complexity of standard DDMs, Latent Diffusion Models (LDMs) [80] have been introduced. While LDMs share the same fundamental principle as standard denoising diffusion models, they operate on a learned, more compact latent representation of the data rather than directly on the images. Training LDMs begins with training an autoencoder, such as VQ-GAN [21], to generate a meaningful low-dimensional latent representation of the data. Subsequently, the diffusion model is trained on this latent representation z instead of the original high-dimensional data x, resulting in a more computationally efficient approach. This principle is illustrated in Fig. 13.5. To generate new samples, the reverse diffusion process is applied starting from random noise $z_T \sim \mathcal{N}(0, I)$ in the latent

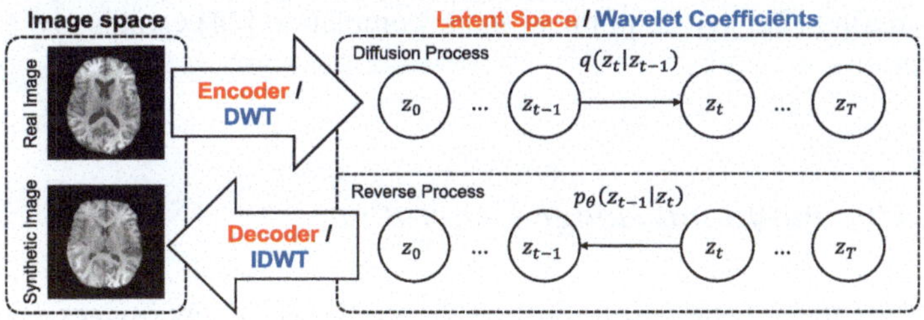

Fig. 13.5 The basic principle of Latent Diffusion Models (red) and Wavelet Diffusion Models (blue)

space, producing a synthetic latent representation z_0. This latent representation is then decoded back into the image space using the trained decoder. Although LDMs effectively reduce the computational complexity of training and sampling from denoising diffusion models, they depend on a well-performing autoencoder. Training such an autoencoder for high-resolution medical volumes is challenging itself and often constrained by computational resources.

13.2.4.2 Wavelet Diffusion Models

Wavelet diffusion models (WDMs) [25, 75], shown in Fig. 13.5, are a promising alternative to LDMs. While both approaches share a similar idea, wavelet diffusion models take a different approach to spatial dimensionality reduction by applying Discrete Wavelet Transform (DWT). This approach is learning-free in the sense that it does not require a pre-trained autoencoder. The diffusion model then operates on the wavelet coefficients z of the images. To generate new images, WDMs start with random noise $z_T \sim \mathcal{N}(0, I)$ and apply the reverse diffusion process to produce synthetic wavelet coefficients z_0. These coefficients can then be transformed back to the image space using Inverse Discrete Wavelet Transform (IDWT). As WDMs do not rely on an autoencoder network, they have an even smaller memory footprint than LDMs, which is particularly important in 3D medical image synthesis tasks that are typically constrained by the available GPU memory.

13.3 Applications in Medical Image Computing

The following section provides an overview of DGMs in 3D medical image synthesis, including unconditional image generation, image-to-image translation and image reconstruction. It is important to note that this only covers a subset of potential applications of DGMs in medicine. Additional tasks, such as image registration [49], classification [59], segmentation [102], anomaly detection [101], image inpainting [20] and anatomical shape completion [24] can also be addressed using generative networks.

13.3.1 Unconditional Image Generation

Unconditional image generation involves the synthesis of new images without any specific condition and simply demonstrates the ability of a generative model to learn the underlying distribution of some given training data. These models can be applied to augment datasets with synthetic images [107] or improve downstream applications fairness under distribution shifts [52]. Unconditional image generation is commonly used to demonstrate the performance of novel architectures, which serve as a foundation for developing methods for conditional generation tasks. An overview of publications that present unconditional 3D medical image synthesis models is given in Table 13.1.

Although VAEs are widely used for modeling 2D medical images, their application to unconditional 3D image generation remains relatively unexplored. Volokitin et al. [94] used 2D slice VAEs to model high-resolution 3D brain MR images by combining a VAE with a Gaussian model that allows for sampling coherent stacks of latent codes that decode into a meaningful volume. Kapoor et al. [45] took a different approach by transforming a reference MRI with multi-scale morphological transformations predicted by a 3D VAE.

GAN-based approaches have been extensively explored for 3D medical image synthesis, with early applications successfully modeling brain MR images. Kwon et al. [54] and Segato et al. [83] adapted the α-GAN framework [65] for this purpose, while Hong et al. [38] presented a 3D version of StyleGAN [46]. While these early approaches were constrained to relatively low resolutions, Chong and Ho [13] were the first to scale GAN-based methods to higher resolutions by applying morphological transformations and texture changes to reference volumes. Sun et al. [89] reached similar resolutions following a hierarchical approach. Liu et al. [63] relied on pretraining 2D models and inflating the 2D convolutions [10] to improve the performance of 3D models.

Dorjsembe et al. [17] were the first to adapt DDPMs [37] for modeling 3D medical data, achieving promising results on brain MR image generation. Despite their success, the computational complexity and long sampling times associated with simple 3D adaptations posed significant challenges. Peng et al. [74] explored a 2.5D approach that models 3D volumes by iteratively predicting 2D slices conditioned on their predecessors and generates new volumes in an autoregressive fashion. Further advances were made by Pinaya et al. [76] and Khader et al. [47], who applied latent diffusion models to high-resolution 3D data, effectively reducing the computational complexity and sampling times. Friedrich et al. [25] proposed to apply discrete wavelet transform for spatial dimensionality reduction, which effectively scaled 3D diffusion models to high resolutions without requiring a pre-trained autoencoder.

Table 13.1 Overview of publications on unconditional 3D medical image synthesis models, the modality of the generated data, public datasets used for training, the maximum image resolution reported in the paper, as well as the utilized network architecture

Study	Model	Modality	Dataset(s)	Resolution	Network(s)
Volokitin et al. [94]	VAE	MRI	HCP	$256 \times 256 \times 256$	2D Slice-VAEs
Kapoor et al. [45]	VAE	MRI	ADNI	$80 \times 96 \times 80$	3D VAE
Kwon et al. [54]	GAN	MRI	ADNI, BRATS, ATLAS	$64 \times 64 \times 64$	3D α-WGAN-GP
Segato et al. [83]	GAN	MRI	ADNI	$64 \times 64 \times 64$	3D α-GAN
Granstedt et al. [31]	GAN	MRI	fastMRI	$256 \times 256 \times 16$	3D GAN
Hong et al. [38]	GAN	MRI	ADNI, ABIDE, ADHD2000, HABS, GSP, MCIC, OASIS, PPMI	$80 \times 96 \times 112$	3D StyleGAN
Chong and Ho [13]	GAN	MRI	HCP	$256 \times 256 \times 256$	3D WGAN-GP + 2D pix2pixGAN
Bergen et al. [7]	GAN	PET	HECKTOR	$64 \times 64 \times 32$	2D TGAN
Mensing et al. [69]	GAN	MRI	German National Cohort	$160 \times 160 \times 128$	3D cGAN (FastGAN)
Sun et al. [89]	GAN	MRI, CT	GSP, COPDGene	$256 \times 256 \times 256$	3D HA-GAN
Liu et al. [63]	GAN	MRI	COCA, ADNI	$64 \times 64 \times 64$	2D StyleGAN2 + 3D StyleGAN2
Kim et al. [50]	GAN	MRI, CT	HCP, CT-ORG	$128 \times 128 \times 128$	3D WGAN-GP
Dorjsembe et al. [17]	DDM	MRI	ICTS	$128 \times 128 \times 128$	3D DDPM
Pinaya et al. [76]	LDM	MRI	UK Biobank	$160 \times 224 \times 160$	3D VAE + 3D DDPM/DDIM
Peng et al. [74]	DDM	MRI	ADNI, UCSF, SRI International	$128 \times 128 \times 128$	2.5D DDPM
Khader et al. [47]	LDM	MRI, CT	DUKE, MRNet, ADNI, LIDC-IDRI	$128 \times 128 \times 128$	3D VQ-GAN + 3D DDPM
Friedrich et al. [25]	WDM	MRI, CT	BRATS, LIDC-IDRI	$256 \times 256 \times 256$	3D WDM (DDPM)

13.3.2 Image-to-Image Translation

Multimodal data plays an important role in medical imaging. However, its accessibility is often limited by challenges such as acquisition time and cost, scanner availability, and the risk of additional radiation exposure. To address these limitations, image-to-image translation models aim to generate synthetic images y of a missing modality given an available source modality image x. In other words, these models try to find a mapping function $F : X \rightarrow Y$ that maps from the source domain X to the target domain Y, such that $y = F(x)$. This problem can be addressed in a paired setting, where training samples $\{x_i, y_i\}_{i=1}^N$ consist of corresponding images $x_i \in X$ and $y_i \in Y$ from the different domains, or in an unpaired setting, where the training data $\{x_i | x_i \in X\}_{i=1}^N$ and $\{y_j | y_j \in Y\}_{j=1}^M$ consists of unrelated samples, requiring different training strategies. Table 13.2 provides an overview of publications on image-to-image translation models for 3D medical images.

A common task in medical image computing is MRI-to-MRI translation (e.g. T1 $\leftrightarrow$ T2, or 1.5T $\leftrightarrow$ 3T), which serves several purposes. First, it provides physicians with different contrasts of the images to aid in diagnosis and treatment planning. Second, it can improve the performance of downstream applications such as segmentation tasks by providing the segmentation model with multiple MRI contrasts to work with. Finally, it allows for harmonizing scans from different MR scanners, reducing potential biases in the acquired datasets. These problems have been tackled using VAE-based [39], GAN-based [77, 90, 110] or DDM/LDM-based approaches [19, 50, 111] and have also been addressed in scientific challenges like the MICCAI 2023 Brain MR Image Synthesis for Tumor Segmentation challenge [4].

Another application involves generating CT or PET scans from MR images. This enables downstream tasks to be performed on the target modalities without exposing patients to additional CT or PET imaging radiation. Graf et al. [30] performed MRI-to-CT translation to enable segmentation networks trained on CT scans to be applied to MR images. Recently, the SynthRAD challenge [41], which aims to provide tools for radiation-free radiotherapy planning by translating MR images to CT scans, has drawn significant attention to this task and highlights the need for well-performing image-to-image translation methods. The task of MRI-to-CT/PET translation has been tackled using different GAN-based [39, 56, 62, 84, 96, 99, 109] and DDM-based approaches [60, 73].

Medical image-to-image translation is not only used to translate between different contrasts and modalities but has also been adapted for other tasks, such as anomaly localization, by transforming pathological images into their pseudo-healthy versions [82, 101]. These approaches, however, have not yet been explored on 3D images.

Image-to-image translation models have proven to be valuable tools for assisting physicians and enabling certain downstream tasks. However, these models have inherent limitations and should not be applied naively. Image-to-image translation models rely on the information present in the input image and the learned prior

Table 13.2 Overview of publications on 3D image-to-image translation frameworks, the translation modalities, public datasets used for training (– for private data), the type of translated data (paired vs. unpaired), as well as the utilized network architecture

Study	Model	Modality	Dataset(s)	Type	Network(s)
Hu et al. [40]	VAE	MRI $\leftrightarrow$ MRI	BRATS	Paired	2D Spatial-VAE
Wei et al. [99]	GAN	MRI $\rightarrow$ PET	–	Paired	3D cGAN
Uzunova et al. [90]	GAN	CT $\leftrightarrow$ CT, MRI $\leftrightarrow$ MRI	COPDGene, BRATS	Unpaired	3D cGAN
Hu et al. [39]	GAN	MRI $\leftrightarrow$ PET, MRI $\leftrightarrow$ CT	ADNI, TCIA	Paired	3D BMGAN
Lan et al. [56]	GAN	MRI $\rightarrow$ PET	ADNI	Paired	3D SC-GAN
Lin et al. [62]	GAN	MRI $\leftrightarrow$ PET	ADNI	Paired	3D RevGAN
Sikka et al. [84]	GAN	MRI $\rightarrow$ PET	ADNI	Paired	3D cGAN
Zhao et al. [110]	GAN	MRI $\leftrightarrow$ MRI	BRATS	Paired	3D CycleGAN
Zhang et al. [109]	GAN	MRI $\rightarrow$ PET	ADNI	Paired	3D BPGAN
Bazangani et al. [6]	GAN	PET $\rightarrow$ MRI	ADNI	Paired	3D E-GAN
Kalantar et al. [43]	GAN	CT $\leftrightarrow$ CT	NCCID	Unpaired	3D CycleGAN
Poonkodi and Kanchana [77]	GAN	PET $\leftrightarrow$ CT, PET $\leftrightarrow$ PET, MRI $\leftrightarrow$ MRI	Lung-PET-CT-Dx	Unpaired	3D CSGAN
Wang et al. [98]	GAN	MRI $\rightarrow$ PET	–	Paired	3D ViT-GAN
Durrer et al. [19]	DDM	MRI $\leftrightarrow$ MRI	–	Paired	2D DDPM
Graf et al. [30]	DDM	MRI $\rightarrow$ CT	MRSpineSeg	Paired	3D DDIM
Pan et al. [72]	DDM	MRI $\leftrightarrow$ MRI	BRATS	Paired	3D DDPM
Zhu et al. [111]	LDM	MRI $\leftrightarrow$ MRI	RIRE	Paired	2D VAE + 2.5D DDPM/DDIM
Zhu et al. [112]	LDM	Mask $\rightarrow$ MRI, Mask $\rightarrow$ CT	BRATS, AbdomenCT-1K	Paired	2D VAE + 2.5D DDIM
Kim and Park [48]	LDM	MRI $\leftrightarrow$ MRI	BRATS, IXI	Paired	3D VQ-GAN + 3D DDPM
Dorjsembe et al. [18]	DDM	Mask $\rightarrow$ MRI	BRATS	Paired	3D DDPM
Pan et al. [73]	DDM	MRI $\rightarrow$ CT	–	Paired	3D DDPM
Li et al. [60]	DDM	MRI $\rightarrow$ PET	ADNI	Paired	2.5D DDPM

knowledge of the target modality. This means that if specific clinically relevant details are missing or poorly represented in the source image, they cannot be accurately generated or inferred in the translated image. In addition, these models tend to hallucinate realistic-looking features that do not necessarily correspond to the actual anatomical structures that should be present in the image. As a result, a translated image may contain elements that falsely appear normal or pathological, leading to potential misdiagnosis if naively assumed to be correct.

13.3.3 Image Reconstruction

Reconstructing high-quality images from sparsely sampled or partial measurements is important in speeding up existing medical imaging tools such as CT, PET, or MRI, reducing examination times, harmful radiation exposure to patients, and acquisition costs of these methods. Typical medical image reconstruction tasks include, but are not limited to: sparse-view computed tomography (SV-CT), limited-angle computed tomography (LA-CT), low-dose CT denoising (LDCT-D), compressed-sensing magnetic resonance imaging (CS-MRI), z-axis super-resolution on MR images (ZSR-MRI), or obtaining standard-dose PET (SPET) scans from low-dose PET (LPET) scans. While these tasks have extensively been explored on 2D images (sliced volumes), research on directly solving these problems on the 3D data is limited. An overview of publications on 3D medical image reconstruction is shown in Table 13.3.

Several scientific challenges have drawn attention to the topic and provided valuable datasets for evaluating different image reconstruction approaches. These challenges include the AAPM 2016 CT Low-Dose Grand Challenge [67], the MICCAI 2021 Brain MRI Reconstruction Challenge with Realistic Noise [68], the MICCAI 2022 Ultra-low Dose PET Imaging Challenge [53], and the MICCAI 2023 Cardiac MRI Reconstruction Challenge [11]. Due to the computational complexity of directly handling 3D data, most presented approaches still operate on 2D slices, highlighting the need for efficient 3D backbones. Existing 3D GAN-based approaches have mostly focused on synthetic SPET image generation with conditional GAN [97], Vision Transformer GANs (ViT-GAN) [64, 98, 108] or Classification-Guided GAN [106] and operate on rather low-resolution volumes. Diffusion-based approaches primarily focused on SV-CT, LA-CT and CS-MRI. They formulate the task as an inverse problem of predicting an unknown image x given limited measurements y. The forward model is denoted as $y = \mathbf{A}x + \epsilon$, with $\mathbf{A}$ being a degradation function (e.g. partial sampling of the sinogram for SV-CT and LA-CT, or k-space for CS-MRI) and the measuring noise ϵ. The inverse task $\hat{x} = G_\theta(y)$ is solved using a DGM G_θ. They address the problem of dealing with high-dimensional 3D data by applying perpendicular 2D models [57, 61], by conditioning the model on adjacent slices to form 2.5D models[105], or by applying 2D models to a triplane representation of the data [35].

Table 13.3 Overview of publications on 3D image reconstruction frameworks, the data modalities, public datasets used for training (– for private data), the solved tasks, as well as the utilized network architecture

Study	Model	Modality	Dataset(s)	Task	Network(s)
Wolterink et al. [103]	GAN	CT	–	LDCT-D	3D GAN
Wang et al. [97]	GAN	PET	–	LPET-SPET	3D cGAN
Luo et al. [64]	GAN	PET	–	LPET-SPET	3D ViT-GAN
Zeng et al. [108]	GAN	PET	–	LPET-SPET	3D ViT-GAN
Xue et al. [106]	GAN	PET	Ultra-low Dose PET Imaging Challenge 2022	LPET-SPET	3D SRGAN
Wang et al. [98]	GAN	PET	–	LPET-SPET	3D ViT-GAN
Lee et al. [57]	DDM	CT, MRI	AAPM 2016 CT Low-Dose Grand Challenge	SV-CT, CS-MRI, ZSR-MRI	2D Score DDMs
Chung et al. [14]	DDM	CT, MRI	AAPM 2016 CT Low-Dose Grand Challenge, BRATS, fastMRI	SV-CT, LA-CT, CS-MRI	2D Score DDM
Xie et al. [105]	DDM	PET	–	LPET-SPET	2.5D DDPM/DDIM
He et al. [35]	DDM	CT, MRI	AAPM 2016 CT Low-Dose Grand Challenge, IXI	SV-CT, LA-CT, CS-MRI, ZSR-MRI	Triplane DDPM
Li et al. [61]	DDM	CT, MRI	AAPM 2016 CT Low-Dose Grand Challenge, BRATS	SV-CT, CS-MRI	2D Score DDMs

Similar to image-to-image translation models, image reconstruction models can hallucinate structures that are not present in the actual anatomy, potentially leading to misdiagnosis. To ensure clinically relevant and reliable images, it is essential to develop robust models, compile comprehensive training datasets, and perform rigorous validation. In addition, these models should be used with caution and an understanding of the potential risks.

13.4 Evaluating Deep Generative Models

Evaluating deep generative models in medical imaging is not trivial and probably deserves its own chapter. Nevertheless, we will give a brief overview of popular metrics and discuss various image quality, diversity, utility, privacy, and other non-image-related metrics that should be considered when evaluating generative models and the data they synthesize.

13.4.1 Image Quality Metrics

The **Fréchet Inception Distance (FID)** [36] is a metric that measures image fidelity by comparing the distribution of real and generated images without requiring image pairs. It has widely been applied to evaluate unconditional image-generation tasks. The FID score is calculated by first extracting high-level features from real and synthetic images using an intermediate activation of a pre-trained neural network, calculating statistics over these features by fitting two multivariate Gaussians to the real $\mathcal{N}(\mu_r, \Sigma_r)$ and synthetic images features $\mathcal{N}(\mu_s, \Sigma_s)$, and computing the Fréchet distance between those distributions:

$$FID = \|\mu_r - \mu_s\|_2^2 + tr(\Sigma_r + \Sigma_s - 2\sqrt{\Sigma_r \Sigma_s}). \tag{13.7}$$

A small FID score indicates that the distributions of real and synthetic images are similar, suggesting that the model effectively learned the data distribution, which results in a good visual appearance. While FID scores are a useful tool for assessing image fidelity in unconditional image generation tasks, comparing these scores across publications is not straightforward and should be done cautiously. This is because FID scores are highly dependent on the choice of feature extraction network and the specific feature layer used. Further, metrics like FID are highly dependent on a sufficiently large number of samples used to approximate the data distributions [12]. Without fulfilling this requirement, these metrics lose their meaningfulness, which is an often overlooked problem within limited data regimes such as medical imaging.

For image generation tasks where a ground truth image is available, such as a paired cross-modality image synthesis task, metrics like Peak Signal-to-Noise-Ratio

(PSNR), Structural Similarity Index Measure (SSIM) or Mean Squared Error (MSE) can be applied to compare generated and ground truth image. The **Peak Signal-to-Noise-Ratio (PSNR)** is a metric originally used to measure the reconstruction quality of lossy compressed images. In the context of evaluating conditional image generation, it measures the fidelity of the synthetic image S compared to the real ground truth R and is defined as

$$PSNR = 10 \cdot \log_{10}\left(\frac{MAX_R^2}{MSE}\right) = 20 \cdot \log_{10}(MAX_R) - 10 \cdot \log_{10}(MSE), \tag{13.8}$$

with MAX_R being the maximum possible intensity value of the images, usually 255 for uint8 grayscale images, and the **Mean Squared Error (MSE)** between real and synthetic image, which is defined over all voxels N of the volume:

$$MSE = \frac{1}{N}\sum_{i=1}^{N}(R_i - S_i)^2. \tag{13.9}$$

While PSNR and MSE are widely applied metrics for assessing image quality, they have several limitations. As pixel-level metrics, they can't capture any structural information that is strongly correlated with good visual perception of the generated images [96]. This drawback led to the development of the **Structural Similarity Index Measure (SSIM)**, which evaluates the perceived change in structural information, luminance, and contrast. It is computed over a shifting window of similar size, e.g. $11 \times 11 \times 11$, denoted as r for a window of R and s for the same window from S. The SSIM is defined as:

$$SSIM = \frac{(2\mu_r\mu_s + c_1)(2\sigma_{rs} + c_2)}{(\mu_r^2 + \mu_s^2 + c_1)(\sigma_r^2 + \sigma_s^2 + c_2)} \tag{13.10}$$

with the mean μ_r and μ_s, and variances σ_r^2 and σ_s^2 over the respective windows pixel intensities, the covariance σ_{rs} between them, as well as two constants c_1 and c_2 to numerically stabilize the score against division with weak denominators. While a small SSIM score indicates that two images significantly differ in structural information, luminance and contrast, a score close to 1 indicates high image similarity. In addition to the classic SSIM score, several variants such as MS-SSIM [95], or 4-(G-)SSIM [58] have been proposed to improve the quality metric further. A competitive evaluation of several SSIM versions on radiology images has been performed in [78], suggesting that 4-MS-G-SSIM provides optimal results and strongly agrees with human perception. Image quality can also be assessed using the **Inception Score** [81], **Precision** [55], or by conduction a **Visual Turing Test** [28].

13.4.2 *Image Diversity Metrics*

While the **Structural Similarity Index Measure (SSIM)** can be used to measure the similarity between image pairs, it has also been applied to assess the diversity of the generated images. In [25] and [76], the authors measure image diversity by averaging the MS-SSIM over generated images by iteratively comparing a reference image to all other generated images. A low SSIM in this case indicates high generation diversity, meaning that the generated images are not similar to each other. Such quantification of diversity can also be carried out in the feature space of pre-trained feature extractors.

Another common way to assess image diversity is the **Recall Score** [55], which measures the fraction of the training data manifold that can be produced by the generative network. Similar to computing the FID score, a feature extraction network is applied to produce a set of high-level features of real Φ_r and synthetic images Φ_s. A feature vector of a single image is denoted as ϕ_r for a real image and as ϕ_s for a synthetic image. The Recall score is then defined as

$$\text{Recall} = \frac{1}{|\Phi_r|} \sum_{\phi_r \in \Phi_r} f(\phi_r, \Phi_s) \tag{13.11}$$

with $|\Phi_r|$ being the number of images to compute the score, and $f(\phi_r, \Phi_s)$ a nearest-neighbor-based binary function that determines whether a real image could be generated by evaluating whether it lays within the approximated synthetic data distribution. A high recall score indicates that the trained network generates diverse samples from the entire data distribution, while a low recall score could be a sign of mode collapse.

13.4.3 *Utility and Privacy Metrics*

Another common way to evaluate the performance of deep generative networks is to assess the utility of the generated data by measuring **performance improvements on relevant downstream tasks** when trained with additional synthetic data. In medical image computing, this has been done by measuring performance improvements of classification [26] or segmentation [1] tasks.

Since deep generative models are known to memorize data [15, 92], assessing the privacy of synthetic images and minimizing the risk of re-identification [22] before sharing images or weights of models trained on non-public data is crucial. To evaluate the privacy of generated images, metrics such as the **Rarity Score** [33] or **Average Minimum Cosine Distance (AMD)** [3], which measures the uncommonness of generated images as the nearest-neighbor distance of real and synthetic data points in a latent space, have been proposed. Other privacy metrics rely on **model-based re-identification** [71] or apply **Extraction Attacks** [9] to measure privacy by trying to extract training images from the trained models.

13.4.4 Non-image Metrics

In addition to the discussed image metrics, other factors such as the model's **Inference Time**, **Computational Efficiency**, usually measured in Floating Point Operations (FLOPs), or **Memory Consumption** must also be considered in the evaluation to ensure the model's applicability to real-world problems. This is especially important for time-critical applications or when the method is to be used in a resource-constrained environment. The **Ethical and Social Impact** of the model, i.e. possible bias and fairness of the model as well as potential misuse, should also be considered.

13.5 Current Challenges and Conclusion

13.5.1 Challenges

High-resolution data is crucial for a thorough and accurate analysis of medical images. However, many current DGMs struggle with scaling to such high-dimensional spaces. Additionally, computational resources are often limited in clinical settings, making in-house training of large-scale generative models challenging. Furthermore, medical image analysis often benefits from longitudinal data, e.g. repeated scans of patients at progressive points in time. Modeling such temporal data with generative models further increases the required compute significantly and is an open and highly relevant research direction [8, 88]. To address these challenges, various methods have been proposed to significantly reduce the number of model parameters, speed up training and inference times, and lower GPU memory requirements. Notable approaches include WDMs [25, 75] and Neural Cellular Automata [44]. Despite these advancements, the **need for scalable and efficient models** continues to drive further research in this area.

The scalability problem also applies to the data itself. Many state-of-the-art generative models are trained on excessive amounts of data that are typically unavailable for most medical problems. Collecting and annotating such data can be a resource/labor-intensive process, further complicated by regulatory issues. In addition, the datasets used to train generative models should be as diverse and representative as possible to avoid the negative effects of bias. One way to mitigate these problems and allow for the development of a robust and useful model is to **provide data in an open access paradigm**. Another way to effectively train generative models and fully capture complex data distributions is to **develop efficient methods**

for federated learning [42] and solve existing problems related. An example of such issues could be the case where a patient—or even an entire institute—opts out of a study and withdraws its samples from the training distribution. The process of unlearning [27], therefore, needs to be addressed in the context of generative models for medical imaging.

Another commonly faced challenge is related to the evaluation of DGMs in the medical domain. Most metrics widely used to evaluate generative models in the natural image domain must only be carefully applied to medical images. These metrics might only provide reliable quantitative results with adequately pre-trained feature extractors [5] and an appropriately large test sample size [12]. In addition, the three-dimensionality of medical imaging data is often not considered in such metrics, e.g. feature extractors for 3D data might not be publicly available and have to be built from scratch. We, therefore, identify the **need for more rigorous quantitative testing of generative models in the medical domain**.

Further challenges arise when it comes to safely deploying these algorithms, as generative models can pose the threat of (unconscious or deliberate) data corruption [34]. Especially when these models are deployed as a data augmentation method for downstream task models, additional curation is needed to minimize the risk of error propagation from the generative to the downstream task model [91]. Additionally, the risk of these models hallucinating can potentially lead to drastic consequences, e.g. for the tasks of reconstruction or inpainting in the medical domain.

Most generative models in the medical domain are developed and trained on publicly available data. In some cases, in which private data cohorts are also considered, privacy protection is an important issue that needs to be taken into account. Even releasing the weights of generative models trained on private data could lead to privacy violations, since the training data can essentially be extracted from these models [9]. The problem of **privacy preserving generative models** needs to be addressed and is an interesting and promising direction for future research.

13.5.2 Conclusion

Deep generative models have achieved significant success in recent years, proving to be a valuable tool for learning complex data distributions and solving medically relevant downstream tasks. We reviewed the background of VAEs, GANs, and DDMs, highlighting their strengths and weaknesses. In addition, we demonstrated their application to unconditional image generation, image-to-image translation, and image reconstruction, and discussed commonly used evaluation metrics as well as pitfalls associated with these metrics.

Despite the mentioned advances in DGMs for 3D medical image synthesis, several open challenges remain that motivate future research in this area. Finding novel, more efficient data representations, developing tools for federated learning, or exploring methods to address unlearning and privacy concerns are critical to advancing the capabilities of DGMs in the medical domain. The goal of these efforts is to create efficient, fair, and reliable algorithms that can provide physicians with valuable insights and ultimately improve personalized medicine, enhance predictive analytics, and facilitate the development of new therapeutic strategies.

Acknowledgments This work was financially supported by the Werner Siemens Foundation through the MIRACLE II project.

Competing Interests The authors have no conflicts of interest to declare that are relevant to the content of this chapter.

References

1. Al Khalil Y, Amirrajab S, Lorenz C, Weese J, Pluim J, Breeuwer M (2023) On the usability of synthetic data for improving the robustness of deep learning-based segmentation of cardiac magnetic resonance images. Med Image Anal 84:102688
2. Arjovsky M, Chintala S, Bottou L (2017) Wasserstein generative adversarial networks. In: International conference on machine learning, PMLR, pp 214–223
3. Bai CY, Lin HT, Raffel C, Kan WCw (2021) On training sample memorization: lessons from benchmarking generative modeling with a large-scale competition. In: Proceedings of the 27th ACM SIGKDD conference on knowledge discovery & data mining, pp 2534–2542
4. Baltruschat IM, Janbakhshi P, Lenga M (2024) Brasyn 2023 challenge: missing MRI synthesis and the effect of different learning objectives. arXiv preprint arXiv:240307800
5. Barratt S, Sharma R (2018) A note on the inception score. arXiv preprint arXiv:180101973
6. Bazangani F, Richard FJ, Ghattas B, Guedj E (2022) FDG-PET to T1 weighted MRI translation with 3d elicit generative adversarial network (e-GAN). Sensors 22(12):4640
7. Bergen RV, Rajotte JF, Yousefirizi F, Klyuzhin IS, Rahmim A, Ng RT (2022) 3D PET image generation with tumour masks using TGAN. In: Medical imaging 2022: image processing, SPIE, vol 12032, pp 459–469
8. Bieder F, Friedrich P, Corbaz H, Durrer A, Wolleb J, Cattin PC (2024) Modeling the Neonatal brain development using implicit neural representations. In: International Workshop on PRedictive Intelligence in Medicine, pp 1–11, Springer
9. Carlini N, Hayes J, Nasr M, Jagielski M, Sehwag V, Tramer F, Balle B, Ippolito D, Wallace E (2023) Extracting training data from diffusion models. In: 32nd USENIX security symposium (USENIX Security 23), pp 5253–5270
10. Carreira J, Zisserman A (2017) Quo vadis, action recognition? a new model and the kinetics dataset. In: Proceedings of the IEEE conference on computer vision and pattern recognition, pp 6299–6308
11. Chengyan W, Xinyu Z, Xutong K, Chen Q, Shuo W, Jun L, Jing Q, Yapeng T, He W, Zhensen C, Xiahai Z, Sha H, Ying-Hua C, Weibo C (2023) Cardiac MRI reconstruction challenge. https://doi.org/10.5281/zenodo.7840229
12. Chong MJ, Forsyth D (2020) Effectively unbiased fid and inception score and where to find them. In: Proceedings of the IEEE/CVF conference on computer vision and pattern recognition, pp 6070–6079
13. Chong CK, Ho ETW (2021) Synthesis of 3D MRI brain images with shape and texture generative adversarial deep neural networks. IEEE Access 9:64747–64760
14. Chung H, Ryu D, McCann MT, Klasky ML, Ye JC (2023) Solving 3D inverse problems using pre-trained 2D diffusion models. In: Proceedings of the IEEE/CVF conference on computer vision and pattern recognition, pp 22542–22551

15. Dar SUH, Seyfarth M, Kahmann J, Ayx I, Papavassiliu T, Schoenberg SO, Engelhardt S (2024) Unconditional latent diffusion models memorize patient imaging data. arXiv preprint arXiv:240201054
16. Dhariwal P, Nichol A (2021) Diffusion models beat GANs on image synthesis. Adv Neural Inf Process Syst 34:8780–8794
17. Dorjsembe Z, Odonchimed S, Xiao F (2022) Three-dimensional medical image synthesis with denoising diffusion probabilistic models. In: Medical imaging with deep learning
18. Dorjsembe Z, Pao H-K, Odonchimed S, Xiao F (2024) Conditional diffusion models for semantic 3D brain MRI synthesis. IEEE J Biomed Health Inf 28(7):4084–4093
19. Durrer A, Wolleb J, Bieder F, Sinnecker T, Weigel M, Sandkuehler R, Granziera C, Yaldizli Ö, Cattin PC (2023) Diffusion models for contrast harmonization of magnetic resonance images. In: Medical imaging with deep learning. Proceedings of machine learning research, vol 227. pp 526–551. PMLR
20. Durrer A, Wolleb J, Bieder F, Friedrich P, Melie-Garcia L, Ocampo-Pineda M, Bercea CI, Hamamci IE, Wiestler B, Piraud M, et al (2024) Denoising diffusion models for 3D healthy brain tissue inpainting. arXiv preprint arXiv:240314499
21. Esser P, Rombach R, Ommer B (2021) Taming transformers for high-resolution image synthesis. In: Proceedings of the IEEE/CVF conference on computer vision and pattern recognition, pp 12873–12883
22. Fernandez V, Sanchez P, Pinaya WHL, Jacenków G, Tsaftaris SA, Cardoso MJ (2023) Privacy distillation: reducing re-identification risk of diffusion models. In: International conference on medical image computing and computer-assisted intervention. Springer, Berlin, pp 3–13
23. Freund Y, Haussler D (1991) Unsupervised learning of distributions on binary vectors using two layer networks. In: Advances in neural information processing systems, vol. 4. Morgan-Kaufmann
24. Friedrich P, Wolleb J, Bieder F, Thieringer FM, Cattin PC (2023) Point cloud diffusion models for automatic implant generation. In: International conference on medical image computing and computer-assisted intervention. Springer, Berlin, pp 112–122
25. Friedrich P, Wolleb J, Bieder F, Durrer A, Cattin PC (2024) WDM: 3d wavelet diffusion models for high-resolution medical image synthesis. arXiv preprint arXiv:240219043
26. Frisch Y, Fuchs M, Sanner A, Ucar FA, Frenzel M, Wasielica-Poslednik J, Gericke A, Wagner FM, Dratsch T, Mukhopadhyay A (2023) Synthesising rare cataract surgery samples with guided diffusion models. In: International conference on medical image computing and computer-assisted intervention. Springer, Berlin, pp 354–364
27. Gandikota R, Materzynska J, Fiotto-Kaufman J, Bau D (2023) Erasing concepts from diffusion models. In: Proceedings of the IEEE/CVF international conference on computer vision, pp 2426–2436
28. Geman D, Geman S, Hallonquist N, Younes L (2015) Visual turing test for computer vision systems. Proc Natl Acad Sci 112(12):3618–3623
29. Goodfellow I, Pouget-Abadie J, Mirza M, Xu B, Warde-Farley D, Ozair S, Courville A, Bengio Y (2014) Generative adversarial nets. In: Advances in neural information processing systems 27
30. Graf R, Schmitt J, Schlaeger S, Möller HK, Sideri-Lampretsa V, Sekuboyina A, Krieg SM, Wiestler B, Menze B, Rueckert D, et al (2023) Denoising diffusion-based MRI to CT image translation enables automated spinal segmentation. Eur Radiol Exp 7(1):70
31. Granstedt JL, Kelkar VA, Zhou W, Anastasio MA (2021) SlabGAN: a method for generating efficient 3D anisotropic medical volumes using generative adversarial networks. In: Medical imaging 2021: image processing, SPIE, vol 11596, pp 329–335
32. Gulrajani I, Ahmed F, Arjovsky M, Dumoulin V, Courville AC (2017) Improved training of Wasserstein GANs. In: Advances in neural information processing systems, vol. 30. Curran Associates, Inc
33. Han J, Choi H, Choi Y, Kim J, Ha JW, Choi J (2022) Rarity score: a new metric to evaluate the uncommonness of synthesized images. In: The eleventh international conference on learning representations

34. Hataya R, Bao H, Arai H (2023) Will large-scale generative models corrupt future datasets? In: 2023 IEEE/CVF international conference on computer vision (ICCV). IEEE, pp 20498–20508
35. He J, Li B, Yang G, Liu Z (2024) Blaze3dm: marry triplane representation with diffusion for 3D medical inverse problem solving. arXiv preprint arXiv:240515241
36. Heusel M, Ramsauer H, Unterthiner T, Nessler B, Hochreiter S (2017) Gans trained by a two time-scale update rule converge to a local nash equilibrium. In: Advances in neural information processing systems, vol. 30. Curran Associates, Inc
37. Ho J, Jain A, Abbeel P (2020) Denoising diffusion probabilistic models. Adv Neural Inf Process Syst 33:6840–6851
38. Hong S, Marinescu R, Dalca AV, Bonkhoff AK, Bretzner M, Rost NS, Golland P (2021) 3D-StyleGAN: a style-based generative adversarial network for generative modeling of three-dimensional medical images. In: Deep generative models, and data augmentation, labelling, and imperfections: first workshop, DGM4MICCAI 2021, and first workshop, DALI 2021, Held in Conjunction with MICCAI 2021, Strasbourg, October 1, 2021, Proceedings 1. Springer, Berlin, pp 24–34
39. Hu S, Lei B, Wang S, Wang Y, Feng Z, Shen Y (2021) Bidirectional mapping generative adversarial networks for brain mr to pet synthesis. IEEE Trans Med Imaging 41(1):145–157
40. Hu Q, Li H, Zhang J (2022) Domain-adaptive 3d medical image synthesis: an efficient unsupervised approach. In: International conference on medical image computing and computer-assisted intervention. Springer, Berlin, pp 495–504
41. Huijben E, Terpstra ML, Galapon Jr A, Pai S, Thummerer A, Koopmans P, Afonso M, van Eijnatten M, Gurney-Champion O, Chen Z, et al (2024) Generating synthetic computed tomography for radiotherapy: Synthrad2023 challenge report. arXiv preprint arXiv:240308447
42. Jothiraj FVS, Mashhadi A (2023) Phoenix: a federated generative diffusion model. arXiv preprint arXiv:230604098
43. Kalantar R, Hindocha S, Hunter B, Sharma B, Khan N, Koh DM, Ahmed M, Aboagye EO, Lee RW, Blackledge MD (2023) Non-contrast ct synthesis using patch-based cycle-consistent generative adversarial network (cycle-GAN) for radiomics and deep learning in the era of covid-19. Sci Rep 13(1):10568
44. Kalkhof J, Kühn A, Frisch Y, Mukhopadhyay A (2024) Frequency-time diffusion with neural cellular automata. arXiv preprint arXiv:240106291
45. Kapoor J, Macke JH, Baumgartner CF (2023) Multiscale metamorphic vae for 3d brain mri synthesis. arXiv preprint arXiv:230103588
46. Karras T, Laine S, Aittala M, Hellsten J, Lehtinen J, Aila T (2020) Analyzing and improving the image quality of StyleGAN. In: Proceedings of the IEEE/CVF conference on computer vision and pattern recognition, pp 8110–8119
47. Khader F, Müller-Franzes G, Tayebi Arasteh S, Han T, Haarburger C, Schulze-Hagen M, Schad P, Engelhardt S, Baeßler B, Foersch S, et al (2023) Denoising diffusion probabilistic models for 3d medical image generation. Sci Rep 13(1):7303
48. Kim J, Park H (2024) Adaptive latent diffusion model for 3d medical image to image translation: multi-modal magnetic resonance imaging study. In: Proceedings of the IEEE/CVF Winter conference on applications of computer Vision, pp 7604–7613
49. Kim B, Han I, Ye JC (2022) Diffusemorph: unsupervised deformable image registration using diffusion model. In: European conference on computer vision. Springer, Berlin, pp 347–364
50. Kim J, Li Y, Shin B-S (2024) 3D-DGGAN: a data-guided generative adversarial network for high fidelity in medical image generation. IEEE J Biomed Health Inf, 28(5):2904–2915
51. Kingma DP, Welling M (2013) Auto-encoding variational bayes. arXiv preprint arXiv:13126114
52. Ktena I, Wiles O, Albuquerque I, Rebuffi SA, Tanno R, Roy AG, Azizi S, Belgrave D, Kohli P, Cemgil T, et al (2024) Generative models improve fairness of medical classifiers under distribution shifts. Nat Med 30:1166–1173

53. Kuangyu S, Rui G, Song X, Axel R, Biao L (2022) Ultra-low dose pet imaging challenge 2022. https://doi.org/10.5281/zenodo.6361846
54. Kwon G, Han C, Kim Ds (2019) Generation of 3d brain MRI using auto-encoding generative adversarial networks. In: International conference on medical image computing and computer-assisted intervention. Springer, Berlin, pp 118–126
55. Kynkäänniemi T, Karras T, Laine S, Lehtinen J, Aila T (2019) Improved precision and recall metric for assessing generative models. In: Advances in neural information processing systems 32
56. Lan H, Initiative ADN, Toga AW, Sepehrband F (2021) Three-dimensional self-attention conditional GAN with spectral normalization for multimodal neuroimaging synthesis. Magn Reson Med 86(3):1718–1733
57. Lee S, Chung H, Park M, Park J, Ryu WS, Ye JC (2023) Improving 3d imaging with pre-trained perpendicular 2d diffusion models. In: Proceedings of the IEEE/CVF international conference on computer vision, pp 10710–10720
58. Li C, Bovik AC (2010) Content-partitioned structural similarity index for image quality assessment. Signal Process Image Commun 25(7):517–526
59. Li AC, Prabhudesai M, Duggal S, Brown E, Pathak D (2023) Your diffusion model is secretly a zero-shot classifier. In: Proceedings of the IEEE/CVF international conference on computer vision, pp 2206–2217
60. Li Y, Yakushev I, Hedderich DM, Wachinger C (2024) Pasta: pathology-aware MRI to pet cross-modal translation with diffusion models. arXiv preprint arXiv:240516942
61. Li Z, Wang Y, Zhang J, Wu W, Yu H (2024) Two-and-a-half order score-based model for solving 3D ill-posed inverse problems. Comput Biol Med 168:107819
62. Lin W, Lin W, Chen G, Zhang H, Gao Q, Huang Y, Tong T, Du M, Initiative ADN (2021) Bidirectional mapping of brain MRI and PET with 3D reversible GAN for the diagnosis of Alzheimer's disease. Front Neurosci 15:646013
63. Liu Y, Dwivedi G, Boussaid F, Sanfilippo F, Yamada M, Bennamoun M (2023) Inflating 2D convolution weights for efficient generation of 3D medical images. Comput Methods Programs Biomed 240:107685
64. Luo Y, Wang Y, Zu C, Zhan B, Wu X, Zhou J, Shen D, Zhou L (2021) 3D transformer-GAN for high-quality pet reconstruction. In: Medical image computing and computer assisted intervention–MICCAI 2021: 24th international conference, Strasbourg, September 27–October 1, 2021, Proceedings, Part VI 24. Springer, Berlin, pp 276–285
65. Lutz S, Amplianitis K, Smolic A (2018) AlphaGAN: generative adversarial networks for natural image matting. arXiv preprint arXiv:180710088
66. Mao X, Li Q, Xie H, Lau RY, Wang Z, Paul Smolley S (2017) Least squares generative adversarial networks. In: Proceedings of the IEEE international conference on computer vision, pp 2794–2802
67. McCollough CH, Bartley AC, Carter RE, Chen B, Drees TA, Edwards P, Holmes III DR, Huang AE, Khan F, Leng S, et al. (2017) Low-dose CT for the detection and classification of metastatic liver lesions: results of the 2016 low dose CT grand challenge. Med Phys 44(10):e339–e352
68. Melanie G, Hannah E (2021) Brain MRI reconstruction challenge with realistic noise. https://doi.org/10.5281/zenodo.4572640
69. Mensing D, Hirsch J, Wenzel M, Günther M (2022) 3D (c) GAN for whole body mr synthesis. In: MICCAI workshop on deep generative models. Springer, Berlin, pp 97–105
70. Miyato T, Kataoka T, Koyama M, Yoshida Y (2018) Spectral normalization for generative adversarial networks. In: International conference on learning representations
71. Packhäuser K, Gündel S, Münster N, Syben C, Christlein V, Maier A (2022) Deep learning-based patient re-identification is able to exploit the biometric nature of medical chest X-ray data. Sci Rep 12(1):14851
72. Pan S, Chang CW, Peng J, Zhang J, Qiu RL, Wang T, Roper J, Liu T, Mao H, Yang X (2023) Cycle-guided denoising diffusion probability model for 3D cross-modality MRI synthesis. arXiv preprint arXiv:230500042

73. Pan S, Abouei E, Wynne J, Chang CW, Wang T, Qiu RL, Li Y, Peng J, Roper J, Patel P, et al (2024) Synthetic CT generation from MRI using 3D transformer-based denoising diffusion model. Med Phys 51(4):2538–2548
74. Peng W, Adeli E, Bosschieter T, Park SH, Zhao Q, Pohl KM (2023) Generating realistic brain MRIs via a conditional diffusion probabilistic model. In: International conference on medical image computing and computer-assisted intervention. Springer, Berlin, pp 14–24
75. Phung H, Dao Q, Tran A (2023) Wavelet diffusion models are fast and scalable image generators. In: Proceedings of the IEEE/CVF conference on computer vision and pattern recognition, pp 10199–10208
76. Pinaya WH, Tudosiu PD, Dafflon J, Da Costa PF, Fernandez V, Nachev P, Ourselin S, Cardoso MJ (2022) Brain imaging generation with latent diffusion models. In: MICCAI workshop on deep generative models. Springer, Berlin, pp 117–126
77. Poonkodi S, Kanchana M (2023) 3D-MedTranCSGAN: 3D medical image transformation using CSGAN. Comput Biol Med 153:106541
78. Renieblas GP, Nogués AT, González AM, Gómez-Leon N, Del Castillo EG (2017) Structural similarity index family for image quality assessment in radiological images. J Med Imaging 4(3):035501–035501
79. Rezende D, Mohamed S (2015) Variational inference with normalizing flows. In: International conference on machine learning, PMLR, pp 1530–1538
80. Rombach R, Blattmann A, Lorenz D, Esser P, Ommer B (2022) High-resolution image synthesis with latent diffusion models. In: Proceedings of the IEEE/CVF conference on computer vision and pattern recognition, pp 10684–10695
81. Salimans T, Goodfellow I, Zaremba W, Cheung V, Radford A, Chen X (2016) Improved techniques for training GANs. In: Advances in neural information processing systems, vol. 29. Curran Associates, Inc
82. Sanchez P, Kascenas A, Liu X, O'Neil AQ, Tsaftaris SA (2022) What is healthy? Generative counterfactual diffusion for lesion localization. In: MICCAI workshop on deep generative models. Springer, Berlin, pp 34–44
83. Segato A, Corbetta V, Di Marzo M, Pozzi L, De Momi E (2020) Data augmentation of 3D brain environment using deep convolutional refined auto-encoding alpha GAN. IEEE Trans Med Robot Bionics 3(1):269–272
84. Sikka A, Virk JS, Bathula DR, et al (2021) MRI to PET cross-modality translation using globally and locally aware GAN (GLA-GAN) for multi-modal diagnosis of Alzheimer's disease. arXiv preprint arXiv:210802160
85. Sohl-Dickstein J, Weiss E, Maheswaranathan N, Ganguli S (2015) Deep unsupervised learning using nonequilibrium thermodynamics. In: International conference on machine learning, PMLR, pp 2256–2265
86. Song J, Meng C, Ermon S (2020) Denoising diffusion implicit models. arXiv preprint arXiv:201002502
87. Song Y, Dhariwal P, Chen M, Sutskever I (2023) Consistency models. In: Proceedings of the 40th international conference on machine learning, pp 32211–32252
88. Stolt-Ansó N, McGinnis J, Pan J, Hammernik K, Rueckert D (2023) Nisf: Neural implicit segmentation functions. In: International conference on medical image computing and computer-assisted intervention. Springer, Berlin, pp 734–744
89. Sun L, Chen J, Xu Y, Gong M, Yu K, Batmanghelich K (2022) Hierarchical amortized GAN for 3D high resolution medical image synthesis. IEEE J Biomed Health Inf 26(8):3966–3975
90. Uzunova H, Ehrhardt J, Handels H (2020) Memory-efficient GAN-based domain translation of high resolution 3D medical images. Comput Med Imaging Graphics 86:101801
91. Van Breugel B, Qian Z, Van Der Schaar M (2023) Synthetic data, real errors: how (not) to publish and use synthetic data. In: International conference on machine learning, PMLR, pp 34793–34808
92. van den Burg G, Williams C (2021) On memorization in probabilistic deep generative models. Adv Neural Inf Process Syst 34:27916–27928

93. Van Den Oord A, Vinyals O, et al (2017) Neural discrete representation learning. In: Advances in neural information processing systems, vol. 30. Curran Associates, Inc
94. Volokitin A, Erdil E, Karani N, Tezcan KC, Chen X, Van Gool L, Konukoglu E (2020) Modelling the distribution of 3D brain MRI using a 2D slice vae. In: Medical image computing and computer assisted intervention–MICCAI 2020: 23rd international conference, Lima, October 4–8, 2020, Proceedings, Part VII 23. Springer, Berlin, pp 657–666
95. Wang Z, Simoncelli EP, Bovik AC (2003) Multiscale structural similarity for image quality assessment. In: The thirty-seventh Asilomar conference on signals, systems & computers, 2003, IEEE, vol 2, pp 1398–1402
96. Wang Z, Bovik AC, Sheikh HR, Simoncelli EP (2004) Image quality assessment: from error visibility to structural similarity. IEEE Trans Image Process 13(4):600–612
97. Wang Y, Yu B, Wang L, Zu C, Lalush DS, Lin W, Wu X, Zhou J, Shen D, Zhou L (2018) 3D conditional generative adversarial networks for high-quality PET image estimation at low dose. Neuroimage 174:550–562
98. Wang Y, Luo Y, Zu C, Zhan B, Jiao Z, Wu X, Zhou J, Shen D, Zhou L (2024) 3D multi-modality transformer-GAN for high-quality PET reconstruction. Med Image Anal 91:102983
99. Wei W, Poirion E, Bodini B, Durrleman S, Ayache N, Stankoff B, Colliot O (2019) Predicting pet-derived demyelination from multimodal MRI using sketcher-refiner adversarial training for multiple sclerosis. Med Image Anal 58:101546
100. Wen Y, Chen L, Deng Y, Zhou C (2021) Rethinking pre-training on medical imaging. J Vis Commun Image Represent 78:103145
101. Wolleb J, Bieder F, Sandkühler R, Cattin PC (2022) Diffusion models for medical anomaly detection. In: International conference on medical image computing and computer-assisted intervention. Springer, Berlin, pp 35–45
102. Wolleb J, Sandkühler R, Bieder F, Valmaggia P, Cattin PC (2022) Diffusion models for implicit image segmentation ensembles. In: International conference on medical imaging with deep learning, PMLR, pp 1336–1348
103. Wolterink JM, Leiner T, Viergever MA, Išgum I (2017) Generative adversarial networks for noise reduction in low-dose ct. IEEE Trans Med Imaging 36(12):2536–2545
104. Xiao Z, Kreis K, Vahdat A (2021) Tackling the generative learning trilemma with denoising diffusion GANs. In: International conference on learning representations
105. Xie H, Gan W, Zhou B, Chen X, Liu Q, Guo X, Guo L, An H, Kamilov US, Wang G, et al (2023) Dose-aware diffusion model for 3D ultra low-dose pet imaging. arXiv preprint arXiv:231104248
106. Xue Y, Peng Y, Bi L, Feng D, Kim J (2023) CG-3DSRGAN: a classification guided 3d generative adversarial network for image quality recovery from low-dose pet images. In: 2023 45th annual international conference of the IEEE engineering in medicine & biology society (EMBC), IEEE, pp 1–4
107. Ye J, Ni H, Jin P, Huang SX, Xue Y (2023) Synthetic augmentation with large-scale unconditional pre-training. In: International conference on medical image computing and computer-assisted intervention. Springer, Berlin, pp 754–764
108. Zeng P, Zhou L, Zu C, Zeng X, Jiao Z, Wu X, Zhou J, Shen D, Wang Y (2022) 3D CVT-GAN: a 3D convolutional vision transformer-GAN for PET reconstruction. In: International conference on medical image computing and computer-assisted intervention. Springer, Berlin, pp 516–526
109. Zhang J, He X, Qing L, Gao F, Wang B (2022) bPGAN: brain PET synthesis from MRI using generative adversarial network for multi-modal Alzheimer's disease diagnosis. Comput Methods Programs Biomed 217:106676
110. Zhao P, Pan H, Xia S (2021) Mri-trans-GAN: 3D MRI cross-modality translation. In: 2021 40th Chinese control conference (CCC). IEEE, pp 7229–7234
111. Zhu L, Xue Z, Jin Z, Liu X, He J, Liu Z, Yu L (2023) Make-a-volume: leveraging latent diffusion models for cross-modality 3d brain mri synthesis. In: International conference on medical image computing and computer-assisted intervention. Springer, Berlin, pp 592–601
112. Zhu L, Codella N, Chen D, Jin Z, Yuan L, Yu L (2024) Generative enhancement for 3D medical images. arXiv preprint arXiv:240312852

Chapter 14
Cross-Modal Attention Fusion Based Generative Adversarial Network for Text-to-Image Synthesis

Xiang Chen and **Xiaodong Luo**

Abstract The synthesis of images from attribute descriptors is an emerging and intricate domain within the realm of computer vision, which has various application potentials in public security and multimedia. Existing attribute vector-to-face (V2F) synthesis methods mainly generate faces based on attribute label vectors that lack rich semantic feature information, which leads to low-quality generated face images. To surmount this limitation, we advocate attribute word-to-face (W2F) synthesis, leveraging sequences of attribute words rich in semantic content. A novel Cross-Modal Attention Fusion Generative Adversarial Network (CMAFGAN) is proposed to generate faces from facial attribute words. CMAFGAN stands out due to its incorporation of two innovative components, CMAF and WFT, which are proposed to explore the correlation between image features and the corresponding attribute word features. Experimental results on the CelebA and LFW datasets demonstrate that our CMAFGAN achieves state-of-the-art performance, effectively improving the quality of the synthesised faces. In particular, the consistency between the predicted images and input attribute words (R-precision) on the CelebA and LFW datasets achieved 61.24% and 64.46% respectively, representing a substantial improvement over prior techniques. Moreover, CMAFGAN achieves comparable or better performance than the current best methods on text-to-image synthesis (R-precision 83.41% on caltech-ucsd birds-200-2011, CUB). Additionally, we explore the application of CMAFGAN for X-ray image synthesis from textual descriptions, yielding finely detailed images that exhibit high fidelity to the ground-truth.

X. Chen (✉)
College of Electrical and Information Engineering, Hunan University, Changsha, China
e-mail: xiangc@hnu.edu.cn

X. Luo
School of Information and Engineering, Sichuan Tourism University, Chengdu, China
e-mail: luoxd@sctu.edu.cn

L. Zhang et al. (eds.), *Generative Machine Learning Models in Medical Image Computing*, https://doi.org/10.1007/978-3-031-80965-1_14

14.1 Introduction

The advent of deep learning, particularly generative adversarial networks (GANs) [7]), has catalyzed face synthesis into a vibrant research frontier within the realm of computer vision. This encompasses a spectrum of innovative applications, such as facial attribute editing [8, 22, 23], text-to-face synthesis [3], and face inpainting [29], sketch-to-face generation [10], and so on. These tasks have enormous potential in public safety, computer-aided design, and multimedia applications [30, 32]. In this paper, we explore a novel task, attribute word-to-face (W2F) synthesis, which aims to achieve face synthesis based on given facial attribute words, as shown in Fig. 14.1. Different from the input of the existing attribute vector-to-face (V2F) synthesis, which is the attribute label vector of the face, the input of W2F is the list of the face attribute words (e.g. hair colour, hairstyle, nose, eyes, mouth, and beard). There are three main goals for W2F approaches: (1) generating realistic faces, (2) ensuring that the generated face images are consistent with input attribute words, and (3) robust face synthesis, invariant to the order of attribute words.

The W2F task holds direct relevance to the tasks of text-to-image and V2F, or it can even be seen as a hybrid of both. Similar to text-to-image/face synthesis [20, 34, 35], W2F is essentially a cross-modal task between language and image. The main difference between these two tasks lies in their input, where the former is a sentence description, and the latter is a sequence of attribute words. Text-to-image/face synthesis has drawn increasing attention in recent years [20, 34, 35]. Based on multistage synthesis [20, 34, 35], with strategies such as attention and dynamic memory [32, 41], they can learn sufficient semantic information from the input sentences to generate realistic images. Nonetheless, the performance of text-to-image generation is easily affected by the phraseology of the input sentence. In contrast, W2F synthesis, which operates on a sequence of attribute words,

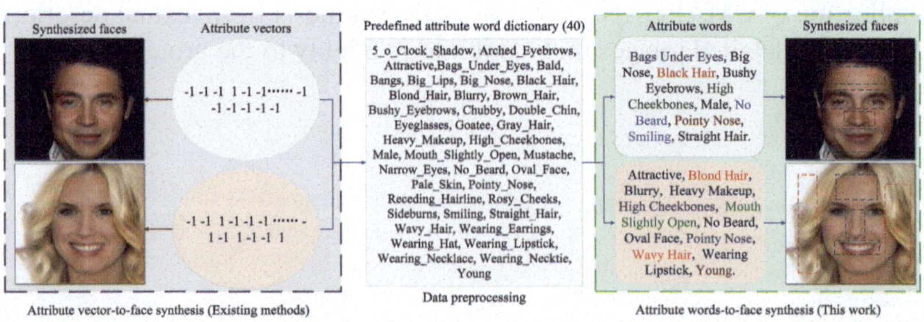

Fig. 14.1 Examples of existing attribute vector-to-face (V2F) and the proposed attribute word-to-face (W2F) synthesis. Given the 40-dimensional attribute vector ('1' means containing this attribute word, while '-1' means without) of each face on the datasets (CelebA [16] and LFW [12]), the attribute words are extracted from the predefined attribute word dictionary of the corresponding dataset. Note that, the attribute words instead of the attributes vector are the input of W2F

demonstrates enhanced resilience to variations in word order, thereby offering a more robust framework for image synthesis.

V2F synthesis represents a closely related yet distinct challenge to W2F synthesis, with the primary distinction lying in the input format. Unlike W2F, which leverages descriptive sentences, V2F relies on a fixed-length attribute vector. Recently, several pieces of research have been proposed to tackle this issue [5, 30, 33]. They generally used conditional generative adversarial networks (GANs), which combine the facial attribute vector with noise (conforming to a normal distribution) to synthesise face images consistent with the given facial attribute vectors. However, the fixed-dimensional attribute vector is too strict for realistic applications and unable to present sufficient semantic information to the network. For example, the attribute vector is generally a 40-dimensional vector (in CelebA and LFW), making it a time-consuming and challenging task for an untrained person to provide such an attribute vector. Instead, W2F synthesis is more flexible, and can be applied to a random number of attribute words, since its input is a list of attribute words. In addition, attribute words can provide more sufficient semantic information from the given attributes, resulting in more realistic and consistent image synthesis. Therefore, instead of using attribute vectors, we propose synthesising face images with attribute words, named attribute word-to-face (W2F) synthesis. Inspired by text-to-image algorithms [32, 35, 41], a novel cross-modal attention fusion based generative adversarial network, CMAFGAN, is designed to directly translate facial attribute words into lifelike face images, leveraging the semantic richness of natural language to transcend the limitations of vector-based methods.

The inherent semantic disparities between attribute word features and image features present a formidable challenge in establishing a direct semantic mapping. To address this challenge, we introduce a novel Word Feature Transformation (WFT) module, crafted to restructure attribute word features, thereby aligning them with the intrinsic structure of image features. Concurrently, to deepen the understanding of the interplay between attribute words and image generation, we have designed an innovative Cross-Modal Attention Fusion (CMAF) module. This module is tasked with uncovering the subtle correlations that exist between visual and linguistic features. The synergistic application of the WFT and CMAF modules allows for the seamless integration of features, which in turn, significantly enhances the network's capacity to produce highly realistic images.

In summary, the contributions of this work are as follows:

- To achieve more efficient and robust face synthesis from given facial attributes, we propose an end-to-end framework, CMAFGAN, to use the corresponding attribute words for face synthesis, instead of the original attribute vectors. To the best of our knowledge, this work is the first work to solve the task of W2F.
- To eliminate the semantic gaps between the word and image domains, a WFT is proposed to transform the structure of the attribute word feature to match the image feature, followed by a CMAF module to explore the correlation between word features and image features. Based on cross-attention, CMAF provides a better approach to fusing word features and image features than previous research.

- The proposed CMAFGAN framework is flexible, which can be easy to apply in realistic applications. CMAFGAN has the advantages of both attribute V2F and text-to-face synthesis, and it can be used for training these two types of datasets, which is not afforded by previous research. Compared to the V2F, it does not require a fixed vector as input. Additionally, our framework establishes a robust face synthesis process that remains consistent, regardless of variations in individual descriptive styles, a common challenge in text-to-face synthesis.
- We comprehensively evaluate the proposed method across two publicly available datasets, CelebA and LFW, and compare it with state-of-the-art V2F methods, showcasing its exceptional performance in terms of image synthesis quality and fidelity. In addition to attribute-to-face synthesis, our method also achieves exciting performance in text-to-image synthesis on the CUB [28] dataset and Open-i X-ray image dataset [4], further underscoring its versatility and efficacy.

14.2 Related Work

W2F synthesis represents a specialized subfield within the broader domain of face synthesis, focusing on the translation of descriptive attribute words into visual representations. Our proposed framework, CMAFGAN, fundamentally operates as a text-to-image synthesis network, distinguished by its integration of cross-modality modules that facilitate the transition between linguistic and visual domains. Therefore, we first summarize the related work on face synthesis, followed by detailed introductions on text-to-image synthesis and cross-modal attention module.

14.2.1 Face Synthesis

Deep learning-based face synthesis aims to generate face images from given conditions (e.g., noise [1], incomplete facial images [2, 17], text, and attribute vectors [5, 30, 33]). In this section, we first discuss those research focusing on general face synthesis and then consider diving into text/attribute-to-face synthesis.

General Face Synthesis Face synthesis is a hot topic in computer vision. Early GANs were proposed to synthesise images by sampling noise vectors from Gaussian distribution [7]. Subsequent research had achieved controllable face synthesis based on conditional GAN, including image-based synthesis (e.g., face in-painting and face reorientation) and semantic-based synthesis [2, 17] (e.g. attribute V2F synthesis and facial attribute editing). Among those tasks, face in-painting and face facial attribute editing were two of the most common applications.

Text-to-Face Synthesis Text-to-face synthesis is a more challenging task compared with the aforementioned tasks, since the inputs (text sentence description of facial attributes) and outputs (facial images) belong to two different modalities.

This topic has drawn some attention in recent research. Gatt et al. [6] constructed a dataset named Face2Text that contains 400 face images, each face of which contained at least 3 sentence descriptions. Although this dataset is built for face description and the corresponding description of faces is not detailed, it is also an early dataset that can be used for text-to-face synthesis. Subsequently, Chen et al. [3] constructed a new dataset SCU-text2face that contains 1000 images based on CelebA [16], where each image contains 5 different refined sentences. They further proposed a novel FTGAN network to substantially improve the quality of text-generated face images. Zhou et al. [39] proposed a cyclic generative adversarial network, and introduced a pre-trained BERT basic model to extract feature vectors of text to generate high-resolution face images, and achieved good results in the FFHQ-Text [38] dataset.

Attribute Vector-to-Face Synthesis Recently, there has been a surge of interest in V2F synthesis [5, 30], a domain closely allied with W2F synthesis. Di et al. [5] proposed a two-stage scheme to synthesise face images according to the given attribute vectors, where the first step was to synthesise facial sketches based on the Gaussian noises and sketch attribute vectors, and the second step was to generate the real-world face images from the synthesised sketch and facial attribute vectors. The fixed-dimensional attribute vector used in V2F synthesis poses limitations in practical scenarios. The rigid structure often falls short of capturing the nuanced semantic information necessary for the network to produce varied and realistic face images. In light of these challenges, we advocate for an alternative approach: utilizing attribute words for face synthesis. This method is capable of extracting comprehensive semantic insights from the given attribute words, thereby enabling a more adaptable and robust synthesis process.

14.2.2 Text-to-Image Synthesis

Our proposed CMAFGAN also draws inspiration from advancements in text-to-image synthesis, which leverage textual descriptions of facial attributes as input. Text-to-image generation methods generally include two categories: single-stage and multistage generation. The single-stage method consists of a single generator and discriminator, such as in [19, 27], in which the generated images were generally at low-resolution. The multistage method mainly adopted the cascade of several generators and discriminators, where low-resolution images were generated in the initial stage, and then, higher-resolution images were synthesised gradually in the subsequent stages. In recent work, multistage synthesis structures have been widely applied in text-to-image synthesis [34, 35, 40]. For example, AttnGAN [32] designed a three-stage generation network, with an attention module to calculate the corresponding region of the word representation in the image. However, existing methods often concatenate independent image and text features for subsequent layers, bypassing a deeper exploration of the semantic interplay between modalities.

14.2.3 Cross-Modal Schemes for Language and Vision

Learning the mapping from input attribute words to generated images necessitates effective integration of information across different modalities—a challenge that has not been fully resolved in prior text-to-image synthesis research. Recently, cross-modal attention mechanisms have emerged as pivotal in bridging the gap between computer vision and natural language processing, as evidenced by a series of influential studies [11, 14, 24, 31]. Li et al. [14] proposed Unicoder-VL to learn joint representations of vision and language in a pretraining manner, which achieved significant improvements in image-text retrieval and visual commonsense reasoning tasks. Similarly, Wang et al. [31] proposed cross-modal adaptive message passing (CAMP) for text-image retrieval. CAMP introduced a language and image cross-modal aggregation module to aggregate the image features and text features, and the cross-fusion feature was used to predict the matching score to improve the accuracy of text-image retrieval. The performance of incorporating cross-modal encoders was also demonstrated in ADCANs [11], and LXMERT [24]. Drawing inspiration from these advances, we design a CMAF module to capture the semantic correlation between synthetic face images and attribute words.

14.3 CMAFGAN

The proposed CMAFGAN is a three-stage generative adversarial network, that synthesises delicate images in three steps, as shown in Fig. 14.2. In the first stage, a decoder composed of four upsampling layers is used to transform the input global feature predicted by a trained Bi-LSTM text-encoder (T_E) into a low-resolution image (64×64). Building upon this foundation, the second and third stages advance the synthesis by taking the low-resolution image features from the preceding stage

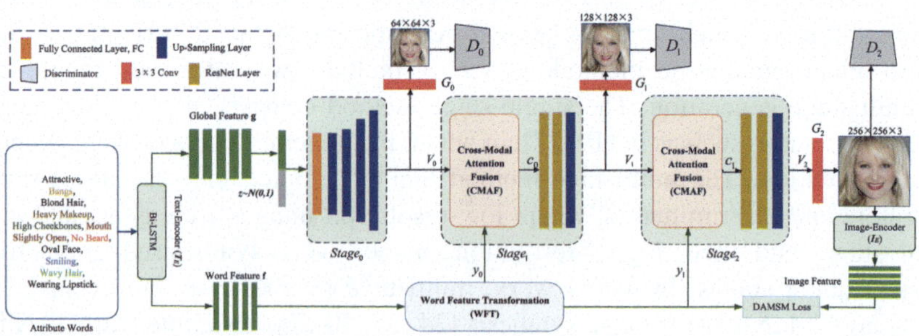

Fig. 14.2 The scheme of our proposed CMAFGAN, which is highlighted by the word feature transformation (WFT) and cross-modal attention fusion (CMAF). The WFT is designed to learn the word features, while the CMAF is proposed to learn the correlation between word features and image features

and leveraging the word features to predict increasingly higher-resolution images. To facilitate a more coherent integration of word features and image features, WFT and CMAF blocks are introduced in the second and third stages. For each stage of image refinement, a corresponding discriminator operates at the resolutions of $64 \times 64, 128 \times 128$, and 256×256 respectively. Furthermore, the loss function is meticulously computed across all three outputs to refine the learning process. Subsequent sections include the overall structure of CMAFGAN, the WFT module, CMAF module, and the design of the loss function.

14.3.1 Three-Stage Generation Network

Different from previous attribute V2F synthesis methods [5, 30, 33] that use the given attribute vector as input directly, we preprocess the original facial attribute vector to a description text (i.e., a text composed of all attribute words, using a comma as a gap, as shown in Fig. 14.1). Consequently, our network aligns more closely with text-to-image synthesis networks, accepting attribute words as input. Then the text of attribute words is fed into the pre-trained T_E to obtain the word feature vector $\mathbf{f}$ and global feature vector $\mathbf{g}$. The $\mathbf{g}$ is the encoding of the entire attribute text, a fixed-dimension feature vector. The $\mathbf{f}$ is the word embedding code for each word, which is a feature vector with variable length, and its dimension is consistent with the number of attribute words. The $\mathbf{g}$ concatenated with random Gaussian noise $\mathbf{z}$ is used as the input of the initial network $Stage_0$. The $\mathbf{f}$ serves as the input of the subsequent $Stage_{(1,2)}$, to further refine and guide the synthesis of high-quality images.

Similar to the previous text-to-image synthesis network [32, 33, 35, 41], our proposed CMAFGAN is based on a conditional generative adversarial network, which includes three cascaded generators G_0, G_1, and G_2, as shown in Fig. 14.2. The G_0, G_1, and G_2 synthesise images at 64×64, 128×128, and 256×256, respectively. Among the three generators, the G_0 is essential, since the initial image plays a dominant contribution in the final image. G_0 takes the concatenation of $\mathbf{g}$ and $\mathbf{z}$ as input and predicts images at 64×64 after the fully-connected layer, reshape, and four upsampling layers. G_1 and G_2 have similar structures, composing a WFT, a CMAF module, two residual module layers, an upsampling layer, and a 3×3 convolution layer. In our three-stage generative adversarial network, each stage G_i has a corresponding discriminator D_i. Similar to DM-GAN [41], in each discriminator, a spectral normalization [18] layer is added after the 3×3 convolution layer to optimize the convergence of gradient descent.

14.3.2 WFT Module

For text/word-to-image synthesis, how to convert language information into image information is a challenging problem. In the proposed three-stage generation

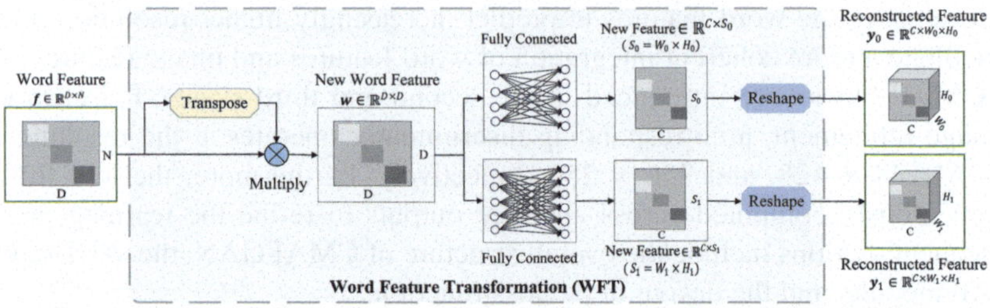

Fig. 14.3 The structure of word feature transformation (WFT) block, where "⊗" is matrix multiplication. WFT transforms the word feature into image space, converting the unfixed length word vectors **f** into the fixed-size image-like feature $\mathbf{y}_i$ $(i = 0, 1)$

solution, the global feature **g** is introduced as conditional input in the initial stage. In the latter two stages, the word feature **f** and image feature $\mathbf{v}_i (i = 0, 1)$ synthesised in the previous stage are fused to guide the image synthesis. The word feature vector and the image feature map originate from distinct domains, each with its unique structure, posing a significant hurdle in establishing a robust semantic link between linguistic and visual information. To bridge this gap, we introduce a WFT module to restructure the word features, aligning their architectural form with that of the image features, thereby facilitating a more coherent semantic association. The variability in the number of input attribute words across the dataset results in a variable-length word feature vector **f**, which introduces complexities in the tensor operations within the network. However, our WFT module adeptly addresses this challenge, enabling seamless integration despite the fluctuating length of the word feature vector. In WFT, we use transpose and self-multiplication operations to fix the length of the word feature. As shown in Fig. 14.3, the new word feature **w** is obtained from the word feature vector **f**, the formula can be given as,

$$\mathbf{w} = \mathbf{f} \times \mathbf{f}^{\mathrm{T}}, \tag{14.1}$$

where $\mathbf{f} \in \mathbb{R}^{D \times N}$, $\mathbf{w} \in \mathbb{R}^{D \times D}$, D is the dimension of word embedding vector, we set $D = 64$ during our model training. N is the number of input words, which is usually variable. The fixed-length word feature **w** is further transformed into a new feature space with the same dimension as the image feature $\mathbf{v}_i (i = 0, 1)$ through a fully connected (FC) and a reshape layer, formulated as,

$$\begin{aligned} \mathbf{y}_0 &= reshape(A_1 * \mathbf{w} + B_1), \\ \mathbf{y}_1 &= reshape(A_2 * \mathbf{w} + B_2), \end{aligned} \tag{14.2}$$

where A_1, B_1, A_2, B_2 are the weights learned automatically by optimisation, $\mathbf{y}_0 \in \mathbb{R}^{C \times W_0 \times H_0}$, $\mathbf{y}_1 \in \mathbb{R}^{C \times W_1 \times H_1}$, where C is the number of channels, $W_0 \times H_0$ and $W_1 \times H_1$ are the sizes of the generated image from $stage_0$ and $stage_1$, respectively. The $reshape(\cdot)$ means reshape operation.

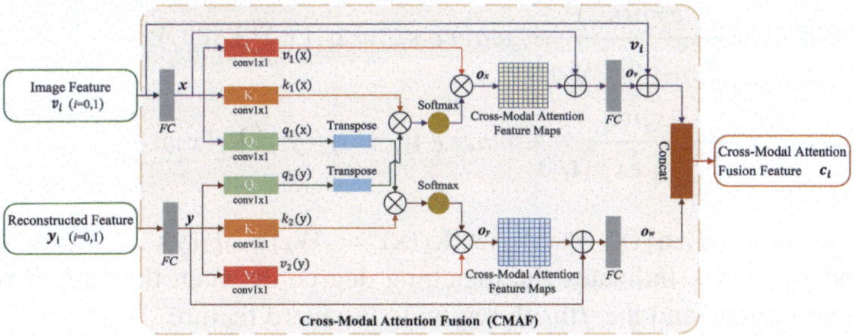

Fig. 14.4 The architecture of our CMAF module. The "⊗" is matrix multiplication, and "⊕" stands for plus. CMAF is used to capture the correlation between visual features and text features by computing cross-modal attention. The incorporation of CMAF helps to generate higher-quality images and advance the consistency between generated images and input text

14.3.3 CMAF Module

Attribute W2F synthesis is a sophisticated task that entails discerning the correlation between descriptive words and facial imagery. Central to this challenge is bridging the semantic chasm between the visual and linguistic domains. Inspired by [24, 36], we propose a CMAF module to jointly learn visual and linguistic information, as shown in Fig. 14.4. The reconstructed feature $\mathbf{y}_i$ $(i = 0, 1)$ is learned by the pretrained Bi-LSTM text encoder and WFT. The image feature $\mathbf{v}_i$ $(i = 0, 1)$ is from the hidden layer of $Stage_0$ and $Stage_1$, respectively. The $\mathbf{y}_i$ and $\mathbf{v}_i$ are used to learn the cross-modal attention map $\mathbf{c}_i$ from each other in the CMAF module. Then the fused feature $\mathbf{c}_i$ is fed into the next generator to generate an image.

In the CMAF, due to the limitations of GPU memory, the size of the features used to calculate the cross-modal attention needs to be reduced, the $\mathbf{v}_i$ and $\mathbf{y}_i$ are transformed into new size features $\mathbf{x}$ and $\mathbf{y}$ by a fully connected (FC) layer, respectively. They are presented as,

$$\begin{aligned} \mathbf{x} &= A_3 * \mathbf{v}_i + B_3, \\ \mathbf{y} &= A_4 * \mathbf{y}_i + B_4, \end{aligned} \tag{14.3}$$

where A_3, B_3, A_4, B_4 are the weights learned automatically by optimisation, $\mathbf{x} \in \mathbb{R}^{C\times W\times H}$ and $\mathbf{y} \in \mathbb{R}^{C\times W\times H}$, $W \times H$ is the new size after dimension reduction.

By 1×1 convolution layers (q_1, k_1, q_2, k_2), the new image features $\mathbf{x}$ and the new word feature $\mathbf{y}$ are transformed into two different feature spaces to calculate the pixel-level cross-modal attention. First, the matching degree between the image feature space and word feature space is calculated, and they can be given as,

$$\beta_{j,i} = \frac{exp(\mathbf{s}_{ij})}{\sum_{i=1}^{S} exp(\mathbf{s}_{ij})}, \; where\; \mathbf{s}_{ij} = \mathbf{q}_1(x_i)^T \mathbf{k}_2(y_j),$$
$$\rho_{j,i} = \frac{exp(\mathbf{t}_{ij})}{\sum_{i=1}^{S} exp(\mathbf{t}_{ij})}, \; where\; \mathbf{t}_{ij} = \mathbf{q}_2(y_i)^T \mathbf{k}_1(x_j), \tag{14.4}$$

where $S = W \times H$, $\mathbf{q}_1(\mathbf{x}) = \mathbf{W}_{q1}\mathbf{x}$, $\mathbf{k}_1(\mathbf{x}) = \mathbf{W}_{k1}\mathbf{x}$, $\mathbf{q}_2(\mathbf{y}) = \mathbf{W}_{q2}\mathbf{y}$, $\mathbf{k}_2(\mathbf{y}) = \mathbf{W}_{k2}\mathbf{y}$, and $\beta_{j,i}$ / $\rho_{j,i}$ indicates the matching degree between the ith/jth region in the generated image and the jth/ith region in the word feature.

Then, the matching degree calculated in the previous step is multiplied by the value of the feature to obtain the cross-modal attention maps $\mathbf{o}_x$ and $\mathbf{o}_y$,

$$\mathbf{o}_x = (\mathbf{o}_{x1}, \mathbf{o}_{x2}, \mathbf{o}_{x3}, \ldots, \mathbf{o}_{xi}, \mathbf{o}_{xj}, \ldots, \mathbf{o}_{xS}) \in \mathbb{R}^{C\times S},$$
$$\mathbf{o}_y = (\mathbf{o}_{y1}, \mathbf{o}_{y2}, \mathbf{o}_{y3}, \ldots, \mathbf{o}_{yi}, \mathbf{o}_{yj}, \ldots, \mathbf{o}_{yS}) \in \mathbb{R}^{C\times S},$$
$$\mathbf{o}_{xj} = \sum_{i=1}^{S} \rho_{j,i}\mathbf{v}_1(x_i), \; where\; \mathbf{v}_1(x_i) = \mathbf{W}_{v1}x_i, \tag{14.5}$$
$$\mathbf{o}_{yj} = \sum_{i=1}^{S} \beta_{j,i}\mathbf{v}_2(y_i), \; where\; \mathbf{v}_2(y_i) = \mathbf{W}_{v2}y_i,$$

in these formulas, $\mathbf{W}_{q1} \in \mathbb{R}^{\overline{C}\times C}$, $\mathbf{W}_{k1} \in \mathbb{R}^{\overline{C}\times C}$, $\mathbf{W}_{v1} \in \mathbb{R}^{C\times C}$ and $\mathbf{W}_{q2} \in \mathbb{R}^{\overline{C}\times C}$, $\mathbf{W}_{k2} \in \mathbb{R}^{\overline{C}\times C}$, $\mathbf{W}_{v2} \in \mathbb{R}^{C\times C}$ are the weight matrices automatically learned by 1×1 convolutions. In our experiments, we use $\overline{C} = \frac{C}{8}$.

The cross-modal attention maps $\mathbf{o}_x$ and $\mathbf{o}_y$ are restored into the same size features as $\mathbf{v}_i$ by linear transformation (FC) layer, the formulas are as,

$$\mathbf{o}_v = A_5 * (\mathbf{o}_x + \mathbf{x}) + B_5,$$
$$\mathbf{o}_w = A_6 * (\mathbf{o}_y + \mathbf{y}) + B_6, \tag{14.6}$$

where A_5, B_5, A_6, B_6 are the weights to be learned automatically in training.

Finally, the new cross-modal attention maps $\mathbf{o}_v$, $\mathbf{o}_w$, and the image feature $\mathbf{v}_i$ obtained in the previous stage are combined as the input (CMAF features $\mathbf{c}_i$) of the subsequent residual layer, expressed as,

$$\mathbf{c}_i = concat(\gamma_1 * \mathbf{o}_v + \mathbf{v}_i, \mathbf{o}_w), \; where\; (i = 0, 1), \tag{14.7}$$

where γ_1 is the weight of $\mathbf{o}_v$ (learned automatically), and $concat(\cdot)$ is concatenation.

14.3.4 Loss Function

The loss function of CMAFGAN includes two parts, the generator loss $\mathcal{L}_{\mathcal{G}}$ and the discriminator loss $\mathcal{L}_{D_i}$. The $\mathcal{L}_{\mathcal{G}}$ further consists of the adversarial loss $\mathcal{L}_{G_i}$ for G_i, Deep Attentional Multimodal Similarity Model (DAMSM) loss $\mathcal{L}_{DAMSM}$ (details can be found in [32]), and conditioning augmentation loss $\mathcal{L}_{CA}$ [41], formulated as,

$$\mathcal{L}_{\mathcal{G}} = \sum_{i=0}^{2} \mathcal{L}_{G_i} + \lambda_1 \mathcal{L}_{DAMSM} + \lambda_2 \mathcal{L}_{CA}, \tag{14.8}$$

where λ_1 and λ_2 are the corresponding weights of DAMSM loss and $\mathcal{L}_{CA}$.

The $\mathcal{L}_{CA}$ is utilized to augment training data and avoid over-fitting by re-sampling the input global feature vectors from an independent Gaussian distribution. The $\mathcal{L}_{CA}$ is obtained by calculating the Kullback-Leibler Divergence between the standard Gaussian distribution and the Gaussian distribution of the input sentence, and its formula can be expressed as,

$$\mathcal{L}_{CA} = \mathcal{D}_{KL}(\mathcal{N}(\mu(\mathbf{g}), \sum(\mathbf{g})) \parallel \mathcal{N}(0, I)), \tag{14.9}$$

where $\mathbf{g}$ is a global feature, $\mu(\mathbf{g})$ and $\sum(\mathbf{g})$ are the corresponding mean and the diagonal covariance matrix. Let G_i be the ith generator and D_i be the ith discriminator, the adversarial loss $\mathcal{L}_{G_i}$ is defined as,

$$\mathcal{L}_{G_i} = \overbrace{-\frac{1}{2}\mathbb{E}_{v_i \sim p_{G_i}}[\log(D_i(v_i)]}^{unconditional\ loss} \overbrace{-\frac{1}{2}\mathbb{E}_{v_i \sim p_{G_i}}[\log(D_i(v_i, \mathbf{g})]}^{conditional\ loss}, \tag{14.10}$$

where v_i is the image feature from the ith generator G_i, and $\mathbf{g}$ stands for the global feature vector of the input. The unconditional loss function serves to discern the authenticity of the images, differentiating between real and synthetic outputs. Concurrently, the conditional loss function assesses the congruence between the generated images and the provided attribute descriptions, ensuring that the synthesized visuals align with the specified characteristics.

CMAFGAN contains three discriminators, each with discriminator loss $\mathcal{L}_{D_i}$,

$$\begin{aligned}\mathcal{L}_{D_i} = & \overbrace{-\frac{1}{2}\mathbb{E}_{r_i \sim p_{data_i}}[\log D_i(r_i)] - \frac{1}{2}\mathbb{E}_{v_i \sim p_{G_i}}[\log(1 - D_i(v_i))]}^{unconditional\ loss} - \\ & \underbrace{\frac{1}{2}\mathbb{E}_{r_i \sim p_{data_i}}[\log D_i(r_i, \mathbf{g})] - \frac{1}{2}\mathbb{E}_{v_i \sim p_{G_i}}[\log(1 - D_i(v_i, \mathbf{g}))]}_{}\end{aligned}, \tag{14.11}$$

(the second line is labelled "conditional loss")

where r_i is from the ground-truth image distribution p_{data_i} at the ith scale.

14.4 Experiments

In this section, we conduct a comprehensive evaluation of our proposed CMAFGAN framework, employing both qualitative and quantitative metrics across three distinct datasets, including two face image datasets (CelebA [16], LFW [12]) and a text-to-image synthesis dataset (CUB [28]). To ensure a robust comparison, we have selected state-of-the-art networks from both the text-to-image synthesis domain and the attribute vector-to-face synthesis domain.

14.4.1 Implementation Details, Datasets and Evaluation Metrics

Implementation Details We implement our CMAFGAN based on Python 3.6, PyTorch 1.7.1 and CUDA 11.2, with a single GeForce RTX 3090 GPU. The hyperparameters λ_1, λ_2, and λ_3 for our model are set as 1.0, 5.0, and 10.0, respectively (the same in all three datasets). The learning rate of all discriminators is 0.0002 and the learning rate for all generators is 0.0001. During training, the batch size is 32. We train the network sufficiently on each dataset, with $\sim$120 epochs on the CelebA, $\sim$1100 epochs on the LFW, and $\sim$1850 epochs on the CUB.

Datasets To assess the efficacy of our proposed approach, we utilize two publicly accessible facial image datasets: CelebA and LFW. Given that each individual in these datasets is represented by a 40-dimensional attribute vector, an initial preprocessing step is necessary to convert these vectors into descriptive attribute words. These words are then concatenated into a single text string, separated by commas, as illustrated in Fig. 14.1. Following this preprocessing, the CelebA dataset, which comprises 202,599 pairs of face images and their corresponding attribute words, is further divided into a training set of 162,080 pairs and a testing set of 40,519 pairs. Similarly, the LFW dataset, consisting of 13,143 face-attribute pairs, is partitioned into training and testing subsets of 10,143 and 3000, respectively. We have also extended the evaluation of our CMAFGAN framework to text-to-image synthesis tasks, using CUB dataset. The CUB dataset encompasses a diverse collection of 11,788 bird images categorized into 200 distinct classes. In our evaluation, 8855 images are allocated for training, with the remaining 2933 images for testing.

Evaluation Metrics For attribute W2F synthesis, we compare the performance of our CMAFGAN with previous methods on the Fréchet inception distance (FID) [9], R-precision [32], face similarity score (FSS), and face similarity distance (FSD) [2]. For text-to-image synthesis, the inception score (IS) [21], FID, and R-precision are used to evaluate the performance. To compute those metrics, each method synthesises 80,000 face images on the CelebA test dataset and 30,000 face images on the LFW test dataset. Consistent with previous methods [13, 15, 25, 26, 32, 37, 41], 30,000 images are synthesised for evaluation on CUB.

14.4.2 Attribute Word-to-Face (W2F) Synthesis

Our CMAFGAN is essentially a text-to-image generation network. Therefore, we choose state-of-the-art text-to-image synthesis methods as the baseline methods for the attribute W2F synthesis. We compared the CMAFGAN model with AttnGAN [32], ControlGAN [13], DFGAN [27] and DM-GAN [41] on the CelebA and LFW datasets. The performance of each method is shown in Tables 14.1 and 14.2.

The experimental results on CelebA are shown in Table 14.1. A discernible enhancement in performance is observed for our CMAFGAN when compared to existing state-of-the-art techniques, particularly in the R-precision metric. Our method achieves an R-precision of 61.24%, surpassing the previous benchmark of 49.63%. This improvement underscores the enhanced alignment between the generated face images and their corresponding input attributes, indicative of a higher degree of consistency. Moreover, CMAFGAN demonstrates superior image quality, as evidenced by a lower Frechet Inception Distance (FID), when juxtaposed with AttnGAN, DFGAN, ControlGAN, and DM-GAN. This comparative analysis further substantiates the efficacy of our approach. While CMAFGAN exhibits a slight deficiency in FSS and FSD metrics in comparison to the state-of-the-art DM-GAN, it is noteworthy that CMAFGAN's R-precision significantly outperforms that of DM-GAN. This underscores the method's capability to predict face images with a heightened degree of consistency relative to the provided attributes.

Table 14.1 Quantitative comparison between current optimal methods and our CMAFGAN on CelebA test dataset. CMAFGAN achieves better FID and R-precision, but its FSD and FSS are marginally weaker than that of DM-GAN

Method	FID ↓	FSD ↓	FSS(%) ↑	R-precision(%) ↑
AttnGAN [32]	56.00	1.286 ± 0.128	58.18 ± 8.17	34.97 ± 0.47
DM-GAN [41]	30.10	**1.263 ± 0.134**	**59.63 ± 8.41**	49.32 ± 0.37
ControlGAN [13]	65.81	1.284 ± 0.131	58.34 ± 8.34	29.88 ± 0.47
DFGAN [27]	31.89	1.277 ± 0.132	58.75 ± 8.37	43.40 ± 0.24
CMAFGAN(Ours)	**29.99**	1.266 ± 0.131	59.47 ± 8.22	**61.24 ± 0.71**

The results highlighted in bold denote the best performance over the rest results in the table

Table 14.2 Quantitative comparison between current optimal methods and our CMAFGAN on LFW test dataset, where CMAFGAN achieves the best performance

Method	FID ↓	FSD ↓	FSS(%) ↑	R-precision(%) ↑
AttnGAN [32]	31.61	1.280 ± 0.129	58.60 ± 8.19	40.01 ± 0.75
DM-GAN [41]	21.00	1.278 ± 0.139	58.64 ± 8.72	61.55 ± 0.89
ControlGAN [13]	43.71	1.288 ± 0.132	58.05 ± 8.39	37.52 ± 0.84
DFGAN [27]	18.19	1.285 ± 0.134	58.21 ± 8.52	50.17 ± 0.13
CMAFGAN(Ours)	**17.77**	**1.272 ± 0.133**	**59.11 ± 8.38**	**64.46 ± 0.81**

The results highlighted in bold denote the best performance over the rest results in the table

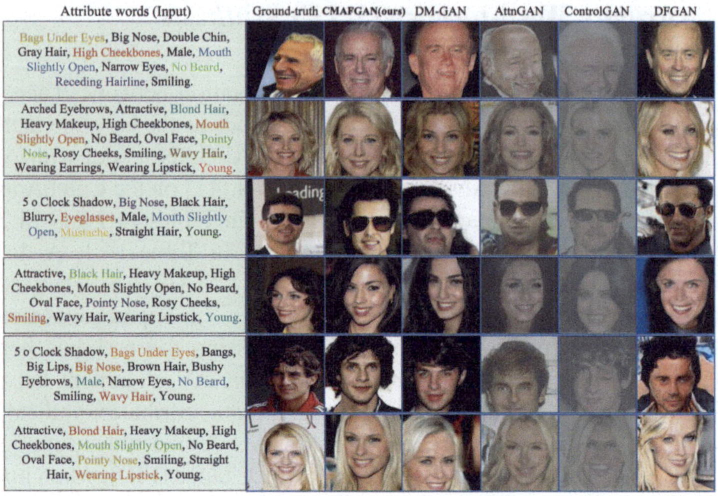

Fig. 14.5 Qualitative comparison between DM-GAN [41], AttnGAN [32], ControlGAN [13], DFGAN [27] and our CMAFGAN on the CelebA dataset. The given attribute words are on the left, with the corresponding ground-truth and generated images on the right. Those attributes corresponding to obvious improvements are highlighted with different colours

The quantitative comparison conducted on the LFW dataset is presented in Table 14.2. Our CMAFGAN model delivers a consistent performance, outperforming state-of-the-art methods across all evaluated metrics. It achieves higher image quality and greater fidelity to the ground-truth, as evidenced by the lowest FID and FSD, and the highest FSS and R-precision. Contrasting the results observed on the CelebA dataset, CMAFGAN excels across the board when tested on LFW, surpassing even the DM-GAN on every metric. This comprehensive outperformance underscores the robustness and superiority of our method, which can generate images that are not only of higher quality but also more closely aligned with the ground-truth.

To further evaluate the performance of each model in attribute W2F synthesis, we also visually present the results of CMAFGAN and state-of-the-art methods in Fig. 14.5. Compared with other methods, the face generated by CMAFGAN mainly has the following advantages: higher fidelity, better fine-grained features, and a higher matching degree with input attributes. Among them, the matching degree with input attributes is especially significant, which is mainly reflected in the beard, hair colour, hairstyle, mouth shape, expression, age, and ornaments (glasses and hats). Although DM-GAN and DFGAN also synthesise some high-quality faces (mainly in terms of high fidelity), some of their synthetic faces are poor at fine-grained features and in the consistency with input attributes (e.g. in the 1st row of Fig. 14.5).

Table 14.3 Quantitative comparison between attribute V2F synthesis methods and our CMAFGAN on CelebA and LFW datasets. The input of attribute V2F synthesis methods is attribute vector, while that of CMAFGAN is attribute words

Dataset	Method	Input	FID ↓	FSD ↓	FSS(%) ↑
CelebA	Di et al. [5]	Attribute vector	35.21	1.277 ± 0.136	58.68 ± 8.57
	AFGAN [33]	Attribute vector	36.76	1.285 ± 0.131	58.11 ± 8.31
	CMAFGAN(Ours)	Attribute words	**29.99**	**1.266 ± 0.131**	**59.47 ± 8.22**
LFW	Di et al. [5]	Attribute vector	25.36	1.289 ± 0.125	57.93 ± 7.26
	AFGAN [33]	Attribute vector	26.31	1.291 ± 0.129	57.12 ± 8.21
	CMAFGAN(Ours)	Attribute words	**17.77**	**1.272 ± 0.133**	**59.11 ± 8.38**

The results highlighted in bold denote the best performance over the rest results in the table

14.4.3 Attribute Vector-to-Face (V2F) Synthesis

To ensure a thorough comparison, we have pitted our CMAFGAN against existing V2F synthesis methods [5, 33] on the CelebA and LFW datasets. Our quantitative analysis is grounded in the FID, FSD, and FSS, which are standard metrics for evaluating the quality of synthesized images. Given that the input for traditional V2F methods is an attribute vector, not descriptive attribute words, it is not feasible to calculate the R-precision metric, which measures the alignment between textual descriptions and generated images. The comparative results are detailed in Table 14.3. It is evident that CMAFGAN outperforms existing methods across all evaluated metrics on both the CelebA and LFW datasets. Specifically, our method has achieved a notable reduction in FID, scoring 7 to 9 points lower than previous V2F methods [5, 33], indicating a significant advancement in the fidelity of the generated images.

14.4.4 Text-to-Image Synthesis

Given that CMAFGAN is fundamentally a text-to-image synthesis network, we deemed it essential to evaluate its efficacy on this task to underscore the network's capabilities. The performance of CMAFGAN on the text-to-image synthesis dataset is presented in Table 14.4. Our model achieves the highest scores in both IS and R-precision, key indicators of the quality and relevance of the synthesized images. Although the FID of CMAFGAN is slightly greater than that of TIME [15], this marginal difference does not detract from the overall performance. The R-precision of CMAFGAN shows a notable increase, with an 11.10% improvement (from 72.31% to 83.41%) over the current leading method [41]. This enhancement underscores CMAFGAN's ability to significantly bolster the alignment between synthetic images and their corresponding textual descriptions, without compromising image quality.

Table 14.4 Quantitative comparison between the state-of-the-art methods and our CMAFGAN on CUB dataset

Method	IS ↑	FID ↓	R-precision(%) ↑
AttnGAN [32]	4.36 ± .03	23.98	67.82 ± 4.43
DM-GAN [41]	4.75 ± .07	16.09	72.31 ± 0.91
SEGAN [25]	4.67 ± .04	18.16	(–)
ControlGAN [13]	4.58 ± .09	(–)	69.33 ± 3.23
KT-GAN [26]	4.85 ± .04	17.32	(–)
DTGAN [37]	4.88 ± .03	16.35	(–)
TIME [15]	4.91 ± .03	**14.30**	71.57 ± 1.20
CMAFGAN(Ours)	**4.91 ± .07**	15.13	**83.41 ± 0.53**

The results highlighted in bold denote the best performance over the rest results in the table

Through rigorous quantitative and qualitative evaluations across two principal tasks, word-to-face and text-to-image generation, the proposed CMAFGAN model has demonstrated several key advantages: (1) In cross-modal tasks involving natural language and image synthesis, CMAFGAN is adept at thoroughly learning semantic information from provided attributes, enabling the generation of fine-grained images. (2) CMAFGAN's images exhibit a higher visual similarity to original images, indicating a superior ability to capture detailed characteristics. (3) Compared to other methods, CMAFGAN constructs a more accurate semantic mapping between natural language descriptions and the corresponding images, ensuring that the synthesized outputs are highly consistent with the given attributes. (4) The model exhibits strong generalization capabilities and application potential, evidenced by its outstanding performance in both attribute-based W2F and text-to-image synthesis tasks. These strengths position CMAFGAN as a robust and versatile framework, well-suited for advancing the field of image synthesis driven by natural language inputs.

14.4.5 Ablation Study

To clearly understand the contribution of the proposed components in image generation, we conduct ablation studies on the WFT and CMAF. Three different networks are constructed: baseline, baseline+WFT, and baseline+WFT+CMAF (CMAFGAN). The baseline is cascaded by three generators, without the WFT and CMAF modules, which use the global feature $\mathbf{g}$ of attribute words and Gaussian noise to guide the network to generate images, without using the word feature vector $\mathbf{f}$. The results on the CelebA, and LFW datasets are shown in Table 14.5. It can be found that, the baseline network shows comparable performance with DM-GAN. Incorporating the WFT into the baseline network, FID, FSD, FSS, and R-precision on CelebA are significantly improved, by 2.81, 0.003, 0.19%, and 2.19%, respectively. Similarly, WFT improves the FID, FSD, FSS, and R-

Table 14.5 Performance of different components in our CMAFGAN on CelebA and LFW datasets. WFT and CMAF represent word feature transformation and cross-modal attention fusion blocks, respectively

Dataset	Method	FID ↓	FSD ↓	FSS(%) ↑	R-precision(%) ↑
CelebA	Baseline	31.99	1.272 ± 0.132	59.08 ± 8.34	59.01 ± 0.85
	+WFT	**29.18**	1.269 ± 0.131	59.27 ± 8.24	61.20 ± 0.51
	+WFT+CMAF (CMAFGAN)	29.99	**1.266 ± 0.131**	**59.47 ± 8.22**	**61.24 ± 0.71**
LFW	Baseline	19.13	1.275 ± 0.116	59.01 ± 7.23	60.03 ± 1.33
	+WFT	18.85	**1.257 ± 0.134**	**59.99 ± 8.36**	61.58 ± 0.68
	+WFT+CMAF (CMAFGAN)	**17.77**	1.272 ± 0.133	59.11 ± 8.38	**64.46 ± 0.81**

The results highlighted in bold denote the best performance over the rest results in the table

precision by 0.28, 0.018, 0.98%, and 0.55% on the LFW dataset, respectively. After further utilising the CMAF block, the overall performance of the network varies in different datasets. On the CelebA dataset, the FSD, FSS, and R-precision metrics are further improved, except of a marginal decrease in FID (from 29.18 to 29.99). In contrast, the FID and R-precision on the LFW dataset increased by 1.08 and 3.88%, respectively, while the FSD and FSS decreased marginally. These findings underscore that the R-precision metric consistently improves, indicating that the CMAF module can effectively enhance the congruence between the generated images and their corresponding input attributes. In summary, the WFT module has been demonstrated to significantly enhance the fidelity of the generated images, particularly in terms of aligning the feature distribution with that of the original images. Furthermore, the CMAF module brings about notable improvements in the fine-grained features of the synthetic images, as well as in the degree of matching between the images and the input attribute words. The synergistic integration of both the WFT and CMAF modules serves to amplify the network's performance. This combined approach harnesses the strengths of each module, leading to a more robust and effective image synthesis process.

14.4.6 Extension to Medical Scenarios

To underscore the efficacy of our proposed approach, we extend the application of CMAFGAN to X-ray image synthesis from descriptive texts, leveraging the Open-i dataset [4]. This dataset encompasses 6423 X-ray images paired with their corresponding caption sentences. In this application, CMAFGAN is employed directly as a text-to-image synthesis network. The resulting synthesized X-ray images, as demonstrated in Fig. 14.6, exhibit high semantic alignment with the input captions and are consistent with the ground-truth X-ray images, capturing fine-grained details. In the immediate term, the synthesis of X-ray images from text has the potential to serve as a data augmentation technique and as an instructional tool for medical students. Looking further ahead, we anticipate more exploration of additional applications for this technology, broadening its utility in this task.

14.5 Conclusions

In this study, we delved into the novel domain of image synthesis driven by attribute words. We deviated from the conventional approach of utilizing attribute vectors and instead opted for input in the form of text composed of descriptive attribute words. This innovative strategy has resulted in higher-quality image synthesis and has introduced a degree of order invariance that is inherently flexible with respect to the arrangement of attribute words. We introduced a pioneering model termed CMAFGAN, which is distinguished by the integration of WFT and CMAF blocks.

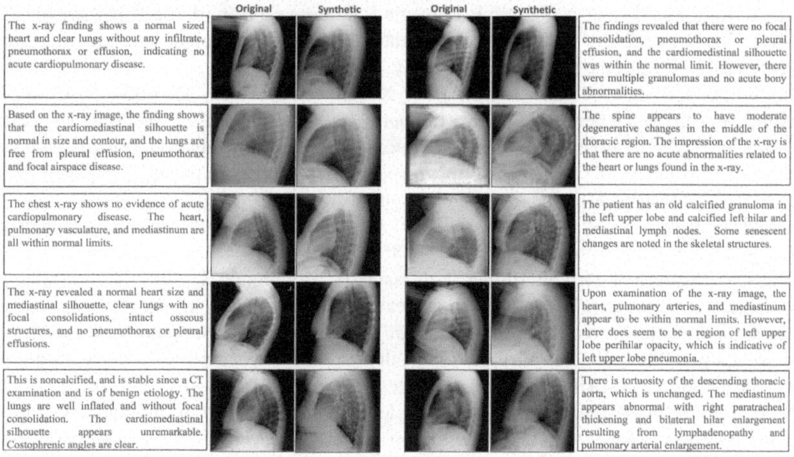

Fig. 14.6 X-ray image synthesis from descriptions

These components were designed to thoroughly investigate the interplay between textual and visual domains, facilitating a more nuanced synthesis process. Our comprehensive experimental evaluation, conducted across the CelebA, LFW, CUB, and Open-i datasets, has conclusively demonstrated that CMAFGAN surpasses current state-of-the-art methods in image quality and fidelity to input attribute words. The results of X-ray image synthesis further demonstrate the efficiency of our proposed CMAFGAN, achieving promising results in terms of high-quality images and high semantic consistency. Despite these advancements, there remain instances of irregularity and ambiguity within the synthesis outcomes generated by our method. Looking ahead, we are committed to further refining the quality of the generated images, aiming to address these challenges and push the boundaries of what is achievable in the realm of attribute-based image synthesis.

References

1. Abdal R, Zhu P, Mitra NJ, Wonka P (2021) Styleflow: attribute-conditioned exploration of stylegan-generated images using conditional continuous normalizing flows. ACM Trans Graphics 40(3):1–21
2. Chen X, Qing L, He X, Su J, Peng Y (2018) From eyes to face synthesis: a new approach for human-centered smart surveillance. IEEE Access 6:14567–14575
3. Chen X, Qing L, He X, Luo X, Xu Y (2019) Ftgan: a fully-trained generative adversarial networks for text to face generation. arXiv preprint arXiv:190405729
4. Demner-Fushman D, Kohli MD, Rosenman MB, Shooshan SE, Rodriguez L, Antani S, Thoma GR, McDonald CJ (2016) Preparing a collection of radiology examinations for distribution and retrieval. J Am Med Inf Assoc 23(2):304–310
5. Di X, Patel VM (2019) Facial synthesis from visual attributes via sketch using multiscale generators. IEEE Trans Biom Behav Identity Sci 2(1):55–67

6. Gatt A, Tanti M, Muscat A, Paggio P, Farrugia RA, Borg C, Camilleri KP, Rosner M, Van der Plas L (2018) Face2text: collecting an annotated image description corpus for the generation of rich face descriptions. arXiv preprint arXiv:180303827
7. Goodfellow I, Pouget-Abadie J, Mirza M, Xu B, Warde-Farley D, Ozair S, Courville A, Bengio Y (2014) Generative adversarial nets. In: Ghahramani Z, Welling M, Cortes C, Lawrence N, Weinberger KQ (eds) Advances in neural information processing systems, vol. 27. Curran Associates, Inc. https://proceedings.neurips.cc/paper_files/paper/2014/file/5ca3e9b122f61f8f06494c97b1afccf3-Paper.pdf
8. He Z, Zuo W, Kan M, Shan S, Chen X (2019) Attgan: facial attribute editing by only changing what you want. IEEE Trans Image Process 28(11):5464–5478
9. Heusel M, Ramsauer H, Unterthiner T, Nessler B, Hochreiter S (2017) Gans trained by a two time-scale update rule converge to a local nash equilibrium. In: Proceedings of the 31st international conference on neural information processing systems, pp 6629–6640
10. Hu M, Guo J (2020) Facial attribute-controlled sketch-to-image translation with generative adversarial networks. EURASIP J Image Video Process 2020(1):1–13
11. Hu W, Hu H (2020) Adversarial disentanglement spectrum variations and cross-modality attention networks for nir-vis face recognition. IEEE Trans Multimedia 23:145–160
12. Huang G, Mattar M, Lee H, Learned-miller E (2012) Learning to align from scratch. In: Pereira F, Burges CJ, Bottou L, Weinberger KQ (eds) Advances in neural information processing systems, vol. 25. Curran Associates, Inc. https://proceedings.neurips.cc/paper_files/paper/2012/file/d81f9c1be2e08964bf9f24b15f0e4900-Paper.pdf
13. Li B, Qi X, Lukasiewicz T, Torr PH (2019) Controllable text-to-image generation. In: Proceedings of the 33rd international conference on neural information processing systems, pp 2065–2075
14. Li G, Duan N, Fang Y, Gong M, Jiang D (2020) Unicoder-vl: a universal encoder for vision and language by cross-modal pre-training. In: Proceedings of the AAAI conference on artificial intelligence, vol 34, pp 11336–11344
15. Liu B, Song K, Zhu Y, de Melo G, Elgammal A (2021) Time: text and image mutual-translation adversarial networks. In: Proceedings of the AAAI conference on artificial intelligence, vol 35, pp 2082–2090
16. Liu Z, Luo P, Wang X, Tang X (2015) Deep learning face attributes in the wild. In: Proceedings of the IEEE international conference on computer vision, pp 3730–3738
17. Luo X, He X, Qing L, Chen X, Liu L, Xu Y (2020) Eyesgan: synthesize human face from human eyes. Neurocomputing 404:213–226
18. Miyato T, Kataoka T, Koyama M, Yoshida Y (2018) Spectral normalization for generative adversarial networks. In: International conference on learning representations
19. Reed S, Akata Z, Mohan S, Tenka S, Schiele B, Lee H (2016) Learning what and where to draw. In: Proceedings of the 30th international conference on neural information processing systems, pp 217–225
20. Reed S, Akata Z, Yan X, Logeswaran L, Schiele B, Lee H (2016) Generative adversarial text to image synthesis. In: International conference on machine learning, pp 1060–1069
21. Salimans T, Goodfellow I, Zaremba W, Cheung V, Radford A, Chen X (2016) Improved techniques for training gans. Adv Neural Inf Process Syst 29:2234–2242
22. Shao M, Zhang Y, Liu H, Wang C, Li L, Shao X (2021) Dmdit: diverse multi-domain image-to-image translation. Knowl Based Syst 229:107311
23. Shen Y, Gu J, Tang X, Zhou B (2020) Interpreting the latent space of gans for semantic face editing. In: Proceedings of the IEEE/CVF conference on computer vision and pattern recognition, pp 9243–9252
24. Tan H, Bansal M (2019) Lxmert: learning cross-modality encoder representations from transformers. arXiv preprint arXiv:190807490
25. Tan H, Liu X, Li X, Zhang Y, Yin B (2019) Semantics-enhanced adversarial nets for text-to-image synthesis. In: Proceedings of the IEEE/CVF international conference on computer vision, pp 10501–10510

26. Tan H, Liu X, Liu M, Yin B, Li X (2020) Kt-gan: knowledge-transfer generative adversarial network for text-to-image synthesis. IEEE Trans Image Process 30:1275–1290
27. Tao M, Tang H, Wu S, Sebe N, Jing XY, Wu F, Bao B (2020) Df-gan: deep fusion generative adversarial networks for text-to-image synthesis. arXiv preprint arXiv:200805865
28. Wah C, Branson S, Welinder P, Perona P, Belongie S (2011) The caltech-ucsd birds-200-2011 dataset. http://www.vision.caltech.edu/visipedia/CUB-200-2011.html
29. Wang Q, Fan H, Sun G, Ren W, Tang Y (2020) Recurrent generative adversarial network for face completion. IEEE Trans Multimedia 23:429–442
30. Wang Y, Dantcheva A, Bremond F (2018) From attribute-labels to faces: face generation using a conditional generative adversarial network. In: Proceedings of the European conference on computer vision (ECCV) workshops
31. Wang Z, Liu X, Li H, Sheng L, Yan J, Wang X, Shao J (2019) Camp: cross-modal adaptive message passing for text-image retrieval. In: Proceedings of the IEEE/CVF international conference on computer vision, pp 5764–5773
32. Xu T, Zhang P, Huang Q, Zhang H, Gan Z, Huang X, He X (2018) Attngan: fine-grained text to image generation with attentional generative adversarial networks. In: Proceedings of the IEEE conference on computer vision and pattern recognition, pp 1316–1324
33. Yuan Z, Zhang J, Shan S, Chen X (2021) Attributes aware face generation with generative adversarial networks. In: 2020 25th international conference on pattern recognition (ICPR). IEEE, pp 1657–1664
34. Zhang H, Xu T, Li H, Zhang S, Wang X, Huang X, Metaxas DN (2017) Stackgan: text to photo-realistic image synthesis with stacked generative adversarial networks. In: Proceedings of the IEEE international conference on computer vision, pp 5907–5915
35. Zhang H, Xu T, Li H, Zhang S, Wang X, Huang X, Metaxas DN (2018) Stackgan++: realistic image synthesis with stacked generative adversarial networks. IEEE Trans Pattern Anal Mach Intell 41(8):1947–1962
36. Zhang H, Goodfellow I, Metaxas D, Odena A (2019) Self-attention generative adversarial networks. In: International conference on machine learning, PMLR, pp 7354–7363
37. Zhang Z, Schomaker L (2020) Dtgan: Dual attention generative adversarial networks for text-to-image generation. arXiv preprint arXiv:201102709
38. Zhou Y (2021) Generative adversarial network for text-to-face synthesis and manipulation. In: Proceedings of the 29th ACM international conference on multimedia, pp 2940–2944
39. Zhou Y, Shimada N (2021) Generative adversarial network for text-to-face synthesis and manipulation with pretrained bert model. In: 2021 16th IEEE international conference on automatic face and gesture recognition (FG 2021). IEEE, pp 01–08
40. Zhu B, Ngo CW (2020) Cookgan: causality based text-to-image synthesis. In: Proceedings of the IEEE/CVF conference on computer vision and pattern recognition, pp 5519–5527
41. Zhu M, Pan P, Chen W, Yang Y (2019) Dm-gan: dynamic memory generative adversarial networks for text-to-image synthesis. In: Proceedings of the IEEE/CVF conference on computer vision and pattern recognition, pp 5802–5810

Chapter 15
CHeart: A Conditional Spatio-Temporal Generative Model for Cardiac Anatomy

Mengyun Qiao, Shuo Wang, Huaqi Qiu, Antonio de Marvao, Declan P. O'Regan, Daniel Rueckert, and Wenjia Bai

Abstract Cardiac image analysis often involves assessing the heart's anatomy and motion from images and understanding their association with clinical factors like gender, age, and diseases. While image segmentation and motion tracking algorithms address the first issue, modeling the second remains challenging. In

---

M. Qiao (✉)
Department of Brain Sciences, Imperial College London, London, UK

Data Science Institute, Imperial College London, London, UK
e-mail: m.qiao21@imperial.ac.uk

S. Wang
Digital Medical Research Center, School of Basic Medical Sciences, Fudan University and Shanghai Key Laboratory of MICCAI, Shanghai, China

H. Qiu
Biomedical Image Analysis Group (BioMedIA), Department of Computing, Imperial College London, London, UK

A. de Marvao
MRC Laboratory of Medical Sciences, Imperial College London, London, UK

The Department of Women and Children's Health, and British Heart Foundation Centre of Research Excellence, School of Cardiovascular and Metabolic Medicine and Sciences, King's College London, London, UK

D. P. O'Regan
MRC Laboratory of Medical Sciences, Imperial College London, London, UK

D. Rueckert
Biomedical Image Analysis Group (BioMedIA), Department of Computing, Imperial College London, London, UK

Klinikum rechts der Isar, Technical University of Munich, Munich, Germany

W. Bai
Department of Computing, Imperial College London, London, UK

Department of Brain Sciences, Imperial College London, London, UK

Data Science Institute, Imperial College London, London, UK
e-mail: w.bai@imperial.ac.uk

L. Zhang et al. (eds.), *Generative Machine Learning Models in Medical Image Computing*, https://doi.org/10.1007/978-3-031-80965-1_15

this work, we propose a novel conditional generative model to describe the 4D spatio-temporal anatomy of the heart and its interaction with non-imaging clinical factors. By integrating these clinical factors as conditions, our model can investigate their influence on cardiac anatomy. We evaluate the model's performance on two main tasks: anatomical sequence completion and sequence generation. It achieves high performance in anatomical sequence completion, comparable to or surpassing state-of-the-art generative models. For sequence generation, the model generates realistic synthetic 4D sequential anatomies that align with real data distributions given clinical conditions. The code and trained generative model are available at https://github.com/MengyunQ/CHeart.

15.1 Introduction

Cardiac imaging is crucial for cardiovascular image diagnosis and management [10]. Techniques like cine cardiac magnetic resonance (CMR) or ultrasound scans reveal the heart's anatomical structure and its contraction and relaxation patterns [24]. A well-established research challenge is to investigate the relationships between three-dimensional (3D) cardiac anatomy and other non-imaging clinical factors, such as age, gender, and diseases [5]. In addition to 3D anatomical data, the heart's temporal dynamic motion also provides valuable information for clinical diagnosis and therapy selection [19, 29, 43]. Developing computational tools to link spatial-temporal imaging features with non-imaging clinical factors is of particular interest. In this study, we aim to enhance our understanding of spatial-temporal cardiac anatomy and clinical factors through a generative modeling approach. We introduce a conditional generative model to capture the interaction between imaging features and clinical factors. Given clinical factors as conditions, the proposed model can generate corresponding 4D spatial-temporal cardiac anatomies. We show that the generated 4D anatomies are realistic and align with the actual data distribution. Recently, the field of conditional generative modeling has seen significant advancements, largely driven by deep learning methods such as conditional generative adversarial networks (GAN) [31], conditional variational autoencoders (VAEs) [27, 44], flow-based models [38], and diffusion models [33]. These methods enable efficient approximation of the underlying conditional distributions and the generation of high-quality samples. Advances in conditional generative models have been marked by numerous developments in various generation tasks: image-to-image translation [13, 22, 25], style and lyrics-to-music generation [16], and text-to-image synthesis [12].

Besides generating static images [33], generative models have also been utilized for sequential data, including videos [42, 48] and music [16]. In these scenarios, it is crucial to develop a model that can capture the intrinsic connections within temporal sequences. To achieve this, long short-term memory (LSTM) [26, 47] and transformers [51] have been investigated to understand the sequential progression of latent representations in samples. Some studies also incorporate spatiotemporal convolution and attention layers to learn temporal dynamics from video collections

[42]. Sequential data encompass both structural variations and motion information. Disentangled representation learning methods like DiSCVAE [54] have been proposed to separate motion features from structural features. In the realm of medical imaging, several studies have examined the integration of non-imaging clinical factors into the image generation process. Dalca et al. [15] introduced a learning framework for constructing deformable brain image templates based on age. Xia et al. [49] developed a model to generate synthetic brain images conditioned on age and Alzheimer's disease status. For cardiac images, Biffi et al. [7] presented LVAE for the interpretable classification of anatomical shapes into different clinical conditions. Krebs et al. [28] proposed a probabilistic motion model for spatio-temporal cardiac image registration. Reynaud et al. [37] introduced a causal generative model to produce synthetic 3D ultrasound videos based on a given input image and an expected ejection fraction. Campello et al. [9] proposed a conditional generative model in cardiac imaging to extract longitudinal patterns related to aging. Duchateau et al. [17] developed a method for synthesizing pathological cardiac sequences from real healthy sequences. Amirrajab et al. [1] created a framework for simulating cardiac MRI with varying anatomical and imaging characteristics. For cardiac temporal modeling, some studies [52, 55, 56] demonstrated that dynamic cardiac data could be represented by low-dimensional latent spaces, such as a conditional autoencoder to capture latent representations [56] or temporal smoothness applied as a regularization term in the reconstruction loss function [55, 56]. These studies offer valuable insights for conditional medical image generation. However, generating sequences of spatio-temporal cardiac anatomies from multiple clinical factors remains underexplored.

In this study, we introduce a conditional generative model capable of producing realistic cardiac anatomical sequences based on non-imaging factors such as age, gender, weight, height, and blood pressure. We refer to this Conditional Heart generation model as CHeart. The model utilizes a variational autoencoder to capture latent representations of cardiac anatomies and a condition encoder to incorporate clinical conditions into a condition latent vector. Subsequently, a *Temporal Module* is crafted to generate the condition-related sequential latent space using the anatomy latent representations and the condition latent vector. The proposed model exhibits high diversity and fidelity in generation, assessed through structural overlaps, surface distance metrics, and clinical measure distributions (ventricular volume and mass). The primary contributions of this work are outlined as follows:

- We introduce a spatio-temporal generative model for 3D cardiac anatomy that considers both spatial and temporal variations, such as motion during the cardiac cycle.
- We utilize both imaging and non-imaging clinical data to train the model, enabling it to generate cardiac anatomical sequences conditioned on multiple clinical factors.
- We incorporate a temporal module into the latent space of cardiac anatomy and conditions to capture the complex sequential patterns of a beating heart.
- We show that the model can produce highly realistic and diverse cardiac anatomical sequences that align with real data distributions.

15.2 Methods

The proposed generative model uses non-imaging clinical factors as input to produce a cardiac anatomical sequence. Figure 15.1 depicts the overall structure. The subsequent sections delve into more technical specifics. Initially, we present the conditional generative model. Next, we explain the temporal module for learning sequential latent representations attributable to cardiac motion. Finally, we showcase two applications of the generative model during the inference phase: *anatomical sequence completion* and *anatomical sequence generation*.

15.2.1 Conditional Generative Model

Consider a dynamic sequence of anatomical data for a subject, x_t $(t = 0, 1, \cdots, T-1)$, where x_t represents the anatomical segmentation at the t-th frame, and T is the total number of frames in the sequence. Additionally, we observe clinical conditions c for this subject, which may include factors such as age, gender, weight, height, blood pressure, etc. Our goal is to learn the probability distribution of the anatomy

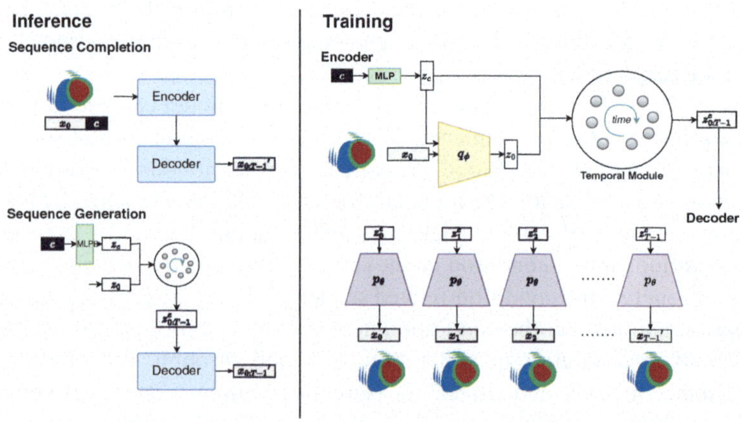

Fig. 15.1 Summary of the CHeart model, detailing both the training and inference phases. During the training phase, an encoder is utilized to capture the latent representations z_c and z_0 corresponding to the clinical conditions c and the anatomy at the initial time frame x_0. A temporal module then tracks the path of $z^c_{0:T-1}$ in the latent space over time, starting from the initial latent vectors z_c and z_0. The decoder reconstructs the 4D cardiac anatomy sequence $x_{0:T-1}$ from these latent vectors along the temporal path. This training process facilitates two inference methods during testing: sequence completion and sequence generation. For sequence completion, the model receives x_0 and c, and predicts the subsequent anatomical sequence in the cardiac cycle. For sequence generation, a random latent code z_0 drawn from the prior distribution and c are provided to the model and the temporal module to create the latent vector sequence $z^c_{0:T-1}$, which is then used to generate a synthetic cardiac anatomical sequence $x'_{0:T-1}$

x conditioned on c using a chosen model, $p_\theta(x|c)$, where θ represents the model parameters. We aim to find a model $p_\theta(x|c)$ that is flexible enough to describe the data x. Deep neural networks are often employed for this modeling due to their complex modeling capacity [20, 27, 44]. Without loss of generality, we first attempt to learn the distribution of anatomy at the initial time frame, $p_\theta(x_0|c)$, which is typically the end-diastolic (ED) frame in cardiac imaging. We utilize the conditional β-VAE model [20, 27, 44] to learn the data distribution. The condition c is embedded as a conditional latent vector z_c by the MLP, which integrates multiple clinical factors and facilitates exploration across the conditional latent space. The model comprises a decoder $p_\theta(x_0|z_0, z_c)$ and an encoder $q_\phi(z_0|x_0, z_c)$. The decoder $p_\theta(x_0|z_0, z_c)$ with parameters θ maps the latent variables z_0, z_c to the anatomy x_0. We assume a prior distribution $p(z_0)$ over the latent variable z_0. The prior and the decoder together define a joint distribution, denoted as $p_\theta(x_0, z_0|z_c)$, parameterized by θ. To make the intractable posterior inference and learning problem tractable, we introduce a parametric encoder model $q_\phi(z_0|x_0, z_c)$ with ϕ as the variational parameters, which approximates the true but intractable posterior distribution $p_\theta(z_0|x_0, z_c)$ of the generative model, given an input x_0 and condition space z_c:

$$q_\phi(z_0|x_0, z_c) \approx p_\theta(z_0|x_0, z_c) \tag{15.1}$$

where $q_\phi(z_0|x_0, z_c)$ often adopts a simpler form, e.g. the Gaussian distribution. By introducing the approximate posterior $q_\phi(z_0|x_0, z_c)$, the log-likelihood of $p_\theta(x_0|z_c)$ can be formulated as:

$$\begin{aligned} \log p_\theta(x_0|z_c) &= \mathbb{E}_{z_0 \sim q_\phi(z_0|x_0, z_c)} \log [p_\theta(x_0|z_c)] \\ &= \mathbb{E}_{z_0 \sim q_\phi(z_0|x_0, z_c)} \log \left[\frac{p_\theta(x_0, z_0|z_c)}{q_\phi(z_0|x_0, z_c)} \right] \\ &+ \mathbb{E}_{z_0 \sim q_\phi(z_0|x_0, z_c)} \log \left[\frac{q_\phi(z_0|x_0, z_c)}{p_\theta(x_0|z_0, z_c)} \right] \end{aligned} \tag{15.2}$$

where the second term denotes the Kullback-Leibler (KL) divergence $D_{KL}(q_\phi \parallel p_\theta)$, between $q_\phi(z_0|x_0, z_c)$ and $p_\theta(z_0|x_0, z_c)$. It is non-negative and zero only if the approximate posterior $q_\phi(z_0|x_0, z_c)$ equals the true posterior distribution $p_\theta(z_0|x_0, z_c)$. Due to the non-negativity of the KL divergence, the first term in Eq. 15.2 is the lower bound of the evidence $\log[p_\theta(x_0|z_c)]$, known as the evidence lower bound (ELBO). Instead of optimising the evidence $\log[p_\theta(x_0|z_c)]$ which is often intractable, we optimise the ELBO:

$$\max_{\theta,\phi} ELBO = \log[p_\theta(x_0|z_c)] - D_{KL} \tag{15.3}$$

To better control the encoding representation capacity and encourage more efficient latent encoding, we adopt β-VAE by modifying VAE with an adjustable hyperparameter β [20]. As a result, the loss function of the generative model is formulated as:

$$\begin{aligned}\mathcal{L}_{\theta,\phi} = &- \mathbb{E}_{z_0 \sim q_\phi(z_0|x_0)} \log[p_\theta(x_0|z_0, c)] \\ &+ \beta \cdot D_{KL}[q_\phi(z_0|x_0, c) \parallel p_\theta(z_0)]\end{aligned} \tag{15.4}$$

where the sign is negated so as we can minimise the loss function.

In practice, we use the reconstruction loss for the first term, i.e. how accurate the generative model $p_\theta(x_0)$ can be for reconstructing the anatomy x_0 from the latent vector z_0 using the decoder. The reparameterization trick is applied to replace the subscript of the expectation and express the random variable $z_0 \sim q_\phi(z_0|x_0, z_c)$ as some differentiable and invertible transformation of another random variable ϵ, so the expectation does not rely on q itself.

15.2.2 Motion Modelling in the Latent Space

In the preceding section, we formulated $q_\phi(z_0|x_0, z_c)$ and $p_\theta(x_0|z_0, z_c)$ for the initial frame x_0 in a sequence. To model the entire anatomical sequence $x_0, x_1, ..., x_{T-1}$ under clinical conditions c, we introduce a *Temporal Module* built using a one-to-many LSTM architecture [34] with parameters ω, which produces the condition-related sequential latent codes based on z_0 and z_c. The detailed architecture of the temporal module is shown in Fig. 15.2. LSTM [13] is a type of recurrent neural network that includes gating mechanisms and cell memory blocks. The first LSTM cell of the module receives the concatenation of the anatomy latent representation z_0 and the condition latent representation z_c as input, denoted as z_0^c. With the hidden state h_0 and cell state $cell_0$ initialized to zero, it infers the latent z_1^c at the next time step. Each subsequent LSTM cell, sharing weights, takes z_{t-1}^c as input, updates the hidden state h_t and cell state $cell_t$, and infers the latent z_t^c. All LSTM cells share weights. Each latent code z_t^c encapsulates information about both the anatomy at time t and the clinical conditions c. The cardiac anatomy of a dynamic sequence forms a temporal sequence z_t^c in the latent space, where $t = 0, 1, \ldots, T$. Once the temporal module computes the latent codes $z_{0:T-1}^c$ across all time frames, the decoder generates the anatomical sequence x_t' from z_t^c, as illustrated in Fig. 15.1. The overall loss function for modelling the anatomical sequence generation is formulated based on Eq. 15.4:

$$\begin{aligned}\mathcal{L}_{\theta,\phi,\omega} = &- \sum_{t=0}^{T-1} \mathbb{E}_{z_0 \sim q_\phi(z_0|x_0)}(\log(p_\theta(x_t|z_t, z_c))) \\ &+ \beta D_{KL}(q_\phi(z_0|x_0, z_c) \parallel p_\theta(z_0))\end{aligned} \tag{15.5}$$

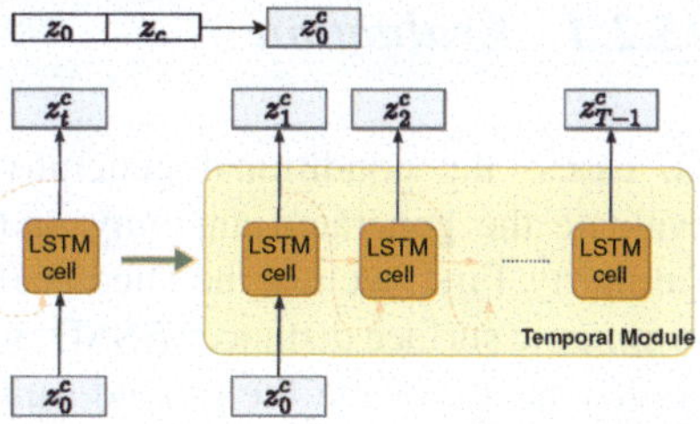

Fig. 15.2 The temporal module for generating the sequential latent codes $z_{0:T-1}$, constructed with a one-to-many long short-term memory (LSTM) structure

The training loss function consists of two components: (1) the reconstruction accuracy across all time frames, evaluated using cross-entropy to assess the performance in reconstructing segmentation maps; (2) the KL divergence term, which penalizes the difference between the learned prior and posterior distributions. The entire training process is conducted end-to-end, with the encoder, temporal module, and decoder being trained simultaneously. The VAE allows the model to learn a low-dimensional latent space that captures the underlying anatomical variations. By integrating the temporal module, the model can effectively capture the temporal dynamics in cardiac images, enabling the generation of anatomically consistent and coherent sequences over time.

15.2.3 Inference

To illustrate the effectiveness of the proposed generative model during inference, we perform two benchmark tasks: anatomical sequence completion and anatomical sequence generation, as depicted in the right panel of Fig. 15.1.

In *anatomical sequence completion*, the model receives the anatomy at the initial time frame x_0 along with clinical conditions c. It is tasked with generating the subsequent sequence of anatomies throughout the cardiac cycle. The model maps x_0 and c to their latent representations z_0 and z_c, predicts the sequential latent codes $z^c_{0:T-1}$ via the temporal module, and ultimately reconstructs the entire sequence of cardiac anatomy $x'_{0:T-1}$ using the shared-weight decoders.

In *anatomical sequence generation*, the model is conditioned solely on the clinical factors c and does not require any anatomical input. Given that the model has learned the distribution of the anatomical latent variable p_{z_0}, we can sample z_0 in the latent space from a Gaussian distribution $\mathcal{N}(0, 1)$ and concatenate it with the clinical latent code z_c. We then feed the concatenated latent code z^c_0 into the temporal module to predict $z^c_{0:T-1}$ and generate the complete anatomical sequence $x'_{0:T-1}$ using the decoder.

15.2.4 Evaluation

To assess the conditional generative model, we utilize quantitative metrics to evaluate the generated anatomy and clinical metrics to examine the distribution similarity. First, we use the Dice coefficient, Hausdorff distance (HD), and average symmetric surface distance (ASSD) to compare the similarity between the generated cardiac anatomy and the ground truth anatomy under the same clinical conditions. Second, we derive five imaging phenotypes: left ventricular myocardial mass (LVM), LV end-diastolic volume (LVEDV), LV end-systolic volume (LVESV), right ventricular end-diastolic volume (RVEDV), and RV end-systolic volume (RVESV). We assess the differences between the generated data and real data with the same clinical conditions, denoted as $d_{\text{phenotype}}$. Additionally, these phenotypes are closely related to age and gender [5]. We compute the distributions of the imaging phenotypes against age and gender and compare the generated data to the real data. The comparison is shown qualitatively using density plots and quantitatively using the Kullback–Leibler (KL) divergence and Wasserstein distance (WD). The KL divergence [14] is an information-theoretic measure of the similarity between two probability mass functions. Similarly, WD [2] quantifies the distance between two probability distributions and can be calculated as:

$$\mathrm{WD} = \inf_{\gamma \sim \prod(P,Q)} \mathbb{E}_{(u,v)\sim\gamma}[\|u - v\|] \tag{15.6}$$

where $\prod(P, Q)$ is the set of all joint distributions over u and v. WD can be seen as the minimum work needed to transform one distribution to another, where work is defined as the amount of mass that must be moved from u to v to transform P to Q and the distance to be moved.

15.3 Experiments

15.3.1 Data Sets

A dataset of 1383 subjects, featuring short-axis 3D cardiac MR images, was obtained from Hammersmith Hospital, Imperial College London. Each cardiac cine image sequence consists of 20 time frames ($T = 20$) that capture a full cardiac cycle, with a spatial resolution of 1.25 mm $\times$ 1.25 mm $\times$ 2 mm. The temporal resolution varies between 0.041 and 0.048 seconds per frame to account for differences in heart rates. The cardiac anatomy is represented by an image segmentation map with four labels: background, left ventricle (LV), myocardium (Myo), and right ventricle (RV). Ground truth segmentation for end-diastolic (ED) and end-systolic (ES) frames was generated using a multi-atlas segmentation method [3], and subsequently quality controlled and manually corrected by an experienced cardiologist using itkSNAP [53]. A state-of-the-art nnU-net model [21] was trained on the ED and ES segmentations and then applied to all time frames to produce the 3D-t segmentations, followed by manual quality control. To remove the influence of image orientations during generation, all 3D-t segmentations were rigidly aligned to a template space using MIRTK [39, 41] and cropped to a standard size of $128 \times 128 \times 64$. This ensures that the generative model focuses on learning subject-specific anatomical variations rather than image orientations. Regarding demographic information, all subjects were healthy volunteers, including 775 females and 608 males, aged 18–73 years, weighing between 33 and 131 kg, with heights ranging from 142 to 195 cm, and systolic blood pressure (SBP) between 79 and 183 mm Hg. Age was represented as a categorical factor with seven age groups in 10-year intervals from 10 to 80 years old for the clinical information incorporated into the model. The dataset was randomly divided into three subsets for training ($n = 968$), validation ($n = 138$), and testing ($n = 277$).

15.3.2 Experimental Setup

15.3.2.1 Implementation

The model was developed using PyTorch [34]. The encoder q_ϕ comprised four 3D convolutional layers, a flatten layer, and a bottleneck layer, producing the latent code z_0. The condition mapping network was designed with an MLP, generating the latent code z_c for the input conditions c. Both z_0 and z_c had a latent dimension of 32, while the concatenated latent vector z_0^c had a dimension of 64. The decoder included a flatten layer and four 3D transposed convolutional layers. All convolutional and transposed convolutional layers in both the encoder and decoder had a kernel size of 4. The temporal module was constructed with one-layer LSTMCells. The regularization weight β in β-VAE was set to 0.001. The model was trained with the Adam optimizer at a learning rate of $5 \cdot 10^{-4}$ and a batch size of 8. Training was conducted for 500 epochs with early stopping based on validation set performance. The training process took 17 hours on an NVIDIA RTX A6000 GPU.

15.3.2.2 Baseline Methods

Currently, there is no other existing work for performing conditional generation of 3D-t cardiac anatomies. For comparison, we implemented the following baseline generation methods developed in other application domains, extending them from 2D image generation to 3D-t data generation:

CGAN A conditional version of the generative adversarial network (GAN) originally developed for MNIST images [31]. Note that the model can only perform cardiac sequence generation, not sequence completion.

CVAE The conditional generative model CVAE [44]. It was modified to adapt to this application. CVAE applied condition incorporation by concatenating conditions and anatomies in both the encoder and decoder.

CVAE-GAN A conditional variational generative adversarial network proposed in [6]. It is a general learning framework that combines a VAE with a GAN for synthesizing natural images in fine-grained categories.

PCA The principal component analysis (PCA) [23]. It is a classical method for dimensionality reduction, which aims to preserve as much of the variation in data as possible using the principal components. Note that the PCA is only used for performing sequence completion, but not for sequence generation.

15.3.3 Sequence Completion

A common challenge in generative modeling is the difficulty in evaluation, as we typically lack access to the ground truth data distribution, such as the distribution of all possible cardiac anatomies in our case. Consequently, we use anatomical sequence completion as a proxy task to evaluate model performance. The sequence completion experiments were carried out to assess the model's ability to capture sequential information given the first frame of a cardiac anatomy sequence. An example of sequence completion is illustrated in Fig. 15.3. The figure shows that the generated anatomies over time maintain the same heart structures as the ED frame and capture the temporal motion pattern, initially contracting and then expanding.

The sequence completion accuracy is assessed by comparing the generated anatomy to the ground truth across the entire sequence using the Dice metric, HD, and ASSD for three structures: LV, Myo, and RV. Table 15.1 presents the sequence completion accuracy of the proposed model and compares it to other generative models, including CVAE-GAN [6], CVAE [44], and PCA [23]. The results indicate that the proposed model achieves a good sequence completion accuracy with an average Dice metric of 0.874, HD of 5.842 mm, and ASSD of 1.462 mm, which is comparable to or outperforms the other three generative models in most metrics.

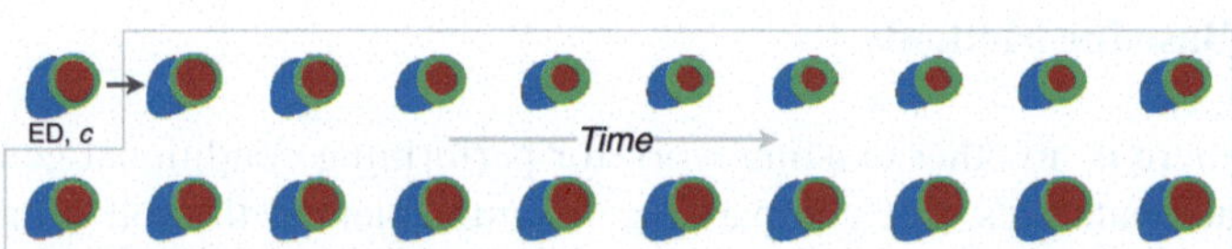

Fig. 15.3 An example of sequence completion, arranged in two rows with the left-to-right and top-to-bottom order. With the end-diastolic (ED) frame in time $t = 0$ and conditions c as input, the model generates the remaining anatomical sequence at time frame $t = 1$–19, shown within the gray box. The top row depicts anatomy images at time frame $t = 0$–9, and the bottom row depicts at time frame $t = 10$–19

Table 15.1 The Sequence Completion Performance of Different Models in terms of Dice, Hausdorff distance (HD), average symmetric surface distance (ASSD). Mean and standard deviation are reported. Asterisks indicate statistical significance (*: $p \leq 0.05$; **: $p < 0.05$) when using a paired Student's *t*-test comparing the performance of the proposed method to other methods

	LV	Myo	RV	Average
	Dice (unit: 1)			
CVAE-GAN [6]	$0.845^{*}_{\pm 0.028}$	$0.697^{*}_{\pm 0.054}$	$0.832^{*}_{\pm 0.028}$	$0.791^{*}_{\pm 0.032}$
CVAE [44]	$0.900_{\pm 0.023}$	$0.800^{*}_{\pm 0.040}$	$0.894_{\pm 0.023}$	$0.864^{*}_{\pm 0.026}$
PCA [23]	$0.906_{\pm 0.022}$	$0.810_{\pm 0.038}$	$0.901_{\pm 0.023}$	$0.872_{\pm 0.025}$
Proposed	$0.908^{**}_{\pm 0.023}$	$0.814^{**}_{\pm 0.037}$	$0.902^{**}_{\pm 0.021}$	$0.874^{**}_{\pm 0.024}$
	HD (unit: mm)			
CVAE-GAN [6]	$10.361^{*}_{\pm 1.475}$	$9.571^{*}_{\pm 1.379}$	$14.070^{*}_{\pm 3.736}$	$11.334^{*}_{\pm 1.849}$
CVAE [44]	$5.920^{*}_{\pm 1.335}$	$5.891^{*}_{\pm 1.055}$	$6.525_{\pm 1.076}$	$6.112^{*}_{\pm 1.049}$
PCA [23]	$5.517^{**}_{\pm 1.029}$	$5.710_{\pm 1.125}$	$6.165^{**}_{\pm 1.072}$	$5.797^{**}_{\pm 0.978}$
Proposed	$5.535_{\pm 1.180}$	$5.576^{**}_{\pm 0.955}$	$6.445_{\pm 1.067}$	$5.842_{\pm 1.017}$
	ASSD (unit: mm)			
CVAE-GAN [6]	$2.120^{*}_{\pm 0.390}$	$1.670^{*}_{\pm 0.236}$	$2.244^{*}_{\pm 0.399}$	$1.983^{*}_{\pm 0.306}$
CVAE [44]	$1.657^{*}_{\pm 0.348}$	$1.376^{*}_{\pm 0.212}$	$1.622_{\pm 0.305}$	$1.461_{\pm 0.280}$
PCA [23]	$1.565_{\pm 0.324}$	$1.319^{*}_{\pm 0.221}$	$1.519^{**}_{\pm 0.301}$	$1.490_{\pm 0.305}$
Proposed	$1.535^{**}_{\pm 0.330}$	$1.298^{**}_{\pm 0.208}$	$1.620_{\pm 0.323}$	$1.462^{**}_{\pm 0.266}$

Additionally, evaluations were conducted at the basal, mid-cavity, and apical slices. The proposed model achieved average Dice metrics of 0.929, 0.927, and 0.878 for LV at these locations, surpassing the corresponding metrics of the other three generative models. We also performed paired Student's t-tests between the results generated by our method and those of competing methods. The performance metrics of the proposed model marked with an asterisk in Table 15.1 were significantly better than other methods at a p value smaller than 0.05. In a different cardiac MR dataset, [4] reports average Dice metrics of 0.94, 0.88, and 0.90 for LV, myocardium, and RV, respectively, for inter-observer variability in manual cardiac image segmentation (Table 3 of [4]). The Dice metric of the proposed generative model is close to this value, indicating its high performance and capability for anatomical sequence completion.

15.3.4 Sequence Generation

In addition to the sequence completion task, we also carry out anatomical sequence generation and assess the similarity between the generated anatomical sequences and the actual data. In this study, we create new synthetic heart anatomies by using clinical conditions as the sole input to the model. Due to the stochastic

Table 15.2 Comparison of sequence generation performance between CGAN, CVAE, CVAE-GAN and the proposed model, in terms of mean and best Dice metric and contour distance metrics for the average performance over LV, RV and Myo. The best value across 20 samples for Dice metric (maximum), HD (minimum) and ASSD (minimum) are reported. Asterisks indicate statistical significance (*: $p \leq 0.05$; **: $p < 0.05$) when using a paired Student's *t*-test comparing the performance of the proposed method to other methods

	Dice (unit: 1)		HD (unit: mm)		ASSD (unit: mm)	
Model	Mean	Best/max	Mean	Best/min	Mean	Best/min
CGAN [31]	$0.713^{**}_{\pm 0.061}$	$0.717^{*}_{\pm 0.061}$	$15.533^{*}_{\pm 2.258}$	$13.956^{*}_{\pm 2.326}$	$3.004^{**}_{\pm 0.714}$	$2.862^{*}_{\pm 0.712}$
CVAE [44]	$0.694_{\pm 0.056}$	$0.789_{\pm 0.049}$	$11.461^{*}_{\pm 1.809}$	$8.321_{\pm 1.536}$	$3.380^{*}_{\pm 0.710}$	$2.317^{*}_{\pm 0.540}$
CVAE-GAN [6]	$0.645^{*}_{\pm 0.052}$	$0.774_{\pm 0.039}$	$16.844^{*}_{\pm 2.008}$	$12.105^{*}_{\pm 1.815}$	$3.693^{*}_{\pm 0.709}$	$2.185_{\pm 0.394}$
Proposed	$0.713^{**}_{\pm 0.058}$	$0.793^{**}_{\pm 0.052}$	$10.940^{**}_{\pm 2.343}$	$8.166^{**}_{\pm 1.621}$	$3.023_{\pm 0.757}$	$2.049^{**}_{\pm 0.521}$

characteristics of VAE generation, multiple anatomical sequences can be produced for each set of input conditions. We extract 20 random samples from the Gaussian distribution of the latent vector and subsequently generate 20 synthetic anatomical sequences for this set of input conditions.

We compare synthetic anatomies to real ones under identical clinical conditions, assessing mean and best similarities across 20 samples using the Dice metric, HD, ASSD, and clinical measure differences. This approach is similar to random average or random best evaluations in recent computer vision studies [35]. Table 15.2 shows that our model achieves a mean Dice of 0.713, HD of 10.940 mm, and ASSD of 3.023 mm. The best values are a Dice of 0.793, HD of 8.166 mm, and ASSD of 2.049 mm, indicating the model's ability to generate anatomies closely resembling real ones. Table 15.3 shows lower clinical measure differences, with mean differences of 25.93 mL, 11.74 mL, 34.63 mL, 15.54 mL, and 17.34 g, and minimum differences of 6.87 mL, 3.54 mL, 6.88 mL, 5.12 mL, and 2.95 g for LVEDV, LVESV, RVEDV, RVESV, and LVM, respectively. These results suggest our model achieves comparable (Dice) or superior (HD, ASSD, clinical measure differences) accuracy relative to other methods. The best metric values highlight the high fidelity of our model, showing how closely generated samples resemble real ones [32, 40]. Note that the model aims to generate plausible anatomies meeting specific conditions, not replicate existing ones.

We visualised two examples of anatomical sequence generation in Fig. 15.4. For each, we show five random synthetic samples sharing the same clinical conditions as the real sample. The LV and RV structures look realistic and similar to real anatomy. The contracting pattern of the ventricles and myocardium from ED to ES frame also appears realistic. This shows our model captures the overall anatomy and temporal dynamics of the heart. The five samples with the same conditions also show variations, demonstrating the diversity of synthetic data. This results from the Gaussian sampling process and reflects individual differences between hearts due to genetic, environmental, lifestyle, and other factors.

Table 15.3 Comparison of sequence generation performance among CGAN, CVAE, CVAE-GAN and the proposed model. The clinical measures derived from each real sample are compared to those derived from 20 synthetic samples of exactly the same conditions. The mean and the minimal differences of the clinical measures are reported here (**: $p < 0.05$)

	d_{LVEDV} (mL)		d_{LVESV} (mL)		d_{RVEDV} (mL)		d_{RVESV} (mL)		d_{LVM} (g)	
Model	Mean	Best/min	Mean	Best/min	Mean	Best/min	Mean	Best/min	Mean	Best/min
CGAN [31]	$35.58_{\pm 20.33}$	$15.66_{\pm 16.67}$	$20.06_{\pm 9.71}$	$19.74_{\pm 9.72}$	$51.47_{\pm 25.25}$	$14.71_{\pm 17.12}$	$17.57_{\pm 12.19}$	$17.04_{\pm 12.18}$	$38.26_{\pm 19.15}$	$10.40_{\pm 11.23}$
CVAE [44]	$35.74_{\pm 16.99}$	$4.91^{**}_{\pm 9.84}$	$13.92_{\pm 6.06}$	$1.87_{\pm 3.46}$	$44.97_{\pm 21.58}$	$6.46^{**}_{\pm 12.92}$	$19.49_{\pm 9.21}$	$2.86_{\pm 5.74}$	$23.07_{\pm 9.96}$	$2.70^{**}_{\pm 4.33}$
CVAE-GAN [6]	$51.32_{\pm 20.40}$	$6.33_{\pm 11.96}$	$19.80_{\pm 6.53}$	$1.69^{**}_{\pm 2.57}$	$48.94_{\pm 28.66}$	$8.28_{\pm 17.52}$	$25.26_{\pm 10.99}$	$2.57^{**}_{\pm 4.11}$	$51.03_{\pm 11.40}$	$8.29_{\pm 7.91}$
Proposed	$25.93^{**}_{\pm 17.47}$	$6.87^{**}_{\pm 12.09}$	$11.74^{**}_{\pm 8.41}$	$3.54_{\pm 6.25}$	$34.63^{**}_{\pm 21.31}$	$6.88_{\pm 12.87}$	$15.54^{**}_{\pm 11.33}$	$5.12_{\pm 9.19}$	$17.34^{**}_{\pm 9.89}$	$2.95_{\pm 5.62}$

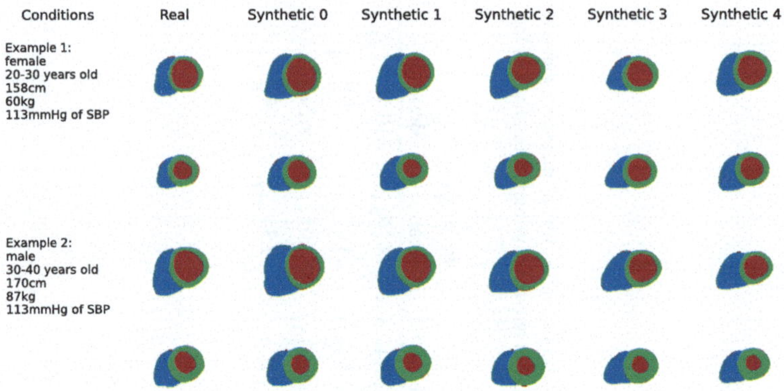

Fig. 15.4 Visualisation of synthetic anatomies (last five columns) generated by the model, compared to the real anatomy (first column) with the same clinical conditions (text annotation). The whole anatomical sequence is generated but only ED and ES frames are shown here. The first and second rows of each example show the ED and ES frames of the cardiac anatomical sequence

To rigorously assess the fidelity and diversity of the generated samples relative to the actual samples, we examine the divergence between their distributions, conditioned on age, a prevalent variable of interest in clinical research. Beyond quantitative evaluations, we performed qualitative comparisons by scrutinizing the distributions of five clinical metrics for both real and synthetic anatomies across age, including LVM, LVEDV, LVEV, RVEDV, and RVEF, as depicted in Fig. 15.5. In comparison to alternative methodologies, the synthetic data distributions produced by our model exhibit a close resemblance to the real distributions and encapsulate the complete variability of the actual samples. Table 15.4 presents the KL divergence and Wasserstein distance between synthetic and real data distributions. The proposed model attains superior KL or WD metrics in the majority of clinical measurements, with KL divergence values of 0.034, 0.043, 0.034, 0.039, 0.031, and WD values of 15.053, 5.773, 12.214, 9.182, 9.215 for LVEDV, LVESV, RVEDV, RVESV, and LVM, respectively. These findings indicate that the synthetic data generated by our model preserves a distribution with respect to age that is analogous to the real data.

15.3.5 Condition Manipulation

Using the conditional generative model, we simulate anatomical changes under varying conditions (e.g., age). Figure 15.6a shows generated anatomies as age increases, with other conditions and latent vectors fixed. The difference map between aged anatomy and that at 10–20 years shows subtle LV and RV changes. We generate 200 random samples of synthetic ageing anatomies and derive clinical measures. Figure 15.6b shows the longitudinal evolution of these measures by

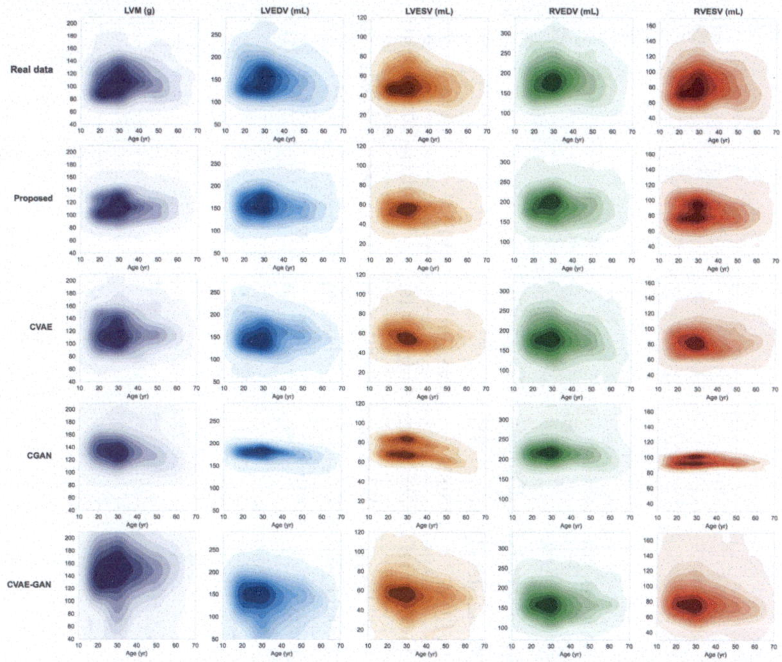

Fig. 15.5 Distributions of clinical measures for real data and synthetic data. Each graph displays a kernel density plot of an imaging phenotype (LVM, LVEDV, LVESV, RVEDV, RVESV) against age. For each plot, the x-axis denotes age and the y-axis denotes the value of the imaging phenotype. Darker areas in the plot indicate the regions where the data is more concentrated. Lighter areas show the regions where the data is sparser

gender. We observe an increasing trend in LVM and a decreasing trend in LVEDV during ageing, consistent with clinical literature [18] (Figure 3 of [18]). This model shows potential for simulating anatomical data distributions. However, caution is needed in interpretation, as our training data is cross-sectional, and cardiac ageing is influenced by more factors (genetics, lifestyle, etc.) than the five conditions used.

15.4 Discussion

The proposed model, based on a β-VAE, learns the latent space of cardiac anatomy. It includes a conditional branch to model clinical factors and a temporal module for anatomical latent vectors during cardiac motion. Experiments show good performance in sequence completion and generation tasks, both qualitatively and quantitatively. The model allows manipulation of conditions to demonstrate clinical factors' impact on anatomical shape variation. Using common clinical measures (ventricular volumes and mass), the generated anatomies' distribution closely

Table 15.4 KL divergence and Wasserstein distance between synthetic data distribution and real data distribution (**: $p < 0.05$)

Distribution	Kullback–Leibler (KL) divergence					Wasserstein Distance (WD)				
similarity	LVEDV	LVESV	RVEDV	RVESV	LVM	LVEDV	LVESV	RVEDV	RVESV	LVM
CGAN [31]	$0.023^{**}_{\pm 0.001}$	$0.019^{**}_{\pm 0.001}$	$0.036_{\pm 0.004}$	$0.022^{**}_{\pm 0.001}$	$0.050_{\pm 0.006}$	$33.687_{\pm 1.173}$	$19.982_{\pm 0.025}$	$41.643_{\pm 4.161}$	$17.434_{\pm 0.036}$	$35.395_{\pm 2.933}$
CVAE [44]	$0.039_{\pm 0.005}$	$0.041_{\pm 0.004}$	$0.042_{\pm 0.004}$	$0.034_{\pm 0.003}$	$0.030_{\pm 0.003}$	$11.929^{**}_{\pm 2.116}$	$7.017_{\pm 0.964}$	$14.680_{\pm 2.869}$	$9.665_{\pm 1.051}$	$10.365_{\pm 1.703}$
CVAE-GAN [6]	$0.153_{\pm 0.025}$	$0.023_{\pm 0.003}$	$0.046_{\pm 0.006}$	$0.064_{\pm 0.008}$	$0.098_{\pm 0.019}$	$27.001_{\pm 2.809}$	$8.425_{\pm 1.771}$	$24.614_{\pm 3.202}$	$9.748_{\pm 2.675}$	$43.251_{\pm 4.566}$
Proposed	$0.034_{\pm 0.002}$	$0.043_{\pm 0.002}$	$0.034^{**}_{\pm 0.002}$	$0.039_{\pm 0.002}$	$0.031^{**}_{\pm 0.002}$	$15.053_{\pm 3.597}$	$5.773^{**}_{\pm 1.358}$	$12.214^{**}_{\pm 2.408}$	$9.182^{**}_{\pm 2.145}$	$9.215^{**}_{\pm 1.713}$

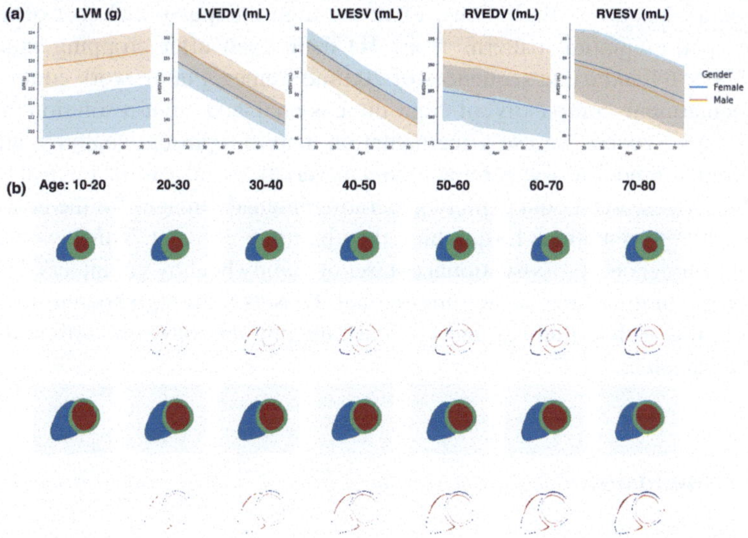

Fig. 15.6 (**a**) The simulated evolution of clinical measures (LVM, LVEDV, LVESV, RVEDV, RVESV) by generating 200 samples of gender-specific ageing cardiac anatomy and plotting their mean measures with 95% confidence interval. (**b**) An example of the synthetic cardiac anatomy during ageing. The first and third rows show the cardiac anatomies at end-systolic (ES) and end-diastolic (ED) frames. The second and fourth rows show the difference maps between the aged anatomy 20–80 years old and the anatomy at 10–20 years old

matches real data visually (Fig. 15.5) and quantitatively (Table 15.4), indicating fidelity and diversity. While the model generates anatomically coherent structures, further improvement is needed to better match the real data distribution. Additionally, exploring the relationship between cardiac motion and clinical conditions is promising.

We foresee several downstream tasks for the generative cardiac anatomy model: discovering patterns in large datasets, facilitating out-of-distribution detection, and generating synthetic data. Training a generative model on a large dataset of cardiac anatomies captures complex patterns and variations associated with clinical factors, aiding in understanding population characteristics, identifying risk factors, and informing public health strategies. By learning the distribution of normal cardiac anatomy and dynamics, the model can detect deviations indicating potential anomalies. As a conditional generative model, it can learn norms for specific conditions (e.g., gender and age group) and evaluate deviations in a personalized manner. The model can also generate synthetic data for tasks like data augmentation for machine learning models [8], creating synthetic fair data to improve prediction model fairness [11, 46], and performing in-silico trials [50]. Diverse and realistic synthetic data will address data scarcity in the medical field, where real data are often limited or hard to share, and support privacy-preserving research [36, 45].

This work has a few limitations. First, the high computational cost of training to learn spatio-temporal patterns from 4D data, even after cropping images to $128 \times 128 \times 64$ and using sequences of 20 time frames. Future work could reduce the computational complexity of high-dimensional and high-resolution medical imaging data. Second, we use a segmentation map to represent anatomy, allowing the generative model to focus on anatomical variations instead of intensity image styles. Future research could explore generating intensity images for the heart [1] or using mesh representations [30], which may be more efficient. Third, we train the generative model on a cross-sectional dataset of mainly healthy volunteers due to the difficulty of curating large-scale longitudinal datasets with high spatial resolution. Extending this to longitudinal and clinical imaging cohorts with cardiac diseases would be valuable.

15.5 Conclusion

We propose a novel conditional generative model to synthesise spatio-temporal cardiac anatomies from clinical factors. It generates realistic 3D-t heart anatomies, capturing anatomical variations and motion. This work paves the way for further research in cardiac imaging, including disease incorporation and mesh representation. It can also be applied to tasks like data augmentation, building condition-specific atlases, and biomechanical heart modelling.

Acknowledgments This work is supported by EPSRC DeepGeM Grant (EP/W01842X/1). SW is supported by Shanghai Sailing Program (22YF1409300), CCF-Baidu Open Fund (CCF-BAIDU 202316) and International Science and Technology Cooperation Program under the 2023 Shanghai Action Plan for Science (23410710400); HQ is supported by EPSRC SmartHeart (EP/P001009/1) and Innovate UK (104691). DO'R is supported by the Medical Research Council (MC_UP_1605/13); National Institute for Health Research (NIHR) Imperial College Biomedical Research Centre; and the British Heart Foundation (RG/19/6/34387, RE/18/4/34215). ADM is supported by the Fetal Medicine Foundation (495237) and Academy of Medical Sciences (SGL015/1006). DR was supported in part by the European Research Council (Grant Agreement no. 884622). We thank Weitong Zhang for helpful discussions on the methodological theory. For the purpose of open access, the authors have applied a creative commons attribution (CC BY) licence to any author accepted manuscript version arising.

References

1. Amirrajab S, Al Khalil Y, Lorenz C, Weese J, Pluim J, Breeuwer M (2023) A framework for simulating cardiac MR images with varying anatomy and contrast. IEEE Trans Med Imaging 42(3):726–738
2. Arjovsky M, Chintala S, Bottou L (2017) Wasserstein generative adversarial networks. In: International conference on machine learning, pp 214–223. https://doi.org/10.48550/arXiv.1701.07875

3. Bai W, Shi W, O'Regan DP, Tong T, Wang H, Jamil-Copley S, Peters NS, Rueckert D (2013) A probabilistic patch-based label fusion model for multi-atlas segmentation with registration refinement: application to cardiac MR images. IEEE Trans Med Imaging 32(7):1302–1315. https://doi.org/10.1109/TMI.2013.2256921
4. Bai W, Sinclair M, Tarroni G, Oktay O, Rajchl M, Vaillant G, Lee AM, Aung N, Lukaschuk E, Sanghvi MM, et al (2018) Automated cardiovascular magnetic resonance image analysis with fully convolutional networks. J Cardiovasc Magn Reson 20(1):65. https://doi.org/10.1186/s12968-018-0471-x
5. Bai W, Suzuki H, Huang J, Francis C, Wang S, Tarroni G, Guitton F, Aung N, Fung K, Petersen SE, et al (2020) A population-based phenome-wide association study of cardiac and aortic structure and function. Nat Med 26(10):1654–1662. https://doi.org/10.1038/s41591-020-0997-7
6. Bao J, Chen D, Wen F, Li H, Hua G (2017) CVAE-GAN: fine-grained image generation through asymmetric training. In: International conference on computer vision, pp 2745–2754. https://doi.org/10.1109/ICCV.2017.297
7. Biffi C, Cerrolaza JJ, Tarroni G, Bai W, De Marvao A, Oktay O, Ledig C, Le Folgoc L, Kamnitsas K, Doumou G, et al (2020) Explainable anatomical shape analysis through deep hierarchical generative models. IEEE Trans Med Imaging 39(6):2088–2099. https://doi.org/10.1109/TMI.2020.2965638
8. Billot B, Greve DN, Puonti O, Thielscher A, Van Leemput K, Fischl B, Dalca AV, Iglesias JE, et al (2023) Synthseg: segmentation of brain mri scans of any contrast and resolution without retraining. Med Image Anal 86:102789. https://doi.org/10.1016/j.media.2022.102789
9. Campello VM, Xia T, Liu X, Sanchez P, Martín-Isla C, Petersen SE, Seguí S, Tsaftaris SA, Lekadir K (2022) Cardiac aging synthesis from cross-sectional data with conditional generative adversarial networks. Front Cardiovasc Med 9. https://doi.org/10.3389/fcvm.2022.850607
10. Cardim N, Galderisi M, Edvardsen T, Plein S, Popescu B, d'Andrea A, Bruder O, Cosyns B, Davin L, Donal E, et al (2015) Role of multimodality cardiac imaging in the management of patients with hypertrophic cardiomyopathy: an expert consensus of the European Association of Cardiovascular Imaging Endorsed by the Saudi Heart Association. Eur Heart J Cardiovasc Imaging 16(3):280. https://doi.org/10.1093/ehjci/jev095
11. Chen RJ, Lu MY, Chen TY, Williamson DFK, Mahmood F (2021) Synthetic data in machine learning for medicine and healthcare. Nat Biomed Eng 5(6):493–497. https://doi.org/10.1038/s41551-021-00751-8
12. Chen Z, Kim VG, Fisher M, Aigerman N, Zhang H, Chaudhuri S (2021) Decor-GAN: 3D shape detailization by conditional refinement. In: IEEE conference on computer vision and pattern recognition, pp 15740–15749. https://doi.org/10.1109/CVPR.2021.01763
13. Choi Y, Choi M, Kim M, Ha JW, Kim S, Choo J (2018) Stargan: unified generative adversarial networks for multi-domain image-to-image translation. In: IEEE conference on computer vision and pattern recognition, pp 8789–8797. https://doi.org/10.1109/CVPR.2018.00916
14. Cover TM (1999) Elements of information theory. John Wiley & Sons. https://doi.org/10.1002/9781119445277
15. Dalca AV, Rakic M, Guttag J, Sabuncu MR (2019) Learning conditional deformable templates with convolutional networks. Neural Inf Process Syst: 806–818. https://doi.org/10.48550/arXiv.1910.12529
16. Dhariwal P, Jun H, Payne C, Kim JW, Radford A, Sutske ver I (2020) Jukebox: a generative model for music. arXiv preprint arXiv:2005.00341
17. Duchateau N, Sermesant M, Delingette H, Ayache N (2018) Model-based generation of large databases of cardiac images: synthesis of pathological cine MR sequences from real healthy cases. IEEE Trans Med Imaging 37(3):755–766. https://doi.org/10.1109/TMI.2017.2756062
18. Eng J, McClelland RL, Gomes AS, Hundley WG, Cheng S, Wu CO, Carr JJ, Shea S, Bluemke DA, Lima JAC (2016) Adverse left ventricular remodeling and age assessed with cardiac MR imaging: the multi-ethnic study of atherosclerosis. Radiology 278(3):714–722. https://doi.org/10.1148/radiol.2015150336

19. Gilbert K, Mauger C, Young AA, Suinesiaputra A (2020) Artificial intelligence in cardiac imaging with statistical atlases of cardiac anatomy. Front Cardiovasc Med 7. https://doi.org/10.3389/fcvm.2020.00121
20. Higgins I, Matthey L, Pal A, Burgess C, Glorot X, Botvinick M, Mohamed S, Lerchner A (2017) beta-VAE: learning basic visual concepts with a constrained variational framework. In: International conference on learning representations
21. Isensee F, Jaeger PF, Kohl SAA, Petersen J, Maier-Hein KH (2021) nnU-Net: a self-configuring method for deep learning-based biomedical image segmentation. Nat Methods 18(2):203–211. https://doi.org/10.1038/s41592-020-01008-z
22. Isola P, Zhu JY, Zhou T, Efros AA (2017) Image-to-image translation with conditional adversarial networks. In: IEEE conference on computer vision and pattern recognition, pp 1125–1134. https://doi.org/10.1109/CVPR.2017.632
23. Jolliffe IT (2002) Principal component analysis for special types of data. Springer, pp 338–372
24. Karamitsos TD, Francis JM, Myerson S, Selvanayagam JB, Neubauer S (2009) The role of cardiovascular magnetic resonance imaging in heart failure. J Am Coll Cardiol 54(15):1407–1424. https://doi.org/10.1016/j.jacc.2009.04.094
25. Karras T, Laine S, Aila T (2019) A style-based generator architecture for generative adversarial networks. In: IEEE conference on computer vision and pattern recognition, pp 4401–4410. https://doi.org/10.1109/CVPR.2019.00453
26. Khamparia A, Pandey B, Tiwari S, Gupta D, Khanna A, Rodrigues JJPC (2020) An integrated hybrid CNN–RNN model for visual description and generation of captions. Circuits Syst Signal Process 39(2):776–788. https://doi.org/10.1007/s00034-019-01229-2
27. Kingma DP, Welling M (2014) Auto-encoding variational Bayes. In: International conference on learning representations
28. Krebs J, Delingette H, Ayache N, Mansi T (2021) Learning a generative motion model from image sequences based on a latent motion matrix. IEEE Trans Med Imaging 40(5):1405–1416. https://doi.org/10.1109/TMI.2021.3052251
29. Mauger CA, Govil S, Chabiniok R, Gilbert K, Hegde S, Hussain T, McCulloch AD, Occleshaw CJ, Omens J, Perry JC, Pushparajah K, Suinesiaputra A, Zhong L, Young AA (2021) Right-left ventricular shape variations in tetralogy of Fallot: associations with pulmonary regurgitation. J Cardiovasc Magn Reson 23(1):1–14. https://doi.org/10.1186/s12968-020-00690-8
30. Meng Q, Bai W, Liu T, O'Regan DP, Rueckert D (2022) Mesh-based 3D motion tracking in cardiac MRI using deep learning. In: International conference on medical image computing and computer-assisted intervention
31. Mirza M, Osindero S (2014) Conditional generative adversarial nets. arXiv preprint, 1411.1784
32. Naeem MF, Oh SJ, Uh Y, Choi Y, Yoo J (2020) Reliable fidelity and diversity metrics for generative models. In: International conference on machine learning, pp 7176–7185. https://doi.org/10.48550/arXiv.2004.05164
33. Nichol A, Dhariwal P, Ramesh A, Shyam P, Mishkin P, McGrew B, Sutskever I, Chen M (2022) Glide: towards photorealistic image generation and editing with text-guided diffusion models. In: International conference on machine learning
34. Paszke A, Gross S, Massa F, Lerer A, Bradbury J, Chanan G, Killeen T, Lin Z, Gimelshein N, Antiga L, et al (2019) PyTorch: an imperative style, high-performance deep learning library. Neural Inf Process Syst 32:8026–8037
35. Petrovich M, Black MJ, Varol G (2022) TEMOS: generating diverse human motions from textual descriptions. In: European conference on computer vision
36. Qian Z, Callender T, Cebere B, Janes SM, Navani N, van der Schaar M (2023) Synthetic data for privacy-preserving clinical risk prediction. medRxiv, 2023-05. https://doi.org/10.1101/2023.05.04.23289513
37. Reynaud H, Vlontzos A, Dombrowski M, Lee C, Beqiri A, Leeson P, Kainz B (2022) D'artagnan: counterfactual video generation. In: Medical image computing and computer assisted intervention, pp 599–609
38. Rezende D, Mohamed S (2015) Variational inference with normalizing flows. In: International conference on machine learning, pp 1530–1538. https://doi.org/10.48550/arXiv.1505.05770

39. Rueckert D, Sonoda LI, Denton ERE, Rankin S, Hayes C, Leach MO, Hill DLG, Hawkes DJ (1999) Comparison and evaluation of rigid and nonrigid registration of breast MR images. In: Medical imaging 1999: image processing, vol 3661, pp 78–88. https://doi.org/10.1117/12.348171
40. Sajjadi MSM, Bachem O, Lucic M, Bousquet O, Gelly S (2018) Assessing generative models via precision and recall. In: Advances in neural information processing systems, vol 31
41. Schuh A, Makropoulos A, Robinson EC, Cordero-Grande L, Hughes E, Hutter J, Price AN, Murgasova M, Teixeira RPAG, Tusor N, et al (2018) Unbiased construction of a temporally consistent morphological atlas of neonatal brain development. Tech. rep. bioRxiv, 251512. https://doi.org/10.1101/251512
42. Singer U, Polyak A, Hayes T, Yin X, An J, Zhang S, Hu Q, Yang H, Ashual O, Gafni O, et al (2022) Make-a-video: text-to-video generation without text-video data, arXiv preprint, 2209.14792
43. Smiseth OA, Torp H, Opdahl A, Haugaa KH, Urheim S (2016) Myocardial strain imaging: how useful is it in clinical decision making? Eur Heart J 37(15):1196–1207. https://doi.org/10.1093/eurheartj/ehv529
44. Sohn K, Lee H, Yan X (2015) Learning structured output representation using deep conditional generative models. Neural Inf Process Syst 28:3483–3491
45. Van Breugel B, van der Schaar M (2023) Beyond privacy: navigating the opportunities and challenges of synthetic data, arXiv preprint, 2304.03722
46. Van Breugel B, Kyono T, Berrevoets J, van der Schaar M (2021) DECAF: generating fair synthetic data using causally-aware generative networks. Adv Neural Inf Process Syst 34:22221–22233
47. Vinyals O, Toshev A, Bengio S, Erhan D (2015) Show and tell: a neural image caption generator. In: IEEE conference on computer vision and pattern recognition, pp 3156–3164. https://doi.org/10.1109/CVPR.2015.7298935
48. Walker J, Razavi A, van den Oord A (2021) Predicting video with VQVAE, arXiv preprint, 2103.01950
49. Xia T, Chartsias A, Wang C, Tsaftaris SA, Initiative ADN, et al (2021) Learning to synthesise the ageing brain without longitudinal data. Med Image Anal 73:102169. https://doi.org/10.1016/j.media.2021.102169
50. Xia Y, Ravikumar N, Lassila T, Frangi AF (2023) Virtual high-resolution MR angiography from non-angiographic multi-contrast MRIs: synthetic vascular model populations for in-silico trials. Med Image Anal 87:102814. https://doi.org/10.1016/j.media.2022.102814
51. Yan W, Zhang Y, Abbeel P, Srinivas A (2021) Videogpt: video generation using VQ-VAE and transformers, arXiv preprint, 2104.10157
52. Yoo J, Jin KH, Gupta H, Yerly J, Stuber M, Unser M (2021) Time-dependent deep image prior for dynamic MRI. IEEE Trans Med Imaging 40(12):3337–3348. https://doi.org/10.1109/TMI.2021.3095394
53. Yushkevich PA, Piven J, Hazlett HC, Smith RG, Ho S, Gee JC, Gerig G (2006) User-guided 3D active contour segmentation of anatomical structures: significantly improved efficiency and reliability. Neuroimage 31(3):1116–1128. https://doi.org/10.1016/j.neuroimage.2006.01.015
54. Zolotas M, Demiris Y (2022) Disentangled sequence clustering for human intention inference. In: International conference on intelligent robots and systems
55. Zou Q, Ahmed AH, Nagpal P, Priya S, Schulte RF, Jacob M (2022) Variational manifold learning from incomplete data: application to multislice dynamic MRI. IEEE Trans Med Imaging 41(12):3552–3561. https://doi.org/10.1109/TMI.2022.3196096
56. Zou Q, Priya S, Nagpal P, Jacob M (2023) Joint cardiac t 1 mapping and cardiac cine using manifold modeling. Bioengineering 10(3):345. https://doi.org/10.3390/bioengineering10030345

Chapter 16
Generative Models for Synthesizing Anatomical Plausible 3D Medical Images

Wei Peng and Kilian M. Pohl

Abstract Deep learning methods trained on 3D medical images typically do not generalize well as training data are relatively homogenous and small. One way to potentially overcome this issue is creating realistic-looking 3D medical images using generative models. This chapter describes the fundamental principles and architectures of generative models used for this purpose, such as those based on generative adversarial networks (GANs) and diffusion probabilistic models (DPMs). The chapter also reviews evaluation techniques for measuring the quality of synthetic medical images, including the evaluation of the biological plausibility of the anatomy displayed.

16.1 Introduction

Medical imaging is indispensable in healthcare, providing valuable insights into human anatomy and facilitating diagnosis, treatment planning, and disease monitoring [51]. However, acquiring medical images is generally expensive, time-consuming, and can pose health risks to patients, such as radiation exposure in CT acquisition [56]. Medical imaging studies are therefore generally quite small in size and homogeneous so that deep-learning models trained on them often do not generalize across different populations and image acquisitions [58]. A promising solution is to create larger and more diverse training data sets by synthetically generating medical images via generative models [34, 35, 37, 53]. Generative models first capture the distribution of the training data and then produce new

W. Peng
Department of Psychiatry & Behavioral Sciences, Stanford University, Stanford, CA, USA
e-mail: wepeng@stanford.edu

K. M. Pohl (✉)
Department of Psychiatry & Behavioral Sciences, Stanford University, Stanford, CA, USA

Department of Electrical Engineering, Stanford University, Stanford, CA, USA
e-mail: kpohl@stanford.edu

L. Zhang et al. (eds.), *Generative Machine Learning Models in Medical Image Computing*, https://doi.org/10.1007/978-3-031-80965-1_16

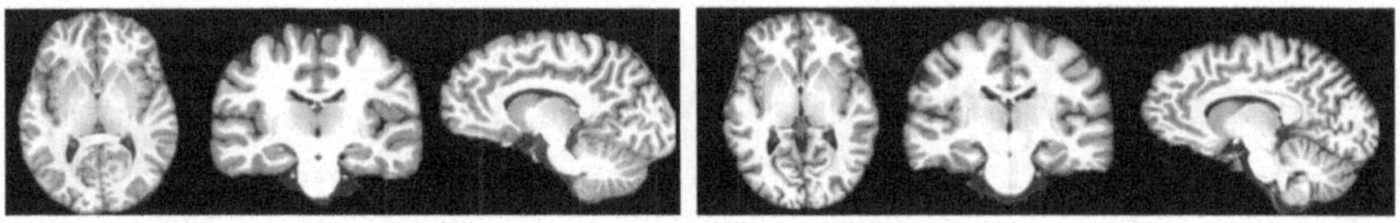

(a) (b)

Fig. 16.1 Axial, coronal, and sagittal view of (**a**) a real MRI and (**b**) a very similar looking synthetic MRI produced by a generative model [35]

samples (such as the magnetic resonance image (MRI) shown in Fig. 16.1) by sampling from that distribution. The generated images can then diversify training data to reduce biases and the influence of confounders [29]. In addition, these models can be used for simulating disease progression [39], which could provide valuable insights about disease dynamics [57] and improve treatment planning [10].

Despite their great potential, the application of generative models in the medical imaging domain has been challenging. Part of the challenge stems from the technology being originally developed for large data sets of natural 2D images [6], which can be easily downloaded from the internet or from large benchmark data sets [5] (>1 Million samples). Compared to those benchmark data sets, publicly available data sets of medical images are rare and small in size (<60K MRIs [50]) as, in addition to the mentioned issues, requires considering ethics and privacy concerns [33]. The issue is further amplified by 3D medical images [37] being relatively noisy and high dimensional [46]. Moreover, synthetic medical images must not only appear visually realistic but also be anatomically plausible [35], i.e., display anatomy and pathology that is biologically accurate. Accounting for all these challenges requires models specifically designed for 3D medical image applications, which is the focus of this chapter.

The next section briefly describes generative models originally developed for the synthesis of 2D natural images and their extensions to 3D medical images. The last section focuses on models generating brain MRIs that display biologically plausible anatomy.

16.2 3D Medical Imaging Generation

Examples of deep learning-based generative models are variational autoencoder (VAE) [23], Normalizing flow [42], generative adversarial networks (GANs) [13], and diffusion probabilistic models (DPMs) [19, 41]. The main objective of these models is to learn the distribution of the given data and later sample from the distribution to produce new samples. Based on how they represent the distribution, generative models can be split into explicit and implicit generative models [55]. Explicit generative models (such as VAEs and DPMs) define cost functions that focus on learning the distribution of the data. These approaches are generally quite stable and theoretically sound [23]. The cost function of implicit models (e.g., GANs) focuses on transforming random noise into a target image. These models are especially suitable for data distributions that are too complex to accurately encode explicitly. Among generative models, GANs and DPMs produce 3D medical images of the highest quality [2]. Their synthetic images have been used for data augmentation, anomaly detection, cross-modality image synthesis, and privacy-preserving data sharing [40]. This section will describe GAN-based and DPM-based models used for the synthesis of 3D medical images.

16.2.1 Generative Adversarial Networks

GANs [13] are a type of generative model that leverages a game-theoretic framework to train two neural networks: a generator that turns random noise into a synthesized image and a discriminator that distinguishes between real and synthetic images. The generator tries to create realistic data that fools the discriminator. This adversarial training process ends once the discriminator cannot reliably differentiate between real and synthetic data.

Originally developed for 2D natural images [13], extending GANs to 3D medical images is challenging [53]. First, GANs often suffer from mode collapse (i.e., only producing images that are similar to each other [15]) as the adversarial training will lead the generator to focus on "easy-to-fake" modes (samples) while neglecting others. The risk of mode collapse increases as the complexity of the task increases (such as from 2D to 3D image synthesis). Furthermore, training normally gets stuck in local minima as it is extremely hard to find the global optimum to the min-max objective function underlying the adversarial training [45]. Finally, a critical challenge is the memory requirement of GANs as the processing of even a single 3D medical volume can often exceed the memory capacity of current GPUs [22]. In the remainder of this section, we review GANs specifically designed for 3D medical images.

16.2.1.1 Auto-Encoding Generative Adversarial Network

One of such approaches makes use of variational autoencoder (VAE) [23], which, unlike GANs, does not suffer from mode collapse as they directly learn the data distribution by training an encoder to map images into a low-dimensional latent space and a decoder to transforms the latent space encoding into an image. However, they generally only produce images of much lower quality (e.g., the images are blurry). By initiating image generation from outputs generated by VAE (instead of from random noise), VAE-GAN [45] aims to address the mode collapse problem and produce high-quality 3D medical images [45].

This is achieved by expanding the adversarial training of the original GAN with a second discriminator that distinguishes between the encoding of the MRI generated by the VAE vs. the GAN. The VAE is then first trained to accurately encode medical images (a.k.a. real code). Next, the goal of the GAN is to produce fake code (from noise) that fools the additional discriminator in believing it is real. Once fooled, the GAN trains the generator to produce images using real and fake code. In addition to feeding those images into the discriminator, the images produced from the real code are also compared to the real images by adding the reconstruction loss (of the VAE) to the objective function of the GAN. This addition avoids mode collapse. Further improving training stability is adding the Wasserstein loss and gradient penalty (WGAN-GP) loss [24] to the objective function, which resulted in the first GAN that was able to produce high-quality 3D medical images.

16.2.1.2 Style-Based GAN

An alternative approach to improving the synthesis of medical images is based on StyleGAN [22], which simplifies the generation of 2D natural images by encoding them by their content (e.g., objects) and style (e.g., visual texture, coloring, lighting). During training, this style-based approach [12] generates low-resolution content, whose resolution is incrementally increased. The generation at each iteration is constrained according to the style of the image. By decoupling style from content, StyleGAN is more stable during training and generates images of significantly higher image quality compared to previous GAN models [22]. Its extension to 3D medical images (called 3D-StyleGAN) is fairly straightforward, i.e., all neural operations (such as convolution) are simply performed in 3D [20].

However, the high dimensionality of 3D medical images and associated memory requirements results in 3D-StyleGAN having feature maps (i.e., features in the middle layers of the generator) and latent vectors (i.e., samples from the latent space) that are significantly smaller than their 2D counterpart. Thus, 3D-StyleGAN [20] can currently only produce realistic-looking 3D t1-weighted MRI of 2 mm isotropic voxel resolution, while MRIs are commonly acquired at higher resolution (i.e., $\leq$1 mm isotropic).

To produce 3D MRIs at higher voxel resolution, one could view 3D images as a sequence of 2D images (i.e., videos), which can be generated by StyleGAN-V [48]. StyleGAN-V generates videos by coupling StyleGAN with a continuous motion representation [48], aiming at improving the temporal consistency. Compared to StyleGAN, its computational cost is only 5% higher, which compares favorably to the 3 times increase by 3D-StyleGAN. However, this approach treats one dimension of the 3D volume differently from the other two dimensions, which is a reasonable assumption for videos but can introduce various artifacts when generating 3D

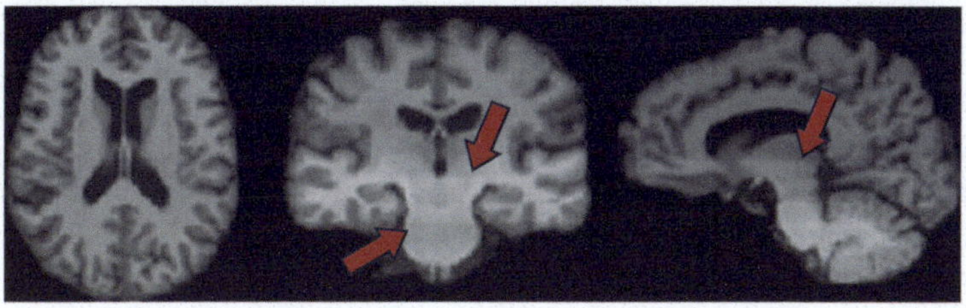

Fig. 16.2 Varying intensities across slices in an MRI generated by a slice-based approach [34]

images [34]. For example, the generated MRI in Fig. 16.2 shows a high quality image of a single slice (left, axial view) but 'stripes' in the other two (out-of-slice) views that are artefacts not found in a real, high quality MRI (such as in Fig. 16.1).

16.2.1.3 Hierarchical Amortized GAN

The computational memory requirements of GANs is generally a bottleneck when applying them to 3D medical images. For example, the size of brain MRI with at least 1mm isotropic voxel resolution is equivalent to a high-resolution 4K image. While running GANs on multiple GPUs could theoretically address this issue, the implementation becomes impractical for 3D medical images (as the memory of a single GPU is not even big enough to store the entire image [34]) so that the model itself or the data would need to be divided and distributed across multiple GPUs. One possible alternative is Hierarchical Amortized GAN (HA-GAN, [53]), which models the generation process using a low-resolution global branch that covers the entire 3D image and a high-resolution local branch, which encodes anatomical details of local patches. In particular, the generator first creates a lower-resolution representation $\hat{Z}$ of the 3D image in the first few network layers. The proceeding layers transform $\hat{Z}$ into a lower-resolution 3D medical image. Simultaneously, $\hat{Z}$ is split into subsets, from which high-resolution image patches are generated. The training now consists of optimizing the entire generator with respect to both tasks. Once trained, the entire $\hat{Z}$ is only fed into the high-resolution branch of the generator, which results in a full-size 3D high-quality medical image. By doing so, HA-GAN distributes the memory requirement across smaller (sub-)volumes during training so that it can generate high-resolution images during inference. Furthermore, the parallel architecture ensures anatomical consistency across the 3D image.

16.2.2 Diffusion Probabilistic Models

An alternative to GANs is diffusion probabilistic models (DPM) [19, 49], which potentially can generate realistic-looking 3D images at 1 mm isotropic voxel resolution. The principle design of the Diffusion Probabilistic Model (DPM) [19, 49] is based on iterating between mapping (1) data (e.g. images) gradually to noise (a.k.a., Forward Diffusion Process (FDP)) and (2) noise back to data (a.k.a., Reverse Diffusion Process(RDP)). Specifically, let $\mathcal{N}(0, I)$ be the Gaussian distribution with zero mean and identity matrix I being the variance. Now, FDP perturbs the real data x_0 into Gaussian noise $x_T \sim \mathcal{N}(0, I)$ after T iterations. This process is formulated as a Markov chain, whose transition kernel $q(x_t|x_{t-1})$ at time step $t \in \{0, \ldots, T\}$ is defined as

$$q(x_t|x_{t-1}) := \mathcal{N}(x_t; \sqrt{1-\beta_t} \cdot x_{t-1}, \beta_t \cdot I). \tag{16.1}$$

The weight $\beta_t \in (0, 1)$ is changed so that the chain gradually enforces drift, i.e., adds Gaussian noise to the data. Let $\alpha_t := 1 - \beta_t$ and $\bar{\alpha}_t := \prod_{s=1}^{t}(1 - \beta_t)$, then x_t is a sample of the distribution conditioned on x_0 as

$$q(x_t|x_0) := \mathcal{N}(x_t; \sqrt{\bar{\alpha}_t} \cdot x_0, (1 - \bar{\alpha}_t) \cdot I). \tag{16.2}$$

Given this closed-form solution, we can sample x_t at any arbitrary time step t without needing to iterate through the entire Markov chain.

The RDP aims to generate realistic data from random noise x_T by approximating the posterior distribution $p(x_{t-1}|x_t)$. It does so by going through the entire Markov chain from time step T to 0, i.e.,

$$p(x_{0:T}) := p(x_T) \prod_{t=1}^{T} p_\theta(x_{t-1}|x_t). \tag{16.3}$$

Defining the conditional distribution $p_\theta(x_{t-1}|x_t) := \mathcal{N}(x_{t-1}; \mu_\theta(x_t, t), \Sigma)$ with fixed variance Σ, then (according to [19]) the mean can be rewritten as

$$\mu_\theta(x_t, t) = \frac{1}{\sqrt{\alpha_t}} \left(x_t - \frac{\beta_t}{\sqrt{(1 - \bar{\alpha}_t)}} \epsilon_\theta(x_t, t) \right), \tag{16.4}$$

with $\epsilon_\theta(\cdot)$ being the estimate of a neural network defined by parameters θ. θ minimizes the reconstructing loss defined by the following expected value

$$\mathbb{E}_{x_0 \sim \mathbf{q}, t \in [0, \ldots, T], \epsilon \sim \mathcal{N}(0, I)} \left[||\epsilon - \epsilon_\theta(x_t, t)||_2^2 \right],$$

where $||\cdot||_2$ is the L2 norm and x_t is inferred from Eq. (16.2) based on x_0. This helps the model to learn the noise distribution at each time step t and thus can remove the noise from the image generated at step $t + 1$.

As for GANs, generating 3D high-resolution medical images is currently constrained by the size of GPU memory [35]. To address this challenge, recent work has explored several memory-efficient approaches, including (1) data re-organization (e.g., wavelet-based processing [36]), and (2) data compression, where the 3D image is compressed into a lower-dimensional latent representation before applying the diffusion process [37]. We now review these two strategies in further detail.

16.2.2.1 Data Re-organization in the Observation Space

Patch-Based Diffusion Model

The traditional diffusion model is based on U-Net architecture [44], which means the model can be trained on different sizes of images as it is a fully convolution network [30]. Patch-based diffusion training [54] takes advantage of this property by training the model based on patches that are much smaller than the final output, thus significantly reducing memory consumption and speeding up the training process. However, training the model directly using the cropped patches results in artifacts across patches in the synthesized images as the patches are defined within fixed grids and the model only learns the distribution of those patches (and not the entire image). One way to address this shortcoming is to add the image position of the patches to the input of the DPM [7]. Thus, for 3D imaging data, three additional channels are added to the input layer of the diffusion model as each coordinate dimension is represented by a separate channel. The model can then be trained on these randomly sampled patches while still being able to generate a full-resolution image during inference.

One limitation of patch-based diffusion is its perception fields [25] being confined to the patches so that dependencies beyond the size of patches are difficult to learn. This could make it hard to model the entire anatomical structure. One solution is to jointly consider global and local interactions by, for example, randomly selecting multiple small patches in the input image [26]. During training, the method then has to learn how to model both global (inter-patches) and local (intra-patches) interactions.

Conditional DPM

Another straightforward approach to reduce the dimensionality of 3D medical images is to view them as a stack of 2D slices. Based on this idea, conditional DPM (cDPM) [34] trains on 2D slices of a 3D volume $x \in \mathbb{R}^{D \times H \times W}$ by defining two sets of arbitrarily chosen slice indices: the 'target' set $\mathcal{P}$, for which the generator aims to produces the slices $x^{\mathcal{P}} \in \mathbb{R}^{\text{len}(\mathcal{P}) \times H \times W}$, and a 'conditional' set C, whose images slices $x^{C} \in \mathbb{R}^{\text{len}(C) \times H \times W}$ guide the generator. Note, the total number of indices of both sets (i.e., $\text{len}(C) + \text{len}(\mathcal{P})$) is chosen so that it does not exceed the computational resources available.

cDPM now learns to generate the target slices $x^{\mathcal{P}}$ conditioned on x^{C} by feeding their index sets C and $\mathcal{P}$ and the corresponding slices (i.e., the real slices x^{C} and noise for $\mathcal{P}$) into an attention network [47]. The goal of the attention network is then to learn the dependencies across slices so that the diffusion process can generate realistic-looking slices for $\mathcal{P}$ conditioned on $x^{\mathcal{C}}$. It does so by repeatability generating random sets of target slices $x^{\mathcal{P}}$ conditioned on random sets of $x^{\mathcal{C}}$. Once trained, a new 3D volume is generated by initiating the process with random noise (i.e., $\mathcal{C}$ is empty) and then using the generated slices as a conditional set for producing the next set of target slices. This process is repeated until all slices of the 3D volume are generated.

As the cDPM can be trained on many different (arbitrary) slice combinations (defined by $\mathcal{C}$ and $\mathcal{P}$), cDPM only requires a relatively small number of 3D medical images for training. Furthermore, it will learn short- and long-range dependencies across slices as the spatial distance between slices from $\mathcal{C}$ and $\mathcal{P}$ varies. Learning these dependencies enables cDPMs to produce 2D slices that, when put together, result in somewhat realistic-looking, high-resolution 3D images. However, one issue with this approach is that the inter-dependency between the slices is not well modeled so the model fails to consistently produce accurate 3D volumes, as shown in Fig. 16.2. To minimize this issue, one can smooth the 3D medical image across slices via, for example, total variation (TV) [27]. TV smooths the images while preserving the contrast of the image by preserving piece-wise constant structures, i.e., the boundaries of anatomical structures.

Diffusion with Wavelet Transformation

Instead of only training on slices [34] or patches [54], wavelet diffusion model (WDM) [36] presents an efficient way to train on a complete volume. As the computional burden is mainly caused by the high dimensionality of the 3D data, WDM reduces the dimension of the medical images by encoding them as wavelet coefficients [38]. Wavelet coefficients capture the essential information of an image at different scales and frequencies. Once the model learns how to produce synthetic wavelet coefficients, medical images are obtained by performing an inverse discrete wavelet transform (IDWT).

In [36], each input image $x \in \mathbb{R}^{D\times H\times W}$ is encoded by 8 wavelet transforms (DWT). The corresponding coefficients are concatenated into a single target matrix $x_w \in \mathbb{R}^{8\times\frac{D}{2}\times\frac{H}{2}\times\frac{W}{2}}$ so that original 1-channel image is now encoded as an 8-channel image with its dimension being an eighth of the original one. The eight sets of coefficients are processed in parallel by neural networks thus significantly reducing the computational burden and memory usage. Based on these wavelet encodes, a 3D diffusion model is trained to produce realistic wavelet coefficients. Finally, the coefficients are transformed into synthetic 3D images using IDWT.

16.2.2.2 Data Compression via the Latent Space

As mentioned, another memory-efficient approach for generating 3D medical images is to first project them to a lower-dimensional latent space before starting the diffusion process. We now review several implementations of this approach.

Extend 2D Pre-trained Diffusion Model for 3D Generation

One way to generate the latent space encoding is to use a pre-trained diffusion model, such as Stable Diffusion (SD) [43]. SD was trained for over 150,000 GPU hours on 5 billion 2D image-text pairs to learn general patterns applicable to a wide range of image-related tasks [4]. One can now apply SD to each slice of a 3D medical image in order to derive the low-dimensional encoding. To ensure consistency across the slices, an extra 'temporal' operation is applied to the slice encoding in order to learn the correlations across slices [28]. One way of doing so is to fully take advantage of the pre-trained model by adding a module enforcing cross-slice consistency to the original 2D SD architecture. Alternatively, one can directly extend the 2D diffusion model to 3D. However, preserving the pre-trained information during this extension is a challenge.

Also expecting to benefit from the knowledge of SD, diffusion transformers (DiT) [32] build a transformer-based diffusion model in SD's latent space. They replace the U-Nets in the diffusion model with a vision transformer (ViT) [7]. As the transformer is in the latent space, the model will process the low-dimensional feature patches instead of image patches. To apply this to 3D medical images, the position embedding should also be extended to 3D. To further reduce the memory cost and improve flexibility, a masking strategy can be applied [11, 17], in which a large part of the patches will be masked out during the training.

Latent Diffusion Model

An extension of Stable Diffusion [43], Latent Diffusion Model (LDM) [37] is currently one of the best methods for generating high quality 3D medical images. This two-stage generative framework first learns a compact latent representation of the high-dimensional data via Vector Quantized Variational Autoencoder (VQVAE) [1, 8]. The core components of VQVAE are the encoder $\mathcal{E}$, a generator $\mathcal{G}$, and a quantizer. Let x be an image, then the quantizer maps the continuous latent space encoding $E(x)$ to a discrete latent space encoding z_q by finding the nearest codebook vector e_k,i.e.,

$$z_q = \text{Quantize}(z) = e_k, \quad k = \arg\min_j \|E(x) - e_j\|. \tag{16.5}$$

During training, the model then tries to jointly minimize the reconstruction and the quantization loss, i.e.,

$$\mathcal{L}(x, z_q) = ||x - \mathcal{G}(z_q)||^2 + \beta||z_q - \mathcal{E}(x)||^2$$

with β being a hyperparameter controlling the weight of the quantization loss. The quantization loss measures the difference between the latent code and its quantized version, which works as an extra regularization term to help the VQVAE training. Once trained, the resulting encoding is a compressed representation of the data while maintaining its key features.

Next, a diffusion model is constructed in this low-dimensional latent space. The architecture of the model is the same as it is in the observation space but the input is now the feature representations from the encoder $\mathcal{E}$. Compared to performing diffusion in the observation space, the model is much more memory efficient as the dimension of the encoding is much smaller (up to 16 times smaller). Furthermore, the sampling speed can be up to 10+ times faster [35]. But as the image quality is determined by the generator from the first stage ($\mathcal{G}$), it is crucial to train a 'perfect' VQVAE, which requires meticulous design (like introducing extra adversarial training loss, e.g., VQGAN [8]) and a substantial number of training samples.

BrainSyn

BrainSyn [35] is a two-stage model that synthesizes high-resolution medical images conditionally dependent on metadata (such as age). The first stage of BrainSyn involves a Variational Autoencoder GAN model (VQGAN) [8], which is VQVAE plus adversarial training. The vector quantization discretizes the feature space derived by the variational autoencoder so that the 3D medical image is represented as a set of indices (a.k.a, code), whose meaning is defined by a code book. This compresses the data over 500 times [35, 43] (compared to 16 times with VQVAE). The code book and the quantized encoding of each 3D image (i.e., the application of the codes to the code book) are the inputs to the second stage, which learns to generate new samples dependent on metadata.

To model the dependency on metadata in the second stage, a Generalized Linear Model (GLM, [31]) disentangles the quantized encoding into a metadata-specific encoding (i.e., the encoding predicted by the metadata) and a subject-specific encoding (i.e., the difference between meta-specific and quantized encoding, a.k.a residual). The subject-specific encoding is then turned into the discrete code (a.k.a., Residual Code or 'R-Code') via the code book of the first stage. This operation is efficient as GLM is a parameter-free model that needs no training. Similar to [1], the discrete diffusion model then learns the (categorical) distribution of R-Codes by learning dependencies of the code throughout the image by using 'masking' [17], i.e., the model has to predict the code of part of the image (masked out region) from the remaining image regions.

After completing training, BrainSyn synthesizes a new "subject" by first generating a (random) R-code, which is transformed into a residual. The residual is combined with the metadata-specific encoding, which is derived from random metadata values. The resulting quantized encoding is finally converted into an MRI using the generator from the first stage.

16.3 Anatomy Plausible Synthesis and Evaluation

Quantitatively evaluating the similarity between synthetic and real images is crucial for using synthetic images in the medical context. Here, we first review metrics commonly used for assessing the perceptual quality of (natural) images, such as structural similarity index (SSIM) [9]. Next, we describe a framework for measuring anatomical plausibility, i.e., whether the anatomy is correctly displayed in the synthetic images. Finally, we will outline strategies for improving the anatomical plausibility of synthetic medical images generated by diffusion models.

16.3.1 Evaluation Metrics

The four metrics commonly used to assess the quality of synthetic 3D medical images are Multi-Scale Structural Similarity (MS-SSIM) [24], peak signal-to-noise ratio (PSNR) [9], Fréchet Inception Distance (FID) [18], and Maximum-Mean Discrepancy (MMD) [14]. Of those four metrics, MS-SSIM and PSNR directly measure the difference between a real and a synthetic image. Specifically, SSIM [9] quantifies the image quality by assessing structural similarity between reference and synthetic images. It divides the images into small windows and then compares the luminance, contrast, and structure across the two image windows between real and synthetic images. The Multi-scale structural similarity (MS-SSIM) [24] extends SSIM to multiple scales (i.e., image resolutions) to incorporate image details at different resolutions.

PSNR [9] is a metric commonly used to quantify the quality of a reconstructed signal compared to a distortion-free original. To apply this concept to image generation, real and synthetic images are randomly paired together. For each pair, the metric then records the ratio between the maximum possible signal value (pixel intensity) and the power of the image differences that affect the image quality. The final outcome is then the average of that ratio across all image pairs.

In contrast, FID and MMD are population-level metrics that are based on the data statistics, e.g., comparing the distributions of synthetic and real data. These metrics can be computed in the observation or latent space. Specifically, Fréchet Inception Distance (FID) [18] first extracts features from the images by using a pre-trained model, such as using a 2D model slice-by-slice [34] or directly using a 3D model like Med3d [3]. Separately for the real ('r') and synthetic ('s') data, the method then determines the multivariate normal distribution $\mathcal{N}(\mu_i, \Sigma_1)$ of the feature vectors. Finally, the Fréchet distance between the resulting two distributions is defined as

$$W(\mu_r, \Sigma_r, \mu_s, \Sigma_s) = \|\mu_r - \mu_s\|^2 + tr(\Sigma_r + \Sigma_s - 2((\Sigma_r^{1/2}\Sigma_s^{1/2})^{1/2})^2)$$

This distance considers both the difference in their means (first term) and the difference in their covariances (second term). Lower FID scores indicate a better overlap between the distribution, i.e., higher quality of the generated medical images.

Maximum-Mean Discrepancy (MMD) [14] also measures the difference in the distribution of real (**X**) and synthetic (**Y**) images. Let k be a kernel function (e.g., Gaussian kernel), then MMD^2 measures how well the distributions align in the feature space by computing

$$\text{MMD}^2(\mathbf{X}, \mathbf{Y}) = \frac{1}{n(n-1)}\sum_{i \neq j}^{n} k(x_i, x_j) + \frac{1}{n(n-1)}\sum_{i \neq j}^{n} k(y_i, y_j) - \frac{2}{n^2}\sum_{i=1}^{n}\sum_{j=1}^{n} k(x_i, y_j).$$

The first two terms of the above measure capture the mean kernel similarities within each set and the third term captures the average kernel similarity between sets. Note, the lower MMD^2 the better generally is the quality of the synthetic images.

However, there are several issues with these four metrics. First, the scores fail to properly assess qualitative differences between generative models. For example in Fig. 16.3, the lower quality MRIs generated by HA-GAN [53] have a lower (i.e., better) FID score (0.080) than the higher quality MRIs generated by cDPM [34] (FID: 0.130). One reason behind this phenomena is that the scores emphasize the semantic meaning (whether this looks like an organ) instead of the anatomical plausibility. Second, metrics are sometimes ambiguous and are hard to interpret. For instance, MS-SSIM measures the similarity of intensity patterns between a real and a synthetic image but neither higher nor lower scores are necessarily better as smaller MS-SSIM also can mean higher diversity. Thus, the metric is only meaningful when also computing the MS-SSIM between real images so that one can tell whether its value is close to the real samples or not. Last, these metrics fail to provide information about the anatomy plausibility, i.e., one can have good scores but the anatomy in the image is unrealistic.

16.3.2 Anatomical Measurements

One can measure anatomy plausibility by measuring the accuracy of human experts correctly distinguishing real from synthetic medical images. One issue with this

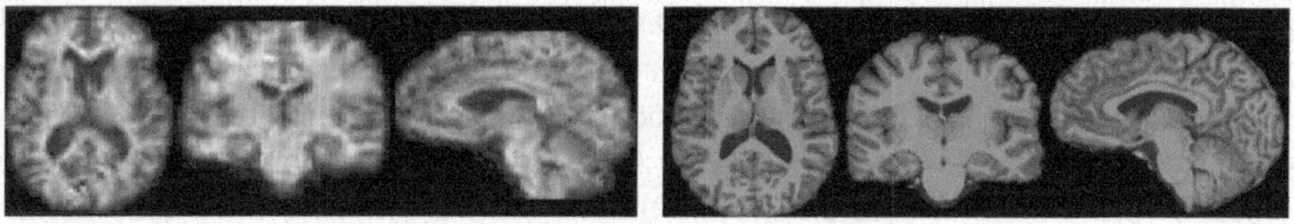

Fig. 16.3 Synthetic brain MRI generated by HA-GAN (FID: 0.080) [53] and cDPM (FID: 0.130) [34]. Even though HA-GAN has a lower FID score, the MRI from HA-GAN is quite blurry, i.e., of much lower quality than the one generated by cDPM

approach is the inconsistency within and across the evaluations performed by human experts. Alternatively, a neural network can be used to evaluate anatomy plausibility. For example, one can train a classifier on the real medical images to identify the sex of a subject [35]. An insignificant difference in the accuracy of the classifier on the synthetic data then indicates the high plausibility of the anatomy displayed in the synthetic images. Another approach to measure anatomical plausibility is to augment the training data with synthetic images and then show a significant reduction in the generalization error of the trained model.

However, this type of assessment is quite indirect and might only focus on certain anatomical regions important to the decision process of the neural networks might only focus on specific anatomical regions for its decision process. Instead, one can first segment all anatomical structures in a set of synthetic medical images and extract regional measurements (such as volume) from the segmentations. For each regional measurement, one then determines its distribution, which is compared to the distribution based on the real medical images using Cohen's d [52] (lower Cohen's d indicates better anatomical plausibility).

16.3.3 Anatomy Enhanced Generation

Creating anatomically plausible images requires models that can capture intrinsic properties of anatomical structures and their complex spatial relationships. The following section introduces several approaches that aim to do so by introducing prior knowledge (such as label maps of anatomical structures) into the generation process.

16.3.3.1 MedGen3D

MedGen3D [16] generates 3D medical images by first creating a label map of the anatomy, which is easier than creating images as one does not have to account for intensity differences between anatomical structures, partial volumes, noise, and, for MRIs, image inhomogeneity. The label map is generated via a conditional diffusion model by dividing the 3D volume into 2D slices and then, as in section "Conditional DPM", producing label maps of those slices from random noise or by conditioning on existing slices. Next, a seq-to-seq model [21] uses the generated label map to synthesize realistic 3D medical images. As the generation is based on slices, the generated 3D image will often show artifacts, such as varying intensities across slices [34]. To add coherence across slices, the model refines the medical images via a diffusion refiner [16]. The diffusion refiner generates the same volume from three views (axial, coronal, and sagittal) and averages the volume to improve the cross-slice coherence. The final outcome is not only a new 3D image but also a segmentation, which eases further analysis.

16.3.3.2 MedSyn

MedSyn [56] was the first text-guided generator of high-resolution (256^3) CT and corresponding label map. Specifically, the input to the generator is a radiology report of a CT image. From that report, the method first generates a low-resolution image and label map in order to minimize memory burden. Conditioned on the low-resolution output, the generator produces the higher-resolution results, which converges faster than directly learning from random noise [19]. In addition, jointly learning to generate image and corresponding label map enables MedSyn to explicitly encode anatomy, which is important for correctly displaying organs in the medical images.

MedSyn is quite versatile as it does not require a training set containing label maps, which is not the case for other joint learning strategies [16, 59]. Furthermore, one can give it a mask outlining anatomy that should not be altered by the generator [59]. Finally, MedSyn can be used as a segmentation tool by keeping the input image fixed.

In conclusion, generative adversarial networks (GANs) and diffusion probabilistic models (DPMs) can produce 3D medical images that not only look realistic but also display anatomy that is biologically plausible. To do so, these models have to account for the high dimensionality of medical images and the relatively small sample size of studies acquiring them. By addressing these challenges they then generate medical images that have the potential to revolutionize medical research and clinical practice.

References

1. Bond-Taylor S, Hessey P, Sasaki H, Breckon TP, and Willcocks CG (2022) Unleashing transformers: parallel token prediction with discrete absorbing diffusion for fast high-resolution image generation from vector-quantized codes. In: European conference on computer vision. Lecture notes in computer science, vol 13683, pp 170–188
2. Celard P, Iglesias EL, Sorribes-Fdez JM, Romero R, Vieira AS, Borrajo L (2023) A survey on deep learning applied to medical images: from simple artificial neural networks to generative models. Neural Comput Appl 35(3):2291–2323

3. Chen S, Ma K, Zheng Y (2019) Med3D: transfer learning for 3D medical image analysis. arXiv preprint arXiv:1904.00625
4. Chung H, Ryu D, McCann MT, Klasky ML, Ye JC (2023) Solving 3D inverse problems using pre-trained 2D diffusion models. In: Proceedings of the IEEE/CVF conference on computer vision and pattern recognition, pp 22542–22551
5. Deng J, Dong W, Socher R, Li L-J, Li K, Fei-Fei L (2009) Imagenet: a large-scale hierarchical image database. In: 2009 IEEE conference on computer vision and pattern recognition, pp 248–255
6. Dhariwal P, Nichol A (2021) Diffusion models beat GANs on image synthesis. In: Advances in neural information processing systems, vol 34, pp 8780–8794
7. Dosovitskiy A, Beyer L, Kolesnikov A, Weissenborn D, Zhai X, Unterthiner T, Dehghani M, Minderer M, Heigold G, Gelly S, Uszkoreit J, Houlsby N (2021) An image is worth 16x16 words: transformers for image recognition at scale. In: International conference on learning representations
8. Esser P, Rombach R, Ommer B (2021) Taming transformers for high-resolution image synthesis. In: IEEE/CVF conference on computer vision and pattern recognition, pp 12873–12883
9. Faragallah OS, El-Hoseny H, El-Shafai W, Abd El-Rahman W, El-Sayed HS, El-Rabaie E-SM, Abd El-Samie FE, Geweid GGN (2020) A comprehensive survey analysis for present solutions of medical image fusion and future directions. IEEE Access 9:11358–11371
10. Feng Z, Wen L, Wang P, Yan B, Wu X, Zhou J, Wang Y (2023) DiffDP: radiotherapy dose prediction via a diffusion model. In: International conference on medical image computing and computer-assisted intervention. Lecture notes in computer science, vol 14225. Springer, Berlin, pp 191–201
11. Gao S, Zhou P, Cheng M-M, Yan S (2023) Masked diffusion transformer is a strong image synthesizer. In: Proceedings of the IEEE/CVF international conference on computer vision, pp 23164–23173
12. Gatys LA, Ecker AS, Bethge M (2016) Image style transfer using convolutional neural networks. In: Proceedings of the IEEE conference on computer vision and pattern recognition, pp 2414–2423
13. Goodfellow I, Pouget-Abadie J, Mirza M, Xu B, Warde-Farley D, Ozair S, Courville A, Bengio Y (2020) Generative adversarial networks. Commun ACM 63(11):139–144
14. Gretton A, Borgwardt KM, Rasch MJ, Schölkopf B, Smola A (2012) A kernel two-sample test. J Mach Learn Res 13(1):723–773
15. Gulrajani I, Ahmed F, Arjovsky M, Dumoulin V, Courville AC (2017) Improved training of Wasserstein GANs. In: Advances in neural information processing systems, vol 30, pp 5769–5779
16. Han K, Xiong Y, You C, Khosravi P, Sun S, Yan X, Duncan JS, Xie X (2023) MedGen3D: a deep generative framework for paired 3D image and mask generation. In: International conference on medical image computing and computer-assisted intervention. Lecture notes in computer science, vol 14220. Springer, Berlin, pp 759–769
17. He K, Chen X, Xie S, Li Y, Dollár P, Girshick R (2022) Masked autoencoders are scalable vision learners. In: IEEE/CVF conference on computer vision and pattern recognition, pp 16000–16009
18. Heusel M, Ramsauer H, Unterthiner T, Nessler B, Hochreiter S (2017) GANs trained by a two time-scale update rule converge to a local Nash equilibrium. In: Advances in neural information processing systems, vol 30
19. Ho J, Jain A, Abbeel P (2020) Denoising diffusion probabilistic models. In: Advances in neural information processing systems, vol 33, pp 6840–6851
20. Hong S, Marinescu R, Dalca AV, Bonkhoff AK, Bretzner M, Rost NS, Golland P (2021) 3D-StyleGAN: a style-based generative adversarial network for generative modeling of three-dimensional medical images. In: Deep generative models, and data augmentation, labelling, and imperfections. Lecture notes in computer science, vol 13003. Springer, Berlin, pp 24–34

21. Isola P, Zhu J-Y, Zhou T, Efros AA (2017) Image-to-image translation with conditional adversarial networks. In: Proceedings of the IEEE conference on computer vision and pattern recognition, pp 1125–1134
22. Karras T, Laine S, Aila T (2019) A style-based generator architecture for generative adversarial networks. In: IEEE/CVF conference on computer vision and pattern recognition, pp 4401–4410
23. Kingma DP, Welling M (2013) Auto-encoding variational Bayes. In: International conference on learning representations, abs/1312.6114
24. Kwon G, Han C, Kim D-s (2019) Generation of 3D brain MRI using auto-encoding generative adversarial networks. In: Medical image computing and computer-assisted intervention. Lecture notes in computer science, vol 11766, pp 118–126
25. LeCun Y, Bengio Y, Hinton G (2015) Deep learning. Nature 521(7553):436–444
26. Leroy V, Revaud J, Lucas T, Weinzaepfel P (2024) Win-win: training high-resolution vision transformers from two windows. In: The twelfth international conference on learning representations
27. Liu J, Sun Y, Xu X, Kamilov US (2019) Image restoration using total variation regularized deep image prior. In: ICASSP 2019-2019 IEEE international conference on acoustics, speech and signal processing (ICASSP). IEEE, pp 7715–7719
28. Liu H, Tam D, Muqeeth M, Mohta J, Huang T, Bansal M, Raffel CA (2022) Few-shot parameter-efficient fine-tuning is better and cheaper than in-context learning. Adv Neural Inf Process Syst 35:1950–1965
29. Liu Q, Chen Z, Wong WH (2024) An encoding generative modeling approach to dimension reduction and covariate adjustment in causal inference with observational studies. Proc Natl Acad Sci 121(23):e2322376121
30. Long J, Shelhamer E, Darrell T (2015) Fully convolutional networks for semantic segmentation. In: Proceedings of the IEEE conference on computer vision and pattern recognition, pp 3431–3440
31. McNamee R (2005) Regression modelling and other methods to control confounding. Occup Environ Med 62(7):500–506
32. Peebles W, Xie S (2023) Scalable diffusion models with transformers. In: Proceedings of the IEEE/CVF international conference on computer vision, pp 4195–4205
33. Peng W, Feng L, Zhao G, Liu F (2022) Learning optimal k-space acquisition and reconstruction using physics-informed neural networks. In: IEEE/CVF conference on computer vision and pattern recognition, pp 20794–20803
34. Peng W, Adeli E, Bosschieter T, Park SH, Zhao Q, Pohl KM (2023) Generating realistic brain MRIs via a conditional diffusion probabilistic model. In: International conference on medical image computing and computer-assisted intervention. Lecture notes in computer science, vol 14227. Springer, Berlin, pp 14–24
35. Peng W, Bosschieter T, Ouyang J, Paul R, Sullivan EV, Pfefferbaum A, Adeli E, Zhao Q, Pohl KM (2024) Metadata-conditioned generative models to synthesize anatomically-plausible 3D brain MRIs. Med Image Anal 98:103325
36. Phung H, Dao Q, Tran A (2023) Wavelet diffusion models are fast and scalable image generators. In: Proceedings of the IEEE/CVF conference on computer vision and pattern recognition, pp 10199–10208
37. Pinaya WHL, Tudosiu P-D, Dafflon J, Da Costa PF, Fernandez V, Nachev P, Ourselin S, Jorge Cardoso M (2022) Brain imaging generation with latent diffusion models. In: MICCAI workshop on deep generative models. Lecture notes in computer science, vol 13609. Springer, Berlin, pp 117–126
38. Pittner S, Kamarthi SV (1999) Feature extraction from wavelet coefficients for pattern recognition tasks. IEEE Trans Pattern Anal Mach Intell 21(1):83–88
39. Pombo G, Gray R, Cardoso MJ, Ourselin S, Rees G, Ashburner J, Nachev P (2023) Equitable modelling of brain imaging by counterfactual augmentation with morphologically constrained 3D deep generative models. Med Image Anal 84:102723

40. Prezja F, Paloneva J, Pölönen I, Niinimäki E, Äyrämö S (2022) Deepfake knee osteoarthritis x-rays from generative adversarial neural networks deceive medical experts and offer augmentation potential to automatic classification. Sci Rep 12(1):18573
41. Radford A, Metz L, Chintala S (2016) Unsupervised representation learning with deep convolutional generative adversarial networks. In: International conference on learning representations
42. Rezende D, Mohamed S (2015) Variational inference with normalizing flows. In: International conference on machine learning, pp 1530–1538. Proceedings of machine learning research
43. Rombach R, Blattmann A, Lorenz D, Esser P, Ommer B (2022) High-resolution image synthesis with latent diffusion models. In: IEEE/CVF conference on computer vision and pattern recognition, pp 10684–10695
44. Ronneberger O, Fischer P, Brox T (2015) U-Net: convolutional networks for biomedical image segmentation. In: Medical image computing and computer-assisted intervention. Lecture notes in computer science, vol 9351, pp 234–241
45. Rosca M, Lakshminarayanan B, Warde-Farley D, Mohamed S (2017) Variational approaches for auto-encoding generative adversarial networks. arXiv preprint arXiv:1706.04987
46. Sagheer SVM, George SN (2020) A review on medical image denoising algorithms. Biomed Signal Process Control 61:102036
47. Shaw P, Uszkoreit J, Vaswani A (2018) Self-attention with relative position representations. In: Proceedings of the 2018 conference of the North American chapter of the association for computational linguistics, vol 2, pp 464–468
48. Skorokhodov I, Tulyakov S, Elhoseiny M (2022) StyleGAN-V: a continuous video generator with the price, image quality and perks of StyleGAN2. In: Proceedings of the IEEE/CVF conference on computer vision and pattern recognition, pp 3626–3636
49. Sohl-Dickstein J, Weiss E, Maheswaranathan N, Ganguli S (2015) Deep unsupervised learning using nonequilibrium thermodynamics. In: International conference on machine learning, pp 2256–2265
50. Sudlow C, Gallacher J, Allen N, Beral V, Burton P, Danesh J, Downey P, Elliott P, Green J, Landray M, Bette L, Paul M, Giok O, Jill P, Alan S, Alan Y, Tim S, Tim P, Rory C (2015) Uk biobank: an open access resource for identifying the causes of a wide range of complex diseases of middle and old age. PLoS Med 12(3):e1001779
51. Suetens P (2017) Fundamentals of medical imaging. Cambridge University Press, Cambridge
52. Sullivan GM, Feinn R (2012) Using effect size—or why the p value is not enough. J Grad Med Educ 4(3):279–282
53. Sun L, Chen J, Xu Y, Gong M, Yu K, Batmanghelich K (2022) Hierarchical amortized GAN for 3D high resolution medical image synthesis. IEEE J Biomed Health Inform 26(8):3966–3975
54. Wang Z, Jiang Y, Zheng H, Wang P, He P, Wang Z, Chen W, Zhou M (2023) Patch diffusion: faster and more data-efficient training of diffusion models. In: Thirty-seventh conference on neural information processing systems, vol 36
55. Wu Q, Gao R, Zha H (2021) Bridging explicit and implicit deep generative models via neural stein estimators. Adv Neural Inf Process Syst 34:11274–11286
56. Xu Y, Sun L, Peng W, Jia S, Morrison K, Perer A, Zandifar A, Visweswaran S, Eslami M, Batmanghelich K (2024) MedSyn: text-guided anatomy-aware synthesis of high-fidelity 3D CT images. IEEE Trans Med Imaging 43(10):3648–3660
57. Zaballa O, Pérez A, Gómez Inhiesto E, Ayesta TA, Lozano JA (2023) Learning the progression patterns of treatments using a probabilistic generative model. J Biomed Inform 137:104271
58. Zhang J, Zhao Q, Adeli E, Pfefferbaum A, Sullivan EV, Paul R, Valcour V, Pohl KM (2022) Multi-label, multi-domain learning identifies compounding effects of HIV and cognitive impairment. Med Image Anal 75:102246
59. Zhang L, Rao A, Agrawala M (2023) Adding conditional control to text-to-image diffusion models. In: Proceedings of the IEEE/CVF international conference on computer vision, pp 3836–3847

Chapter 17
Diffusion Probabilistic Models for Image Formation in MRI

Şaban Öztürk, Alper Güngör, and Tolga Çukur

Abstract Diffusion probabilistic modeling has recently emerged as a state-of-the-art framework in MRI image-formation tasks. Two mainstream tasks in this domain are image reconstruction from undersampled k-space acquisitions with the purpose of accelerating MRI exams, and image translation to impute missing sequences for broadening the scope of multi-contrast MRI protocols. Diffusion models, known for their exquisite capability to generate high-fidelity images, have demonstrated great promise in solving the ill-posed inverse problems associated with these tasks. In the context of reconstruction, diffusion models have shown prowess in recovering high-quality MR images from heavily undersampled acquisitions, to enable significant reductions in scan times. In the context of translation, they have shown superior quality in imputed images of missing sequences, to ensure availability of comprehensive multi-contrast MRI protocols without the need for additional exams per patient. This chapter provides a comprehensive overview of the theoretical foundations, practical implementations, and recent advancements in the use of diffusion models for these pivotal MRI tasks, highlighting the potential of this deep learning framework to transform clinical imaging practices. Through detailed discussions and illustrative examples, we explore how diffusion models can bridge existing gaps in MRI technology, paving the way for faster, more accurate, and comprehensive imaging solutions.

Ş. Öztürk
Department of Management Information Systems, Ankara Hacı Bayram Veli University, Ankara, Turkey
e-mail: saban.ozturk@hbv.edu.tr

A. Güngör · T. Çukur (✉)
Department of Electrical-Electronics Engineering, Bilkent University, Ankara, Turkey
e-mail: alperg@ee.bilkent.edu.tr; cukur@ee.bilkent.edu.tr

L. Zhang et al. (eds.), *Generative Machine Learning Models in Medical Image Computing*, https://doi.org/10.1007/978-3-031-80965-1_17

17.1 Introduction

Magnetic Resonance Imaging (MRI) is a powerful and versatile imaging modality widely used in clinical assessments and research studies. Yet, MRI characteristically suffers from prolonged scans and limited signal-to-ratios, which limit the amount of data that can be acquired within practically reasonable exam times [1]. This limitation has driven MRI physicists to seek approaches to improve scan efficiency. A mainstream approach for efficient MRI scans rests on undersampling k-space acquisitions to only capture a subset of measurements that would be required for fully-sampled acquisitions [30]. Images linearly recovered from such undersampled acquisitions suffer from aliasing artifacts as MRI reconstruction is an ill-posed inverse problem. Another approach is to prioritize sequences within a multi-contrast protocol and acquire only those with high priority as exam time permits [22]. To impute the images for omitted sequences, an ill-posed inverse problem must then be solved to non-linearly map the tissue signals in acquired sequences to those in omitted sequences. In both problems, powerful image priors that emphasize desirable attributes of high-quality MR images are key in obtaining accurate and efficient solutions.

In the past decade, deep learning (DL) models have been established as gold standard to capture image priors that aid in solution of MRI inverse problems [26]. Traditional methods often employ hand-constructed image priors that have limited power in describing the complex visual attributes embodied in medical images [22, 30]. In contrast, DL-based image priors can learn a hierarchy of nonlinear features from large training sets of MRI data. These rich, data-driven features can facilitate solution of inverse problems as they offer a more accurate representation of visual attributes of MRI images [2, 7]. Generative DL models have shown particular promise in MRI image formation tasks, due to their ability to produce a diverse collection of images [13, 47]. Such representational diversity has been shown to enhance reliability and performance in image reconstruction [10, 31] and image translation [23, 36, 41]. Until the last couple of years, generative adversarial networks (GAN) were arguably the prime approach in generative modeling of MRI images [15, 24]. Relying on a game theoretic interplay between two agents, i.e., the generator and the discriminator, GAN models can offer exceptional realism and structural detail during image generation. Unfortunately, the two-agent games are susceptible to instabilities that can cause premature convergence in GAN models, and hence severely compromise image quality and diversity [32].

As an emerging paradigm, diffusion probabilistic models (DPM) have gained growing attention in the field as a powerful substitute for previous generative modelling frameworks [44]. Instead of employing a two-agent game to implicitly learn the data likelihood, DPMs provide an explicit characterization of the likelihood to avoid training instabilities and other common pitfalls associated with GANs. To do this, conventional DPMs cast a diffusion process to map between image samples from the desired data distribution and random noise samples from a Gaussian distribution [46]. In the forward direction of the process, image samples are degraded with modest amounts of Gaussian noise over many time steps, until a start-point of pure noise. In the reverse direction, a recovery network is used to progressively denoise intermediate image samples to arrive at an end-point of clean images that serve as ground-truth. The advent of DPMs in MRI image formation have set new standards for image quality based on these fundamental ideas, offering high image quality and fidelity all at once [21, 38].

In this chapter, we will explore the application of DPMs in MRI image formation tasks. We begin with a preliminary overview of DPMs, including the forward and reverse processes, training methodologies, and sampling procedures. Following this, we take a look at the basics of MRI image reconstruction, discussing how diffusion models can help enhance recovery of images from undersampled data. Next, we cover MRI image translation, illustrating how diffusion models facilitate the imputation of missing sequences in multi-contrast protocols. Finally, we conclude with a discussion on potential future directions to further boost the performance and reliability of diffusion-based MRI image formation, highlighting ongoing research and emerging trends in the field.

17.2 Preliminary: Diffusion Probabilistic Models

In this preliminary section, we provide a detailed overview of diffusion probabilistic models, focusing on the foundational aspects of the forward diffusion process and the degradation operator, the reverse diffusion process and the recovery operator, the training objectives for the network-based recovery operator, and the sampling procedures used to generate images from trained models.

17.2.1 Forward Diffusion Process

In conventional DPMs, the forward diffusion process is devised to map between the data distribution and a pure Gaussian noise distribution [44]. Starting with a clean image sample drawn from the training set, intermediate samples in the forward direction are obtained by adding a small amount of Gaussian noise. The forward transition probability in between consecutive time steps can then be described as [18]:

$$q(\mathbf{x}_t \mid \mathbf{x}_{t-1}) = \mathcal{N}(\mathbf{x}_t; \sqrt{1-\beta_t}\mathbf{x}_{t-1}, \beta_t \mathbf{I}), \tag{17.1}$$

where $t \in [0, T]$ denotes the current time step, $\mathbf{x}_0$ is the original clean image, β_t is the noise variance scheduled across time steps, and $\mathcal{N}(\cdot; \mu, \sigma^2)$ denotes a Gaussian distribution with mean μ and variance σ^2. Over a total of T time steps, the clean image becomes increasingly noisy, essentially transforming the original data distribution into a simple Gaussian distribution. Based on these forward transition probabilities, the cumulative distribution of the forward process from the original image to any time step t can be written as:

$$q(\mathbf{x}_t \mid \mathbf{x}_0) = \mathcal{N}(\mathbf{x}_t; \sqrt{\bar{\alpha}_t}\mathbf{x}_0, (1 - \bar{\alpha}_t)\mathbf{I}), \tag{17.2}$$

where $\bar{\alpha}_t = \prod_{i=1}^{t}(1 - \beta_i)$. This cumulative formulation allows us to express the state of the intermediate image sample at any time step t directly in terms of the clean image $\mathbf{x}_0$. The forward diffusion process in DPMs can be viewed as a Markov chain, where transitions between states involve adding a small amount of noise to the image sample. The noise schedule $\{\beta_t\}$ is typically chosen such that it gradually increases over time, ensuring a progressive transition from the clean image to pure noise.

17.2.2 Reverse Diffusion Process

The reverse diffusion process aims to conduct transitions between image samples in the opposite direction, i.e., starting at time step T and moving towards time step 0. In conventional DPMs based on a Gaussian-noise degradation operator, these reverse transitions naturally involve progressive denoising of image samples, and this is exactly where the power of deep learning comes into play [45]. The recovery operator that performs reverse transitions is implemented as a neural network G_θ parameterized by θ. Given the image sample x_t at time step t, the recovery network can be used to estimate either the incremental noise $\epsilon_\theta(\mathbf{x}_t, t)$ between consecutive time steps or the clean image at $t = 0$. Afterwards, these estimates can be used to draw a less-noisy sample at time step $t - 1$.

For instance, the network-operationalized reverse transition probability based on incremental noise estimates can be described via the following equation [18]:

$$p_\theta(\mathbf{x}_{t-1} \mid \mathbf{x}_t) = \mathcal{N}(\mathbf{x}_{t-1}; \mu_\theta(\mathbf{x}_t, t), \sigma_t^2\mathbf{I}), \tag{17.3}$$

where $\mu_\theta(\mathbf{x}_t, t)$ is the predicted mean, and σ_t^2 can be either learned or assumed to be fixed. Note that this reverse transition probability assumes that the denoising transformation that must be implemented to obtain the less-noisy image sample is governed by a Gaussian distribution as well [45]. This approximation is valid when the step sizes are sufficiently small (i.e., a larger T on the order of thousands is prescribed to discretize the diffusion process). The predicted mean $\mu_\theta(\mathbf{x}_t, t)$ can then be derived from the network's estimation of incremental noise as follows:

$$\mu_\theta(\mathbf{x}_t, t) = \frac{1}{\sqrt{\alpha_t}}\left(\mathbf{x}_t - \frac{\beta_t}{\sqrt{1 - \bar{\alpha}_t}}\epsilon_\theta(\mathbf{x}_t, t)\right). \tag{17.4}$$

Afterwards, posterior sampling can be performed based on a Gaussian distribution as follows:

$$\mathbf{x}_{t-1} = \mu_\theta(\mathbf{x}_t, t) + \sigma_t \mathbf{z}, \tag{17.5}$$

where $\mathbf{z} \sim \mathcal{N}(\mathbf{0}, \mathbf{I})$. This iterative process gradually denoises intermediate image samples, leveraging the network's predictions to move step-by-step towards the original clean image.

17.2.3 Training Objective

The forward diffusion process in conventional DPMs can be emulated via simple Monte Carlo simulations, where the clean images from a training set are progressively degraded with increasing levels of noise. This emulation will yield a set of intermediate image samples $\mathbf{x}_{0,1,\ldots,T}$ across time steps. Afterwards, the network-based recovery operator can be trained in order to estimate either the incremental noise in between consecutive steps or the clean image at step 0, as mentioned before. Assuming that the incremental noise is estimated, the naive objective for learning the parameters of the recovery operator can be formulated as [44]:

$$\mathcal{L}_{\text{simple}} = \mathbb{E}_{t,\mathbf{x}_0,\epsilon}\left[\|\epsilon - \epsilon_\theta(\mathbf{x}_t, t)\|^2\right], \tag{17.6}$$

where $\mathbb{E}$ is expectation that is typically computed via a Monte-Carlo estimator over a set of training samples, ϵ is the true noise that can be derived as $(\mathbf{x}_t - \mathbf{x}_{t-1})$, and $\epsilon_\theta(\mathbf{x}_t, t)$ is the noise predicted by the model. This simple yet effective loss function directly trains the model to predict the noise added in between steps t and $t-1$. Yet, pioneering studies on DPMs have suggested that a mean-squared error loss on the noise can occasionally suffer from instabilities and thereby suboptimal learning. To address these issues, a variational lower bound (VLB) loss is commonly adopted [43]:

$$\mathcal{L}_{\text{vlb}} = \mathbb{E}_q\left[\sum_{t=1}^{T} D_{\text{KL}}\left(q(\mathbf{x}_{t-1} \mid \mathbf{x}_t, \mathbf{x}_0) \parallel p_\theta(\mathbf{x}_{t-1} \mid \mathbf{x}_t)\right) - \log p_\theta(\mathbf{x}_0 \mid \mathbf{x}_1)\right], \tag{17.7}$$

where D_{KL} denotes the Kullback-Leibler divergence between the true posterior probability $q(\mathbf{x}_{t-1} \mid \mathbf{x}_t, \mathbf{x}_0)$ and the model's estimate for the posterior $p_\theta(\mathbf{x}_{t-1} \mid \mathbf{x}_t)$. This objective ensures that the model not only learns to denoise effectively but also aligns its approximate posterior distribution closely with the true posterior distribution of the data.

17.2.4 Sampling Procedures

A trained DPM can be used to synthesize random images from the learned data distribution through progressive denoising transformations mediated by the recovery operator. For this purpose, a pure Gaussian noise sample $\mathbf{x}_T \sim \mathcal{N}(\mathbf{0}, \mathbf{I})$ is drawn, and the recovery operator is applied iteratively to perform reverse diffusion steps as outlined below [18]:

Initialize $\mathbf{x}_T \sim \mathcal{N}(\mathbf{0}, \mathbf{I})$
For $t = T, T-1, \ldots, 1$:

$$\mathbf{x}_{t-1} = \mu_\theta(\mathbf{x}_t, t) + \sigma_t \mathbf{z}, \quad \mathbf{z} \sim \mathcal{N}(\mathbf{0}, \mathbf{I})$$

By following this iterative denoising process, the model generates a high-quality image $\mathbf{x}_0$ that approximates a sample from the original data distribution. The gradual refinement ensures that the generated images are both diverse and of high fidelity, making diffusion models particularly suitable for complex image generation tasks.

In sum, DPMs offer a robust framework for generating high-quality images through well-defined forward and reverse processes, stable training objectives, and effective sampling procedures. These models have shown great promise in various applications, including challenging MRI image formation tasks. The explicit characterization of data likelihood, stability during training, and avoidance of mode collapse make them an attractive alternative to other generative models like GANs, particularly in the field of medical imaging where reliability and accuracy are paramount.

17.3 Diffusion-Based MRI Reconstruction

Accelerated MRI constitutes a significant area of investigation in the domain of medical imaging, primarily focused on mitigating characteristic aliasing artifacts while reconstructing images from undersampled k-space data [10]. The inverse problem involved in this reconstruction task can be formulated based on the physical signal model for MRI acquisitions:

$$\mathcal{A}\mathbf{x} = \mathbf{y}, \tag{17.8}$$

where $\mathcal{A} = \Omega \mathcal{F} B$ represents the imaging operator that accounts for the k-space undersampling pattern (Ω) and coil sensitivities (B), with $\mathcal{F}$ denoting the Fourier transform. Due to the ill-posed nature of the inverse problem described in Eq. 17.8, prior information has to be leveraged in order to obtain a high-quality reconstruction $\breve{x}$:

$$\breve{\mathbf{x}} = \min_{\mathbf{x}} \|\mathcal{A}\mathbf{x} - \mathbf{y}\|_2 + R(\mathbf{x}, \mathbf{y}), \tag{17.9}$$

where the first term enforces data consistency and $R(\mathbf{x}, \mathbf{y})$ denotes a regularization term that modifies the optimization objective for MRI reconstruction by enforcing the assumed image prior [13].

DPMs have recently emerged as a promising approach to tackle MRI reconstruction, promising enhanced image fidelity and improved generalization capabilities [8, 16]. In essence, a trained DPM model can be used to compute the posterior probability $p(\mathbf{x}|\mathbf{y})$ of the MR image $\mathbf{x}$ given undersampled k-space data $\mathbf{y}$. To do this, reverse diffusion steps are taken with the trained DPM starting from a pure Gaussian noise image. To ensure that the DPM does not simply reconstruct a random MRI image that doesn't belong to the actual subject, reverse diffusion steps must be guided by the physical signal model and the acquired data. Using Bayes' theorem, this can be achieved by multiplying the distribution of each intermediate image sample $p(\mathbf{x}_i)$ with the likelihood term $p(\mathbf{y}|\mathbf{x}_i)$ [14]. Assuming $\tilde{p}(\mathbf{x}_i) \propto p(\mathbf{x}_i)p(\mathbf{y}|\mathbf{x}_i)$, an unadjusted Langevin algorithm can be cast for sampling images:

$$\mathbf{x}_i^{k+1} \leftarrow \mathbf{x}_i^k + \frac{\gamma}{2}\nabla_{\mathbf{x}_i} \log \tilde{p}(\mathbf{x}_i^k \mid \mathbf{x}_{i+1}) + \sqrt{\gamma}\mathbf{z}, \tag{17.10}$$

where $\mathbf{z}$ denotes standard complex Gaussian noise, and γ controls noise scale. Note that the DPM has not been trained to capture $\tilde{p}(\mathbf{x}_i^k \mid \mathbf{x}_{i+1})$, yet the score function for $\tilde{p}_\theta(\mathbf{x}_i \mid \mathbf{x}_{i+1})$ parameterized by θ can be derived by computing its log-gradient:

$$\nabla_{\mathbf{x}_i} \log \tilde{p}_\theta(\mathbf{x}_i \mid \mathbf{x}_{i+1}) = \nabla_{\mathbf{x}_i} \log p_\theta(\mathbf{x}_i \mid \mathbf{x}_{i+1}) + \nabla_{\mathbf{x}_i} \log p(\mathbf{y} \mid \mathbf{x}_i). \tag{17.11}$$

The first term reflects the reverse transition probabilities as learned by the trained DPM, whereas the second term reflect likelihood of measured data given the underlying intermediate image sample. The influence of this second term on the derived intermediate samples can be formulated based on the physical signal model of accelerated MRI acquisitions, i.e., by performing data consistency projections as in traditional MRI reconstruction [14]. As such, the overall sampling equation can be expressed as follows:

$$\mathbf{x}_i^{k+1} \leftarrow \mathbf{x}_i^k + \frac{\gamma}{2\tau_{i+1}^2}\left(\sigma_{i+1}^2 - \sigma_i^2\right) s_\theta\left(\mathbf{x}_i^k, i\right) - \frac{\gamma}{2\sigma_\eta^2}\left(\mathcal{A}^H\mathcal{A}\mathbf{x}_i^k - \mathcal{A}^H\mathbf{y}\right) + \sqrt{\gamma}\mathbf{z}, \tag{17.12}$$

where $s_\theta\left(\mathbf{x}_i^k, i\right)$ denotes the recovery operator that receives the intermediate image sample at the current time step to produce an estimate of the clean image, $\mathcal{A}^H$ denotes the Hermitian transpose of the operator $\mathcal{A}$.

While MRI reconstruction based on the above formulation has been suggested to attain high image fidelity, it can suffer from poor generalization under domain shifts, e.g., when the training and test sets contain MRI data acquired under different protocols or scanners. Adaptive diffusion priors (AdaDiff) [16] have been developed to address this challenge in DPM-based MRI reconstruction. AdaDiff learns an unconditional diffusion prior for high-fidelity image generation (Fig. 17.1) and adapts this prior during inference to enhance generalization performance compared to static DPMs. Accordingly, MRI reconstruction with AdaDiff involves two phases: a rapid-diffusion phase that quickly produces an initial reconstruction using the trained prior, and an adaptation phase that refines this reconstruction by updating the prior to minimize data-consistency loss on the acquired k-space data of the given test subject (Fig. 17.1).

Note that traditional DPMs generate images through a lengthy sequence of inference steps, resulting in prolonged image sampling times [18], thus building AdaDiff based on these DPMs would be computationally prohibitive. To overcome this barrier, AdaDiff instead employs an adversarial diffusion model that enables generation in a few large reverse diffusion steps, significantly speeding up image sampling during the rapid-diffusion phase. The primary reason that traditional DPMs require a large number of diffusion steps is that they rely on approximating $q(\mathbf{x}_t|\mathbf{x}_{t+1})$ with an auxiliary Gaussian distribution. In contrast, Adadiff employs a rapid adversarial diffusion model with a large step size k without the need to assume normality, following the approach described by [46]. The training process involves optimizing both a discriminator and a generator, D_{θ_D} and G_{θ_G} parameterized by θ_D and θ_G respectively. The discriminator loss L_D is defined as follows:

$$L_D = \sum_{t\geq 0} \Big(\mathbb{E}_{q(\mathbf{x}_0,\mathbf{x}_t)}\mathbb{E}_{q(\mathbf{x}_{t+k}|\mathbf{x}_t)}\left[-\log(D_{\theta_D}(\mathbf{x}_t,\mathbf{x}_{t+k},t+k))\right]$$
$$+\,\mathbb{E}_{q(\mathbf{x}_{t+k})}\mathbb{E}_{\mathcal{N}_{\theta_G}(\mu,\gamma)}\left[-\log(1-D_{\theta_D}(\hat{\mathbf{x}}_t,\mathbf{x}_{t+k},t+k))\right] \tag{17.13}$$
$$+\,\mathbb{E}_{q(\mathbf{x}_0,\mathbf{x}_t)}\mathbb{E}_{q(\mathbf{x}_{t+k}|\mathbf{x}_t)}\left[\frac{1}{2}\|\nabla_{\mathbf{x}_t}D_{\theta_D}(\mathbf{x}_t,\mathbf{x}_{t+k},t+k)\|^2\right]\Big)$$

where $\hat{\mathbf{x}}_t$ is the generated image from the reverse diffusion process. Meanwhile, the generator loss L_G is defined as:

$$L_G = \sum_{t\geq 0} \mathbb{E}_{q(\mathbf{x}_{t+k})}\mathbb{E}_{\mathcal{N}_{\theta_G}(\mu,\gamma)}\left[-\log(D_{\theta_D}(\hat{\mathbf{x}}_t,\mathbf{x}_{t+k},t+k))\right] \tag{17.14}$$

Given the trained diffusion prior, an initial reconstruction ($\mathbf{x}_{\text{init}}$) is obtained in the rapid-diffusion phase by balancing between the image sets defined by the imaging operator and the trained diffusion prior. This balance is maintained by alternating between data-consistency projections and reverse diffusion projections. Data-consistency projections ensure alignment with the imaging operator, while reverse diffusion projections ensure conformity with the trained diffusion prior. Starting from $\mathbf{x}_T$ at the final time step T, drawn from a Gaussian noise distribution, the data-consistency projection at time step $t+k$ is implemented as [39]:

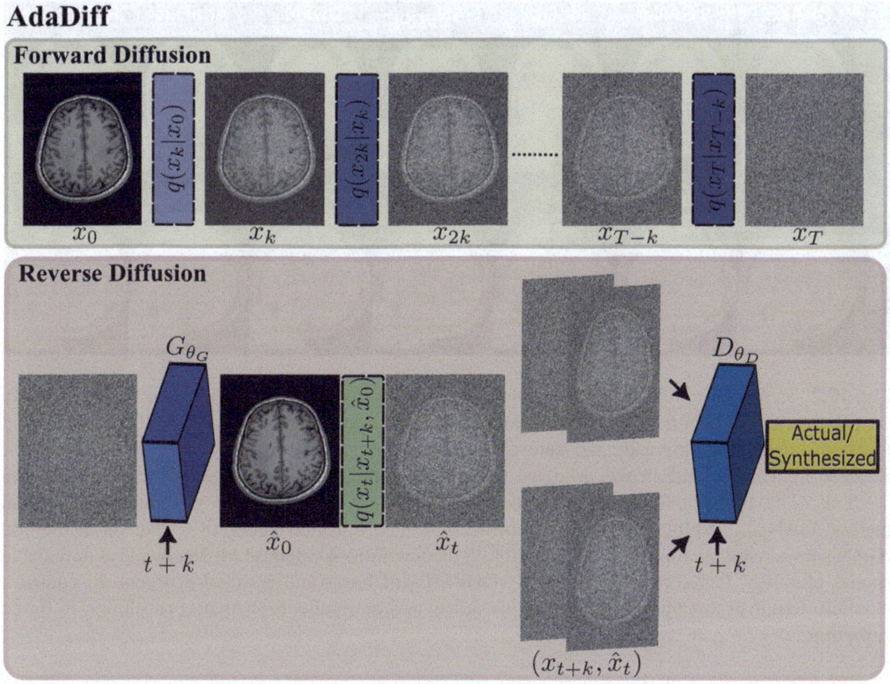

Fig. 17.1 DPMs synthesize an image ($\mathbf{x}_0$) starting from a white Gaussian noise sample ($\mathbf{x}_T$) by going through a sequential process. In a forward step of this process, scaled Gaussian noise is added to the previous sample $\mathbf{x}_{t-1}$, resulting in a noisier sample $\mathbf{x}_t$. In a reverse step of the process, noise introduced to $\mathbf{x}_{t+1}$ during forward sampling is suppressed to obtain $\mathbf{x}_t$. This reverse mapping is modeled as a projection through a neural-network operator, $p_\theta(\mathbf{x}_t|\mathbf{x}_{t+1})$. Conventional DPMs use small step sizes to preserve the approximate normality of the reverse transition probability $q(\mathbf{x}_t|\mathbf{x}_{t+1})$, which leads to long sampling times. AdaDiff employs a rapid adversarial diffusion model that enables sampling under large step size k, thus allowing transitions between $\mathbf{x}_0$ and $\mathbf{x}_T$ in fewer steps. The increased noise in each step, due to the larger step size, disrupts the normality assumption for the reverse transition probability $q(\mathbf{x}_t|\mathbf{x}_{t+k})$. To address this, AdaDiff utilizes an adversarial mapper that implicitly models the distribution of the reverse diffusion steps. The generator estimates denoised image samples, while the discriminator distinguishes real samples obtained via the forward diffusion process from the synthetic samples produced by the generator

$$\dot{\mathbf{x}}_{t+k} = \left(\mathbf{x}_{t+k} + \mathcal{A}^H(\mathbf{y} - \mathcal{A}\mathbf{x}_{t+k})\right), \tag{17.15}$$

where $\mathcal{A}$, $\mathcal{A}^H$ are the imaging operator and its Hermitian. The reverse diffusion projection refines $\dot{\mathbf{x}}_{t+k}$ to align it with the support of the diffusion prior:

$$\mathbf{x}_t = \dot{\mathbf{x}}_{t+k} + \beta_t(\hat{\mathbf{x}}_t - \dot{\mathbf{x}}_{t+k}), \tag{17.16}$$

where β_t is a blending factor, and $\hat{\mathbf{x}}_t$ is generated by the reverse diffusion process.

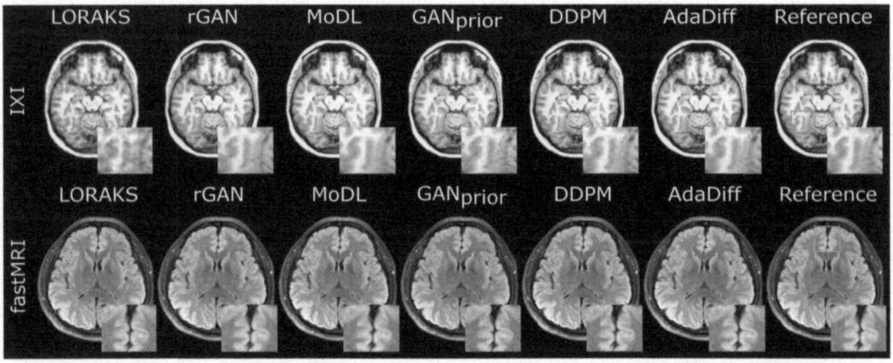

Fig. 17.2 Reconstructions from undersampled acquisitions with an acceleration factor of R=4x are presented. The results include data from both the IXI and fastMRI datasets. Each reconstructed image is displayed alongside the reference image obtained from fully-sampled acquisitions. Zoomed-in sections and arrows are used to emphasize the differences among the reconstruction methods. The traditional low-rank method LORAKS and the adaptive generative adversarial method $\text{GAN}_{\text{prior}}$ exhibit high noise amplification. The unrolled generative adversarial method rGAN shows residual aliasing, while the unrolled convolutional method MoDL displays noticeable spatial blurring. The conventional DPM (DDPM) still has some residual artifacts. In contrast, AdaDiff demonstrates minimal artifacts and noise, and maintains high spatial resolution in tissue depiction

Next, a prior adaptation phase is executed to further refine the reconstruction by adapting the diffusion prior to the individual test subject's data distribution as closely as possible. For this purpose, an inference optimization is performed where the parameters of the prior are updated to minimize a data-consistency loss between the generated and measured k-space data:

$$L_{\text{dc}} = \|\mathbf{y} - \mathcal{A}\mathbf{x}\|_2^2, \tag{17.17}$$

where $\mathbf{x}$ is the reconstructed image. Parameter updates are performed iteratively to minimize this data-consistency loss, leading to an improved reconstruction:

$$\theta_{\text{new}} = \theta_{\text{old}} - \eta \nabla_\theta L_{\text{dc}} \tag{17.18}$$

where θ represents the parameters of the diffusion prior, and η is the learning rate. This iterative optimization ensures that the final reconstruction is both data-consistent and aligns with the adapted prior.

Illustrative reconstructions using standard DPMs, adaptive diffusion priors, and other renowned MRI reconstruction techniques are shown in Fig. 17.2. The methods LORAKS [17] and $\text{GAN}_{\text{prior}}$ [34] exhibit significant noise amplification. Although rGAN and MoDL present lower noise levels, rGAN [11] displays residual reconstruction artifacts, and MoDL [2] experiences spatial blurring due to its pixel-wise loss function. Among the diffusion models, DDPM [18] is characterized by relatively high noise levels. Conversely, AdaDiff adjusts its diffusion prior to align more closely with the distribution of the test data, allowing it to produce superior quality reconstructions that depict tissues with minimal artifacts and noise.

17.4 Diffusion-Based MRI Translation

Image translation is a pervasive task in multi-modal medical imaging that involves converting images from one modality to another, such as generating CT images from MRI data or synthesizing missing contrasts in a multi-contrast MRI protocol. This enables imputation of missing modalities without the need to run additional scans, so it can lower costs of comprehensive imaging exams [3]. While translation is attempted between images of the same underlying anatomy, medical image translation is still a challenging task since the tissue signals in different modalities are related to each other through hard to characterize, nonlinear relationships. As such, employing data-driven regularization priors to help improve predictions is key for the translation task, as it is for the single-modality reconstruction tasks.

DPMs have shown significant potential in medical image translation as they are highly adept in learning the underlying data distribution and generating high-fidelity image samples through a gradual denoising process [42]. Early adoption of DPMs have shown significant promise for this family of deep learning models in difficult translation tasks such as synthesizing missing MRI contrasts, mapping MRI to CT images, and converting PET onto MRI images, which can all increase the diagnostic utility of multi-modal imaging protocols [38]. Among within-modality translation tasks, conversion between MRI sequences, such as T1-weighted to T2-weighted images, allows for curation of comprehensive protocols even when additional scans are prohibited by time constraints or patient conditions [38]. Among cross-modality translation tasks, generation of CT images from MRI data and generation to MRI images from PET data are two prominent examples. Note that these cross-modality tasks help provide more divergent tissue information than would be possible by either modality alone. For instance, MRI provides excellent soft tissue contrast, while CT offers detailed structural information regarding bone tissue. Analogously, PET images provide metabolic information to help locate tumor formation in the body, whereas MRI serves to do a more detailed mapping of healthy tissue in the surroundings of the tumor site [8].

Taken together, findings in recent reports suggest that DPMs provide a robust framework for image translation in medical imaging by capturing intricate relationships between different modalities. Their ability to generate high-quality synthetic images can significantly enhance diagnostic evaluation by imputation of comprehensive multi-modal imaging protocols. Yet, to learn these translation tasks, conventional DPMs commonly require training on paired datasets of source and target modalities, which require spatially-registered source and target images from the same set of subjects [35, 44]. As such, conventional DPMs for translation tasks rely on supervised learning setups. This reliance of supervision can be limiting in cases where spatially-misaligned source and target images are available, or when source and target images cannot be acquired from the same set of subjects due to practical limitations. Unsupervised diffusion models can be a promising solution to this problem by facilitating the use of unpaired datasets of source-target images.

In a recent study, SynDiff [38], an adversarial diffusion model has been introduced to enable unsupervised training for multi-contrast MRI and multi-modal translation tasks, while benefiting from high-fidelity synthesis capabilities of DPMs (Fig. 17.3). Unlike conventional DPMs, SynDiff employs a rapid diffusion process with large step sizes to improve computational efficiency while preserving accuracy, with similar motivations to AdaDiff introduced for MRI reconstruction. However, while AdaDiff uses an inherently unconditional DPM that maps Gaussian noise samples onto target images, SynDiff aims to maps Gaussian noise samples onto target images under source image guidance that is received via a conditional DPM architecture. At the core of SynDiff thus lies a novel source-conditional adversarial projector that enhances target image generation by leveraging information from the source image. For unsupervised learning, SynDiff incorporates a cycle-consistent architecture that integrates diffusive and non-diffusive processes to map back and forth between the source and target modalities.

The diffusive component of SynDiff utilizes a source-conditioned adversarial projector to enhance reverse diffusion sampling efficiency. Regular diffusion models use large T to ensure small step sizes for normality, but this can be inefficient. SynDiff proposes a fast diffusion process where the noise variance γ_t is set as:

$$\gamma_t = 1 - \exp\left(\frac{\beta_{\min}k}{T} - \frac{(\beta_{\max} - \beta_{\min})2tk - k^2}{2T^2}\right). \tag{17.19}$$

In the reverse diffusion direction, a conditional process is proposed due to available guidance from a source image $\mathbf{y}$. A source-conditional adversarial projector captures the transition probability $q(\mathbf{x}_{t-k}|\mathbf{x}_t, \mathbf{y})$, and a conditional generator $G_\theta(\mathbf{x}_t, \mathbf{y}, t)$ performs gradual denoising in each reverse step:

$$\hat{\mathbf{x}}_{t-k} \sim p_\theta(\mathbf{x}_{t-k}|\mathbf{x}_t, \mathbf{y}) \tag{17.20}$$

To synthesize target-modality images, reverse diffusion steps require guidance from source-modality images. Given a training set of unpaired source and target modality images, SynDiff first produces paired estimates so that pseudo-supervised learning can then be performed. To obtain these estimates, a non-diffusive component is employed that is essentially a cycle-consistent GAN model, known for its effective and efficient translation capabilities [23]. This non-diffusive module estimates source images paired with each target image in the training set, and it employs two generator-discriminator pairs (G_{ϕ^A}, D_{ϕ^A}) and (G_{ϕ^B}, D_{ϕ^B}) with parameters $\phi^{A,B}$ [23]. The generators produce source image estimates $\tilde{\mathbf{y}}^{A,B}$:

$$\tilde{\mathbf{y}}^B = G_{\phi^B}(\mathbf{x}_0^A), \tag{17.21}$$

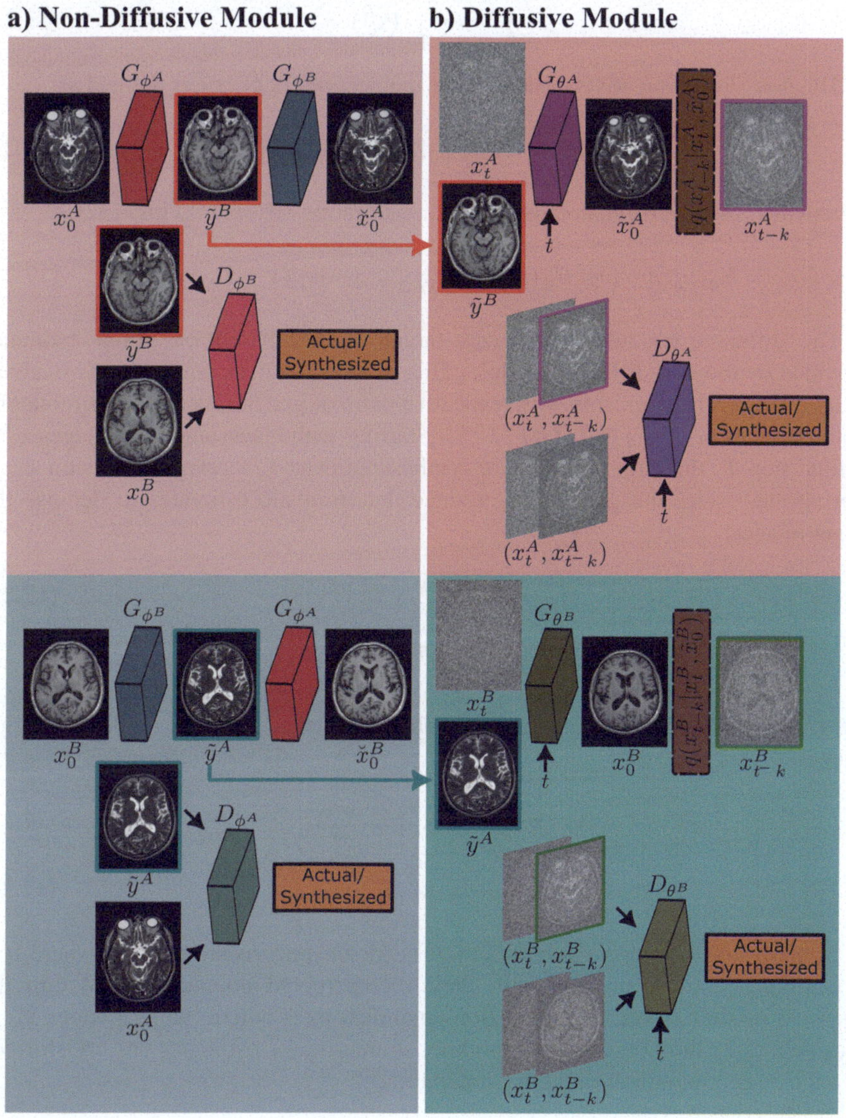

Fig. 17.3 For unsupervised learning, SynDiff utilizes a cycle-consistent approach that translates bidirectionally between two modalities (A and B). To synthesize a target image $\hat{\mathbf{x}}_0^A$ in modality A, the diffusion module depends on a source image $\mathbf{y}^B$ from modality B of the same anatomy for guidance. However, training data may not always include paired source images of the same anatomy. To enable training with unpaired images, SynDiff incorporates a non-diffusion module to initially estimate a paired source image $\tilde{\mathbf{y}}^B$ from $\hat{\mathbf{x}}_0^A$. Likewise, to produce a target image $\hat{\mathbf{x}}_0^B$ in modality B, the non-diffusion module first estimates a paired source image $\tilde{\mathbf{y}}^A$ from $\hat{\mathbf{x}}_0^B$. The non-diffusion module consists of two generator-discriminator pairs $(G_{\phi^{A,B}}, D_{\phi^{A,B}})$ that generate initial translation estimates for $\hat{\mathbf{x}}_0^A \rightarrow \tilde{\mathbf{y}}^B$ and $\hat{\mathbf{x}}_0^B \rightarrow \tilde{\mathbf{y}}^A$. These initial translation estimates $\tilde{\mathbf{y}}^A, \tilde{\mathbf{y}}^B$ are then used as source-modality guides in the diffusion module. For cycle-consistent learning, the diffusion module includes two generator-discriminator pairs $(G_{\theta^{A,B}}, D_{\theta^{A,B}})$ to produce denoised image estimates for $(\mathbf{x}_t^A, \tilde{\mathbf{y}}_t^B) \rightarrow \hat{\mathbf{x}}_{t-k}^A$ and $(\mathbf{x}_t^B, \tilde{\mathbf{y}}_t^A) \rightarrow \hat{\mathbf{x}}_{t-k}^B$

$$\tilde{\mathbf{y}}^A = G_{\phi^A}(\mathbf{x}_0^B). \tag{17.22}$$

The non-saturating adversarial loss for the generators $G_{\phi^{A,B}}$ is defined as:

$$L_{G_\phi} = \mathbb{E}_{p_\phi(\mathbf{y}|\mathbf{x}_0)}[-\log(D_\phi(\mathbf{y}))]. \tag{17.23}$$

Meanwhile, the discriminators adopt a non-saturating adversarial loss [32]:

$$L_{D_\phi} = \mathbb{E}_{q(\mathbf{y}|\mathbf{x}_0)}[-\log(D_\phi(\mathbf{y}))] + \mathbb{E}_{p_\phi(\mathbf{y}|\mathbf{x}_0)}[-\log(1 - D_\phi(\mathbf{y}))]. \tag{17.24}$$

The diffusive module synthesizes target images based on initial estimates provided by the non-diffusive module. This process involves employing two adversarial diffusion mechanisms with respective pairs of generators and discriminators, denoted as $(G_{\theta^A}, D_{\theta^A})$ and $(G_{\theta^B}, D_{\theta^B})$. Starting with Gaussian noise images $\mathbf{x}_T^{A,B}$ at time step T, the target images are synthesized over T/k reverse diffusion steps. During each step, the generators produce deterministic estimates to denoise the target images:

$$\tilde{\mathbf{x}}_0^A = G_{\theta^A}(\mathbf{x}_t^A, \mathbf{y} = \tilde{\mathbf{y}}^B, t), \tag{17.25}$$

$$\tilde{\mathbf{x}}_0^B = G_{\theta^B}(\mathbf{x}_t^B, \mathbf{y} = \tilde{\mathbf{y}}^A, t). \tag{17.26}$$

Next, the denoising distribution for each modality is used to synthesize target images:

$$\hat{\mathbf{x}}_{t-k}^A \sim q(\mathbf{x}_t^A | \mathbf{x}_t^A, \tilde{\mathbf{x}}_0^A), \tag{17.27}$$

$$\hat{\mathbf{x}}_{t-k}^B \sim q(\mathbf{x}_t^B | \mathbf{x}_t^B, \tilde{\mathbf{x}}_0^B). \tag{17.28}$$

SynDiff employs cycle-consistency loss for unsupervised learning, where true target images are compared with their reconstructed counterparts. Within the diffusive module, these reconstructions manifest as synthetic target images $\hat{\mathbf{x}}_0^{A,B}$. Meanwhile, in the non-diffusive module, source-image estimates are transformed into the target domain through the generators:

$$\check{\mathbf{x}}_0^A = G_{\phi^A}(\tilde{\mathbf{y}}^B), \tag{17.29}$$

$$\check{\mathbf{x}}_0^B = G_{\phi^B}(\tilde{\mathbf{y}}^A). \tag{17.30}$$

Given these definitions, the aggregated cycle-consistency loss is defined as:

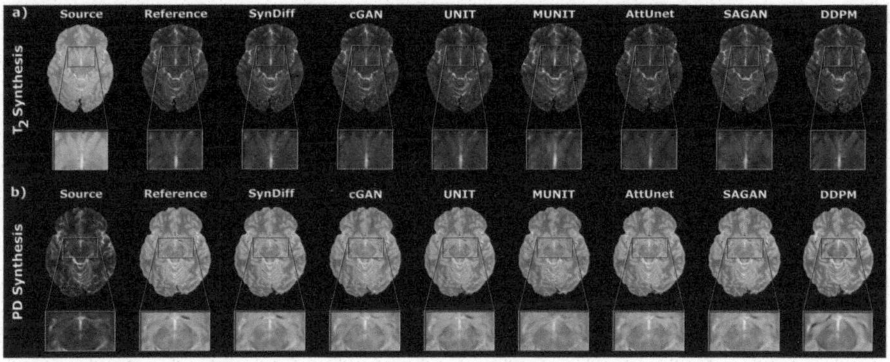

Fig. 17.4 SynDiff was evaluated on the IXI dataset for translating between different MRI contrasts. Representative synthesized images for (**a**) T1 →T2 and (**b**) T2 →PD translation tasks are shown alongside the source and ground-truth target (reference) images. Compared to other methods, SynDiff produces images with reduced noise and artifacts, while preserving higher anatomical accuracy

$$L_{\text{cyc}} = \mathbb{E}_{t,q(\mathbf{x}_0^{A,B}),q(\mathbf{x}_t^{A,B}|\mathbf{x}_0^{A,B})}\Big[\lambda_{1\phi}(\|\mathbf{x}_0^A - \check{\mathbf{x}}_0^A\|_1 + \|\mathbf{x}_0^B - \check{\mathbf{x}}_0^B\|_1) + \lambda_{1\theta}(\|\mathbf{x}_0^A - \hat{\mathbf{x}}_0^A\|_1 + \|\mathbf{x}_0^B - \hat{\mathbf{x}}_0^B\|_1)\Big] \tag{17.31}$$

where $\lambda_{1\phi}$ and $\lambda_{1\theta}$ are the weights for cycle-consistency loss terms from the non-diffusive and diffusive modules, respectively. The overall generator loss is:

$$L_{\text{total}}^{G} = \lambda_{2\phi}(L_{G_{\phi A}} + L_{G_{\phi B}}) + \lambda_{2\theta}(L_{G_{\theta A}} + L_{G_{\theta B}}) + L_{\text{cyc}}, \tag{17.32}$$

where $\lambda_{2\phi}$ and $\lambda_{2\theta}$ are the weights for adversarial loss terms from the non-diffusive and diffusive modules, respectively [16, 35, 42].

Representative target-modality images synthesized diffusion-based and GAN-based methods for multi-contrast MRI protocols are displayed in Fig. 17.4. Specifically, SynDiff is compared against the following techniques: cGAN [23], UNIT [27], MUNIT [19], AttUnet [37], SAGAN [48], and DDPM [18]. GAN methods exhibit noise and local inaccuracies in tissue contrast. Traditional DPMs often suffer from spatial warping and blurring. UNIT-DDPM demonstrates relatively lower anatomical accuracy, occasionally losing tissue features. In contrast, SynDiff exhibits reduced noise and artifacts, and achieves superior accuracy in tissue depiction.

17.5 Emerging Directions in MRI Image Formation

Diffusion probabilistic models have already started to transform how we approach image formation tasks in the realm of MRI applications. We have showcased prominent use cases of DPMs for reconstructing MRI images from undersampled k-space acquisitions, and for translating source onto target contrasts in multi-contrast MRI protocols. In these tasks, DPMs have been reported to significantly outperform previous state-of-the-art in the field in terms of image quality. That said, DPMs are not without limitation, and several lines of technical development are currently sought after to push the envelope of performance and efficiency.

One of the critical challenges faced by current DPMs is their slow sampling speed, which can hinder their practical applicability in real-time scenarios. The primary cause of inefficiency in diffusion models is that they rely on small step sizes (equivalently a large number of time steps) to ensure that the denoising transformations in the reverse direction approximately follow a Gaussian distribution. Several promising approaches have been introduced in the literature to cope with this challenge. On one hand, distillation techniques have been proposed that transfer the representations learned by a teacher DPM with a large number of time steps (e.g., T=1000), onto a student DPM with a much smaller number of time steps (e.g., T=10) [40]. Alternatively, implicit sampling techniques have been suggested to reduce the number of sampling steps through a teacher DPM without transferring representations onto a separate model [43]. While these techniques enable mimicking the behavior of the original, inefficient DPM to speed up inference, they inevitably cause losses in image quality. One potential reason that has been suggested to mediate these losses is that the denoising transformations that have to be performed at different time steps in the diffusion process can show divergent characteristics, thus a single denoising network may have difficulty in maintaining sample quality especially when under acceleration [5]. To mitigate these losses, a practical strategy is to split the diffusion process into multiple non-overlapping time fractions, and to train independent denoising networks for each fraction so as to ensure high performance following acceleration [6]. One the other hand, adversarial mechanisms have been suggested to improve the efficiency of DPMs directly during the training phase so as to lower the number time steps required [38, 46]. This approach corresponds to setting a hybrid adversarial-diffusion model, wherein there is an outer diffusion sampling loop with few time steps, and an inner adversarial sampling loop that enables accurate sample generation over large step sizes without the need to assume a Gaussian distribution for denoising transformations. It is possible that by integrating these various approaches, researchers can significantly enhance the efficiency of diffusion models, making them more viable for real-time applications.

A second group of developments concern the neural network architecture used to implement the recovery operator. Starting on with the earliest studies introducing DPMs, UNet-based convolutional architectures have been mainstream in the literature. This can be attributed in part to the prowess of this particular architecture in performing denoising transformations, and in part to the practical challenges in hyperparameter optimization in deep neural networks that have likely discouraged many practitioners from adopting other architectures to build DPMs. Still, there is a growing interest in exploring alternative architectures such as transformers and more recent state-space models. Transformers, with their self-attention mechanisms, offer superior capabilities in capturing long-range dependencies, which can enhance the denoising capabilities of diffusion models [9, 24]. Several bodies of work have already reported performance improvements by building DPMs on transformers as opposed to convolutional backbones [25]. While the contextual sensitivity offered by transformers is desirable in medical imaging, self-attention-based architectures often suffer from high model complexity, which can compromise learning especially in domains where the training sets are relatively compact such as medical imaging [12]. As a remedy, recent selective state-space models, a prime example being the Mamba architecture, enable efficient processing with reduced model complexity, all the while enabling capture of long-range context [29, 49]. Early studies for adopting Mamba in image formation tasks [4, 20] suggest that, with further research to optimize architectures, we can pave the way for enhanced efficiency and accuracy in diffusion models.

Another important group of developments involve the design of the diffusion process that inherently characterizes image generation capabilities of DPMs. In conventional DPMs, the diffusion process is designed with a Gaussian noise distribution at the start-point and the clean data distribution at the end-point. This process is highly adept if the aim is to learn the marginal distribution of clean image samples. However, when these conventional DPMs are deployed in inverse problem solutions, where the aim is to map degraded measurements onto clean images, information regarding the measurement model and measured data have to be injected during inference via a dedicated optimization procedure. This common approach seeks a compromise solution between the support set of the trained diffusion model and the support set of the measurements. In certain cases, these sets might only weakly intersect, causing conventional DPMs to yield suboptimal solutions or poor convergence. Recently, diffusion bridges have been introduced with the aim to address this fundamental limitation. Diffusion bridges present an innovative approach to embed task-specific information directly into model training, by setting the start-point of the diffusion process as the distribution of measurements and the end-point as the clean data distribution [28]. This allows integration of task-specific knowledge about the inverse problem that must be solved into the training of the recovery operator. Several studies in MRI image reconstruction and translation have already reported performance benefits with diffusion bridges over common DPMs [3, 33]. Future research should focus on refining diffusion bridge methodologies to fully harness their advantages over conventional approaches.

17.6 Conclusion

DPMs hold immense potential, particularly in the realm of MRI image formation tasks such as reconstruction and translation. Their ability to generate high-fidelity images and capture intricate details makes them well-suited for clinical and research applications of MRI. The ongoing developments underscore the transformative potential of DPMs in these domains, heralding a new era of innovation and efficiency. Therefore, as advancements continue in accelerating sampling speeds, devising powerful backbones, and embedding task-specific information within the diffusion process, diffusion models are poised to revolutionize MRI imaging.

Competing Interests The authors have no conflicts of interest to declare that are relevant to the content of this chapter.

References

1. Adam A, Dixon A, Gillard J, Schaefer-Prokop C, Grainger R, Allison D (2014) Grainger & Allison's diagnostic radiology. Elsevier, Amsterdam
2. Aggarwal HK, Mani MP, Jacob M (2019) MoDL: model-based deep learning architecture for inverse problems. IEEE Trans Med Imaging 38(2):394–405
3. Arslan F, Kabas B, Dalmaz O, Ozbey M, Çukur T (2024) Self-consistent recursive diffusion bridge for medical image translation. arXiv:240506789
4. Atli OF, Kabas B, Arslan F, Yurt M, Dalmaz O, Çukur T (2024) I2I-Mamba: multi-modal medical image synthesis via selective state space modeling. arXiv:240514022
5. Balaji Y, Nah S, Huang X, Vahdat A, Song J, Kreis K, Aittala M, Aila T, Laine S, Catanzaro B, et al (2022) ediffi: text-to-image diffusion models with an ensemble of expert denoisers. arXiv:221101324
6. Bedel HA, Çukur T (2023) DreaMR: diffusion-driven counterfactual explanation for functional MRI. arXiv:230709547
7. Chartsias A, Joyce T, Dharmakumar R, Tsaftaris SA (2017) Adversarial image synthesis for unpaired multi-modal cardiac data. In: Simul Synth Med Imaging, pp 3–13
8. Chung H, Ye JC (2022) Score-based diffusion models for accelerated MRI. Med Image Anal 80:102479
9. Dalmaz O, Yurt M, Çukur T (2022) ResViT: residual vision transformers for multi-modal medical image synthesis. IEEE Trans Med Imaging 44(10):2598–2614
10. Dar SU, Yurt M, Karacan L, Erdem A, Erdem E, Cukur T (2019) Image synthesis in multi-contrast MRI with conditional generative adversarial networks. IEEE Trans Med Imaging 38(10):2375–2388
11. Dar SU, Yurt M, Shahdloo M, Ildız ME, Tınaz B, Çukur T (2020) Prior-guided image reconstruction for accelerated multi-contrast MRI via generative adversarial networks. IEEE J Sel Top Signal Process 14(6):1072–1087
12. Dosovitskiy A, Beyer L, Kolesnikov A, Weissenborn D, Zhai X, Unterthiner T, Dehghani M, Minderer M, Heigold G, Gelly S, Uszkoreit J, Houlsby N (2021) An image is worth 16x16 words: transformers for image recognition at scale. arXiv:201011929
13. Elmas G, Dar SU, Korkmaz Y, Ceyani E, Susam B, Özbey M, Avestimehr S, Çukur T (2023) Federated learning of generative image priors for MRI reconstruction. IEEE Trans Med Imaging 42(7):1996–2009

14. Fan Y, Liao H, Huang S, Luo Y, Fu H, Qi H (2024) A survey of emerging applications of diffusion probabilistic models in MRI. Meta-Radiology 2(2):100082
15. Goodfellow I, Pouget-Abadie J, Mirza M, Xu B, Warde-Farley D, Ozair S, Courville A, Bengio Y (2014) Generative adversarial networks. In: Adv Neural Inf Process Syst, vol 24
16. Güngör A, Dar SU, Öztürk Ş, Korkmaz Y, Bedel HA, Elmas G, Ozbey M, Çukur T (2023) Adaptive diffusion priors for accelerated MRI reconstruction. Med Image Anal 88:102872
17. Haldar JP, Zhuo J (2016) P-loraks: low-rank modeling of local k-space neighborhoods with parallel imaging data. Magn Reson Med 75(4):1499–1514
18. Ho J, Jain A, Abbeel P (2020) Denoising diffusion probabilistic models. In: Adv Neural Inf Process Syst, vol 33, pp 6840–6851
19. Huang X, Liu MY, Belongie S, Kautz J (2018) Multimodal unsupervised image-to-image translation. In: European Conf Comput Vis, pp 172–189
20. Huang J, Yang L, Wang F, Wu Y, Nan Y, Aviles-Rivero AI, Schönlieb CB, Zhang D, Yang G (2024) Mambamir: an arbitrary-masked mamba for joint medical image reconstruction and uncertainty estimation. arXiv:240218451
21. Jalal A, Arvinte M, Daras G, Price E, Dimakis AG, Tamir J (2021) Robust compressed sensing MRI with deep generative priors. In: Adv. Neural Inf. Process. Sys., vol 34, pp 14938–14954
22. Jog A, Carass A, Roy S, Pham DL, Prince JL (2017) Random forest regression for magnetic resonance image synthesis. Med Image Anal 35:475–488
23. Kabas B, Arslan F, Nezhad VA, Ozturk S, Saritas EU, Cuku T (2024) Physics-driven autoregressive state space models for medical image reconstruction. arXiv:2412.09331
24. Korkmaz Y, Dar SUH, Yurt M, Ozbey M, Cukur T (2022) Unsupervised MRI reconstruction via zero-shot learned adversarial transformers. IEEE Trans Med Imaging 41(7):1747–1763
25. Korkmaz Y, Cukur T, Patel V (2023) Self-supervised MRI reconstruction with unrolled diffusion models. In: Med. Imag. Comput. Comput. Assist. Int., pp 491–501
26. Litjens G, Kooi T, Bejnordi BE, Setio AAA, Ciompi F, Ghafoorian M, van der Laak JA, van Ginneken B, Sánchez CI (2017) A survey on deep learning in medical image analysis. Med Image Anal 42:60–88
27. Liu MY, Breuel T, Kautz J (2017) Unsupervised image-to-image translation networks. In: Adv Neural Inf Process Syst, vol 30
28. Liu GH, Vahdat A, Huang DA, Theodorou EA, Nie W, Anandkumar A (2023) I^2SB: image-to-Image Schrödinger Bridge. In: Int. Conf. Mach. Learn., pp 22042–22062
29. Liu Y, Tian Y, Zhao Y, Yu H, Xie L, Wang Y, Ye Q, Liu Y (2024) Vmamba: visual state space model. arXiv:240110166
30. Lustig M, Donoho D, Pauly JM (2007) Sparse MRI: the application of compressed sensing for rapid MR imaging. Magn Reson Med 58(6):1182–1195
31. Mardani M, Gong E, Cheng JY, Vasanawala S, Zaharchuk G, Xing L, Pauly JM (2019) Deep generative adversarial neural networks for compressive sensing MRI. IEEE Trans Med Imaging 38(1):167–179
32. Mescheder L, Geiger A, Nowozin S (2018) Which training methods for gans do actually converge? In: Int Conf Mach Learn, pp 3481–3490
33. Mirza MU, Dalmaz O, Bedel HA, Elmas G, Korkmaz Y, Gungor A, Dar SU, Çukur T (2023) Learning Fourier-constrained diffusion bridges for MRI reconstruction. arXiv:230801096
34. Narnhofer D, Hammernik K, Knoll F, Pock T (2019) Inverse GANs for accelerated MRI reconstruction. In: Proceedings of SPIE, vol 11138, pp 381–392
35. Nichol AQ, Dhariwal P (2021) Improved denoising diffusion probabilistic models. In: Int. Conf. Mach. Learn., pp 8162–8171
36. Nie D, Shen D (2020) Adversarial confidence learning for medical image segmentation and synthesis. Int J Comput Vis 128(10):2494–2513
37. Oktay O, Schlemper J, Folgoc LL, Lee MJ, Heinrich M, Misawa K, Mori K, McDonagh SG, Hammerla N, Kainz B, Glocker B, Rueckert D (2018) Attention U-Net: learning where to look for the pancreas. arXiv:180403999
38. Özbey M, Dalmaz O, Dar SU, Bedel HA, Özturk Ş, Güngör A, Çukur T (2023) Unsupervised medical image translation with adversarial diffusion models. IEEE Trans Med Imaging 42(12):3524–3539

39. Peng C, Guo P, Zhou SK, Patel V, Chellappa R (2022) Towards performant and reliable undersampled MR reconstruction via diffusion model sampling. arXiv:220304292
40. Salimans T, Ho J (2022) Progressive distillation for fast sampling of diffusion models. arXiv:220200512
41. Sharma A, Hamarneh G (2020) Missing MRI pulse sequence synthesis using multi-modal generative adversarial network. IEEE Trans Med Imaging 39:1170–1183
42. Sohl-Dickstein J, Weiss E, Maheswaranathan N, Ganguli S (2015) Deep unsupervised learning using nonequilibrium thermodynamics. In: Int Conf Mach Learn, pp 2256–2265
43. Song J, Meng C, Ermon S (2020) Denoising diffusion implicit models. arXiv:201002502
44. Song Y, Sohl-Dickstein J, Kingma DP, Kumar A, Ermon S, Poole B (2020) Score-based generative modeling through stochastic differential equations. arXiv:201113456
45. Song Y, Shen L, Xing L, Ermon S (2022) Solving inverse problems in medical imaging with score-based generative models. In: Int Conf Learn Represent
46. Xiao Z, Kreis K, Vahdat A (2022) Tackling the generative learning trilemma with denoising diffusion GANs. In: Int Conf Learn Represent
47. Yi X, Walia E, Babyn P (2019) Generative adversarial network in medical imaging: a review. Med Image Anal 58:101552
48. Zhang H, Goodfellow I, Metaxas D, Odena A (2019) Self-attention generative adversarial networks. In: Int Conf Mach Learn, vol 97, pp 7354–7363
49. Zhu L, Liao B, Zhang Q, Wang X, Liu W, Wang X (2024) Vision mamba: efficient visual representation learning with bidirectional state space model. arXiv:240109417

Chapter 18
Embedding 3D CT Prior into X-ray Imaging Using Generative Adversarial Networks

Han Li, Zhen Huang, and S. Kevin Zhou

Abstract There is clinical evidence that suppressing the bone structures in X-rays (e.g., Chest X-rays (CXRs), pelvic X-rays (PXRs)) improves diagnostic value, either for radiologists or computer-aided diagnosis. However, bone-free CXRs are not always accessible. In this chapter, we explore the integration of 3D CT prior knowledge into X-ray imaging using generative adversarial networks (GANs) to address challenges posed by 2D projection superposition and improve diagnostic accuracy. **First,** we introduce the Decomposition GAN (DecGAN) designed for the anatomical decomposition of CXR images, leveraging unpaired CT data. DecGAN utilizes decomposition loss, adversarial loss, cycle consistency loss, and mask loss to ensure realistic anatomical separation of components such as bone, lung, and soft tissue. We can remove the bone components and get the bone-suppressed CXRs. **Next,** we propose a coarse-to-fine High-Resolution CXRs Suppression (HRCS) approach to suppress bone structures in high-resolution CXRs. By leveraging digitally reconstructed radiographs (DRRs) and domain adaptation techniques, this method mitigates domain differences between CXRs and CT-derived images. Experiments on benchmark datasets show that this method outperforms existing unsupervised bone suppression techniques and significantly reduces false-negative rates in lung disease diagnoses. **Finally,** we address the superposition problem in PXRs by introducing the Pelvis Extraction (PELE) module. This module, comprising a decomposition network, a domain adaptation network, and an

---

H. Li (✉)
Computer Aided Medical Procedures (CAMP), School of Computation, Information and Technology, Technische Universitaet Muenchen (TUM), Munich, Germany

Medical Imaging, Robotics, Analytic Computing Laboratory and Engineering (MIRACLE), School of Biomedical Engineering & Suzhou Institute for Advanced Research, University of Science and Technology of China (USTC), Suzhou, China
e-mail: hanli21@mail.ustc.edu.cn

Z. Huang · S. K. Zhou
Medical Imaging, Robotics, Analytic Computing Laboratory and Engineering (MIRACLE), School of Biomedical Engineering & Suzhou Institute for Advanced Research, University of Science and Technology of China (USTC), Suzhou, Suzhou

L. Zhang et al. (eds.), *Generative Machine Learning Models in Medical Image Computing*, https://doi.org/10.1007/978-3-031-80965-1_18

enhancement module, utilizes 3D anatomical knowledge from CT scans to isolate the pelvis from PXR images, enhancing landmark detection. Evaluations of public and private datasets demonstrate that the PELE module significantly improves landmark detection accuracy, achieving state-of-the-art performance across several metrics. These approaches are based on similar principles but evaluated across different scenarios. The results demonstrate the potential to improve X-ray diagnosis at no extra cost by leveraging generative models enriched with CT knowledge.

18.1 Introduction

X-ray (e.g., Chest X-rays (CXRs), pelvic X-rays (PXRs)), which is reconstructed from a series of X-ray projections, is one of the most common imaging modalities employed in the diagnosis. However, its utility is often limited by the 2D nature of the projection, where important anatomical structures may be obscured. For instance, in CXR imaging, bones such as ribs can obscure the lung area, making accurate diagnosis difficult [4, 11]. Similarly, in PXRs, soft tissue such as the bladder and intestines can overlap with the pelvis, complicating landmark detection. To address these challenges, we explore the integration of 3D computed tomography (CT) priors into 2D X-ray imaging to overcome the challenges posed by structural overlaps and ambiguous anatomical details inherent in X-ray images. In this chapter, we propose three different methods that utilize CT-derived prior to improve X-ray analysis.

First, for CXRs, we introduce a Decomposition Generative Adversarial Network (DecGAN) [12], which leverages CT-derived anatomical priors to decompose X-rays into distinct components (e.g., bones, lungs, and soft tissue) using unpaired data. We can remove the bone components and get the bone-suppressed CXRs. This unsupervised method does not rely on dual-energy (DE) images, making it more accessible for clinical use. DecGAN achieves superior unsupervised CXR bone suppression and improves the prediction accuracy of lung diseases.

Second, we further develop a coarse-to-fine **High-Resolution** CXRs Suppression (HRCS) [13] that utilizes digitally reconstructed radiographs (DRRs) derived from CT data. By using DRRs as a bridge between CT and CXR, and employing domain adaptation techniques, we are able to perform high-resolution bone suppression without requiring paired data or manual annotations. This method enhances diagnostic accuracy by reducing the false-negative rate of lung disease detection.

Third, we tackle the challenge of soft tissue overlap in pelvic X-rays by introducing the PELvis Extraction (PELE) module [8]. This method explicitly extracts the pelvis bone from PXRs using unpaired 3D CT priors. The extracted pelvis is enhanced and then used for landmark detection, significantly improving the accuracy of computer-assisted diagnosis and surgical planning.

Through these approaches, we demonstrate that embedding 3D CT priors into X-ray analysis can significantly enhance the diagnostic value of 2D X-rays, providing a robust solution to the challenges posed by anatomical superposition.

The structure of the chapter is as follows. Sections 18.2–18.4 introduce DecGAN, HRCS, and PELE respectively, followed by the conclusion in Sect. 18.5. We add more discussion in the end of each section to help readers to be inspired by our book and explore this direction, potentially creating something meaningful.

18.2 Decomposition Generative Adversarial Network (DecGAN)

DecGAN is built on the backbone of CycleGAN with latent space disentanglement, as illustrated in Fig. 18.1. Given a CXR input X, our goal is to construct a function F that generates the modulated reconstruction X_m, where different chest components can be adjusted by modifying the corresponding factors $[\alpha_b, \alpha_l, \alpha_o]$:

$$X_m = F(X, \alpha_b, \alpha_l, \alpha_o) = G_X(G_{Dec}(G_D(X, \alpha_b, \alpha_l, \alpha_o))), \tag{18.1}$$

To address the challenge of CXR decomposition, we contribute in three key ways: (1) We design an additional latent space decomposition discriminator, D_{Dec}, to facilitate the embedding of prior CT decomposition knowledge and ensure the separation of different components in the generated DRR. (2) The DRR decomposition network, G_{Dec}, is incorporated into the CycleGAN backbone, providing the decoder with sufficient knowledge to manage the decomposition information in the latent space. (3) A soft bone mask $\mathcal{M}$, generated from the bone components in the latent space, is used as an additional constraint to ensure the separation and realism of the reconstructed components. We primarily introduce the DRR Decomposition Network G_{Dec} and the Mask Loss here, as the other components are similar to those in CycleGAN. For more details, please refer to the original paper.

18.2.1 DRR Decomposition Network

The decomposition network G_{Dec} is built upon the U-Net architecture [18]. The components of a 3D CT volume are projected using consistent parameters and concatenated into channels, serving as the ground truth for DRR decomposition:

$$I_{Dec} = [I_{bone}, I_{lung}, I_{other}], \tag{18.2}$$

where I_{bone}, I_{lung} and I_{other} are the components of DRR for bone, lung and other soft-tissue, respectively.

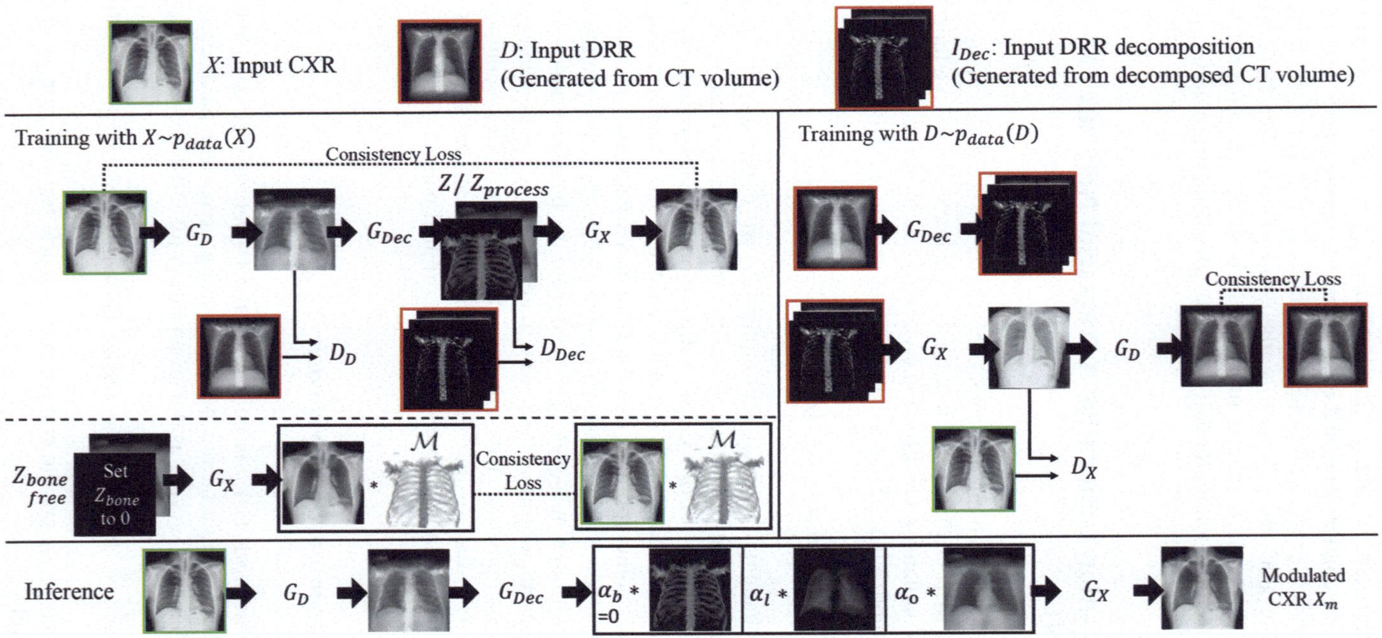

Fig. 18.1 Illustration of the proposed method. **Training phase:** The decomposition network G_{Dec} and the decomposition discriminator D_{Dec} are integrated into the CycleGAN backbone, which bridges the domains of CXR and digitally reconstructed radiograph (DRR). A mask loss is applied to ensure that non-bone components maintain consistent correspondence between the latent space and the reconstructed images. **Inference phase:** The reconstructed CXR components can be adjusted by modifying the weights of the probability maps within the latent space

Based on the input DRR image D and its separated components I_{Dec}, the decomposition network can be trained in a supervised way by the decomposition loss:

$$\mathcal{L}_{Dec}(G_{Dec}) = \mathbb{E}_{D\sim p_{data}(D)}[\|G_{Dec}(D) - I_{Dec}\|_2^2]. \tag{18.3}$$

18.2.2 Mask Loss

In early experiments with DecGAN, we observed that the reconstruction results lacked fidelity when modifying the probability maps $Z_{process}$. This issue arises because G_X has limited prior knowledge for generating outputs with altered $Z_{process}$. To address this, we introduce additional constraints on the generative model for CXR decomposition. The bone component is particularly well-suited for this purpose, as it only appears in specific regions of the CXR and is easily distinguishable from other components. Moreover, the bone component is generally irrelevant to lung disease diagnosis. Thus, we aim to improve the generative model by placing less emphasis on bone structures.

Unlike the complete probability maps $Z_{process}$, we first remove the bone components from the latent space:

$$Z_{bonefree} = [0, Z_{lung}, G_D(X) - Z_{bone} - Z_{lung}]. \tag{18.4}$$

A soft mask $\mathcal{M}$ is subsequently generated from the bone probability map, using a confidence threshold of 95%. Since the images are normalized to a range of [0,1], the soft mask is defined as:

$$\mathcal{M} = 1 - (Z_{bone} - t)/(1 - t) * \delta[Z_{bone}], \tag{18.5}$$

where t is a threshold (we set $t = 0.95$) and the binary function $\delta[Z_{bone}]$ is defined:

$$\delta[Z_{bone}] = \begin{cases} 0 & Z_{bone} < t; \\ 1 & Z_{bone} \geq t. \end{cases} \tag{18.6}$$

Using the mask $\mathcal{M}$ from (18.5), the reconstruction results—without bone components or with suppressed bone structures—are constrained by the input CXRs. The mask loss encourages the non-bone regions of the reconstructed images to resemble the original images more closely:

$$\mathcal{L}_{mask}(G_X) = \mathbb{E}_{X\sim p_{data}(X)}[\|G_X(Z_{bonefree}) * \mathcal{M} - X * \mathcal{M}\|_1]. \tag{18.7}$$

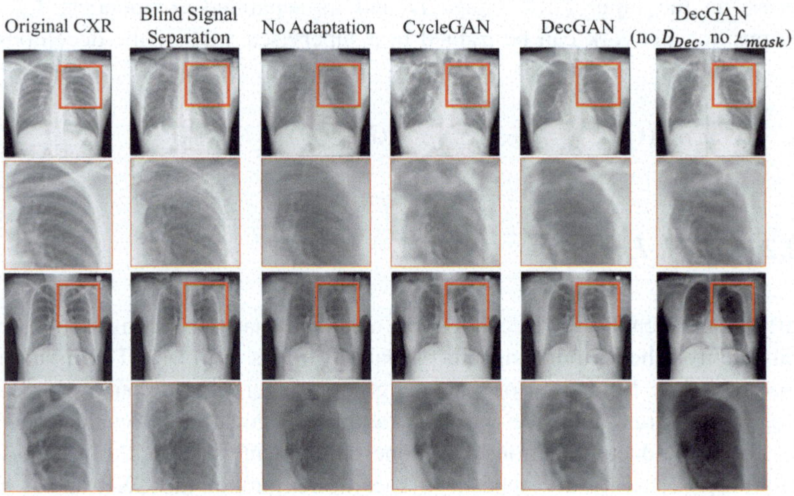

Fig. 18.2 Qualitative results of CXR bone suppression. In DecGAN, we implement multiple constraints that allow for the separate decomposition of various components while ensuring realistic output. DecGAN effectively suppresses bone components to a high degree while maintaining the integrity and realism of the non-bone regions

18.2.3 Inference and Modulation

During the inference phase, since the CXR components are separated within the latent space and the generative model is trained to decode this information, we can modulate specific components (e.g., lung) by adjusting the weights of the probability maps, $[\alpha_b, \alpha_l, \alpha_o]$, to generate the modulated CXR reconstruction as follows:

$$X_m = G_X([\alpha_b * Z_{bone}, \alpha_l * Z_{lung}, \alpha_o * (G_D(X) - Z_{bone} - Z_{lung})]). \tag{18.8}$$

Clearly, setting α_b to 0 results in bone-suppressed CXRs (Fig. 18.2).

18.2.4 Experiments of DecGAN

18.2.4.1 Datasets

We collected 246 CT volumes from LIDC-IDRI [1]. The bone regions in the 3D CT volumes were manually labeled, while the lung regions were segmented based on intensity and dilation techniques. DRRs were generated from these 246 CT volumes with augmentation through rotation and rescaling. Additionally, 662 CXRs from the Shenzhen Hospital X-ray Set [9] and 112,120 CXRs from ChestX-ray14 [22] were collected. For testing, 99 cases were randomly selected from the Shenzhen Hospital X-ray Set, and the official split of ChestXray14 was used for our experiments.

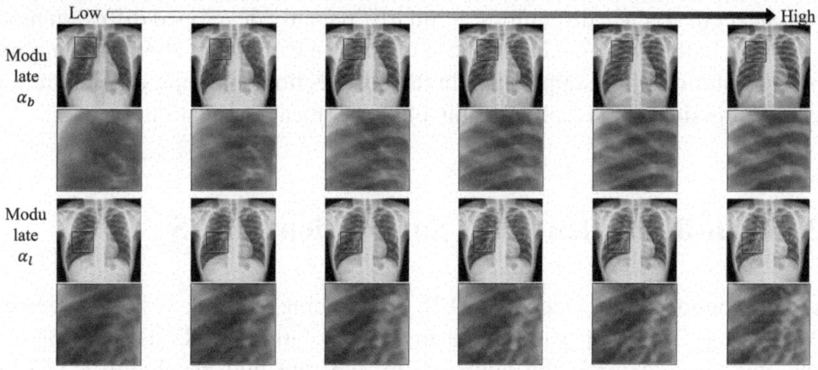

Fig. 18.3 Illustration of CXR modulation. DecGAN allows targeted modulation of specific components while keeping other regions unaffected

18.2.4.2 DecGAN Bone-Suppressed CXRs for Automatic Disease Classification

The components of a CXR can be modulated by adjusting the weights of $Z_{process}$, as described in (18.8). Figure 18.3 shows the results of modulating the components. The weights α_b and α_l are varied while keeping the other weights constant. It is evident that the bone and lung components can be either suppressed or enhanced without affecting the other components.

To directly demonstrate the effectiveness of DecGAN for lung disease diagnosis, the decomposition results are fed into a lung disease prediction system based on DenseNet-121. The lung enhancement results are generated with weights $[\alpha_b, \alpha_l, \alpha_o]$ set to [1,2,1]. These enhanced lung images are concatenated with the original CXRs and used as inputs for the pretrained DenseNet-121 model [7]. The quantitative prediction results are summarized in the next section Table 18.1.

18.2.5 Conclusion of DecGAN

In this section, we present DecGAN, a model trained *in an unpaired setting* to decompose CXR images into different components by leveraging prior CT anatomical knowledge. We demonstrate the effectiveness of DecGAN in unsupervised bone suppression and lung disease diagnosis tasks, achieving state-of-the-art performance. We believe DecGAN has the potential to significantly enhance the diagnostic utility of CXR images.

However, DecGAN's low-resolution output limits its clinical applicability. Built on CycleGAN, DecGAN requires significant GPU resources, making it challenging to process high-resolution CXRs (e.g., 1024 $\times$ 1024) due to both memory constraints and convergence difficulties. Similarly, recently developed diffusion models face similar challenges. To address these issues, we explore an alternative approach for high-resolution bone suppression in the next section, enabling efficient removal of bone impressions at a resolution suitable for clinical application.

18.3 High-Resolution CXRs Suppression (HRCS)

This work builds upon DecGAN [12], introducing several key advancements: (1) While DecGAN [12] was limited to low-resolution CXRs as both input and output, this study extends the approach to generate high-resolution CXRs with bone suppression, which is more relevant for clinical use; (2) Unlike the previous approach, which directly produced bone-suppressed CXRs via a learning-based model [12], this work separates the process by first computing bone decomposition and then subtracting it from the original high-resolution CXR, thereby preserving non-bone regions. This distinction is critical for clinical diagnostic accuracy; (3) We introduce bone decomposition in the Laplacian of Gaussian (LoG) domain instead of the conventional image domain, which helps to reduce the domain discrepancy between DRR and CXR; (4) Finally, we assess the approach by having experienced radiologists utilize the high-resolution, bone-free CXRs for diagnostic purposes, confirming the clinical value of the improved resolution and accuracy.

Our method starts with a high-resolution CXR input and aims to produce a high-resolution bone-suppressed CXR by extracting structural knowledge from unpaired CT scans. This knowledge serves as a structural prior in our framework. As depicted in Fig. 18.4, the proposed approach is composed of two main stages. In the initial stage, we conduct a low-resolution decomposition of the CXR to obtain bone decomposition results. This is achieved by utilizing unpaired CT structural priors in combination with a decomposition network and domain adaptation techniques. In the second stage, the low-resolution bone decomposition results are upsampled to match the size of the high-resolution CXR. These results are then normalized to ensure that their intensity distributions are consistent with the original CXR. The bone components are subsequently subtracted from the original CXR to achieve bone suppression.

The two stages of our method can be further divided into four key steps: (1) The first step involves employing multi-task learning [5, 21] to train a decomposition network. This network is used to break down a given DRR image into a bone component, $\triangle_g I_{bone}$, and a lung mask, $I_{lungmask}$, within the LoG-DRR domain; (2) In the second step, the low-resolution CXR image I_X is transformed into the LoG domain, where the decomposition network F_{MT} is applied to generate the bone decomposition $\triangle_g I_{predbone}$ and the predicted lung mask $M_{predlung}$ using domain adaptation techniques; (3) The third step focuses on obtaining a high-resolution bone decomposition result. Histogram matching is then applied to adjust its intensity distribution, aligning it with that of the original high-resolution CXR

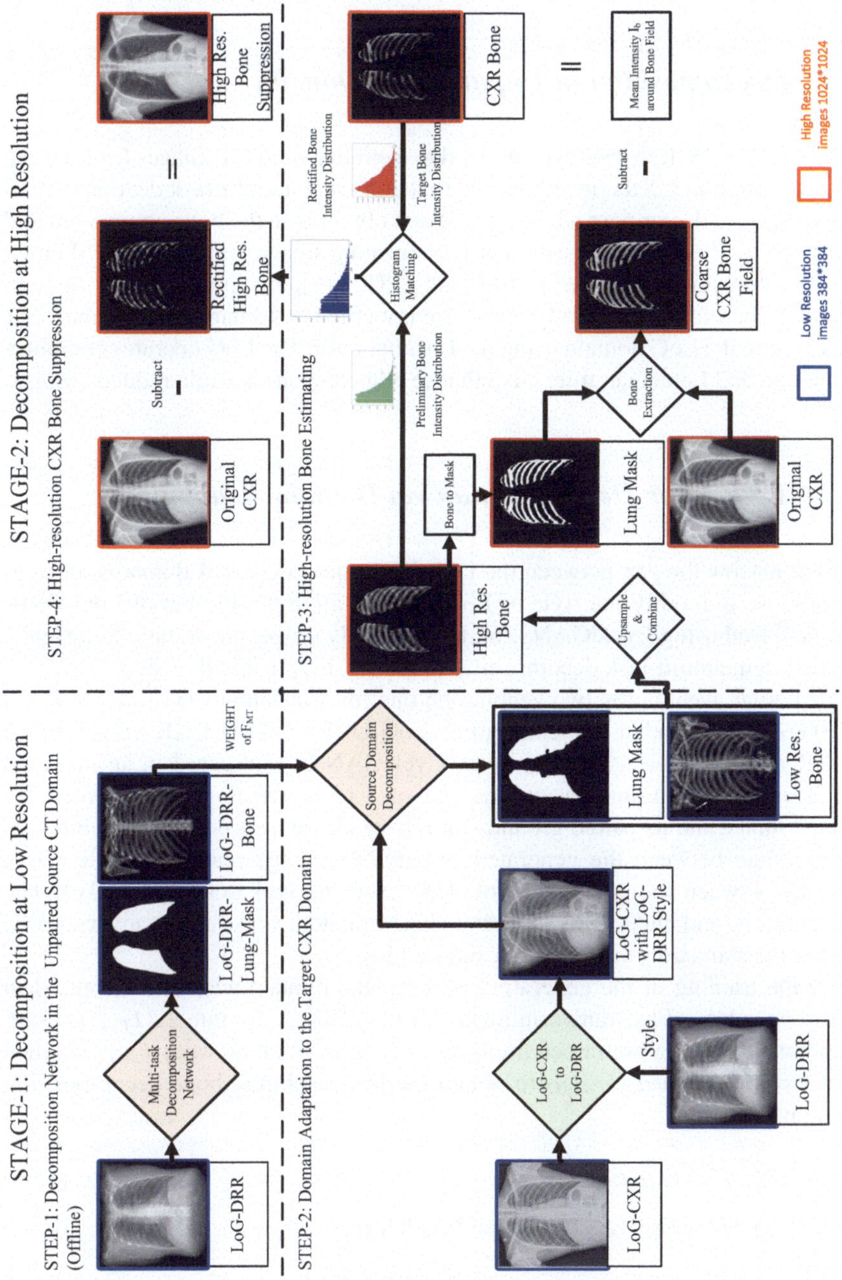

Fig. 18.4 Our method consists of two main stages: low-resolution decomposition and high-resolution decomposition, further divided into four distinct steps

image; (4) Finally, the rectified bone component is subtracted from the original CXR to produce the final bone-suppressed result.

18.3.1 Decomposition in Unpaired CT Domain

As shown in Fig. 18.4, to leverage knowledge from unpaired CT images for accurate bone suppression in CXRs, in step-1, we first construct a multi-task decomposition network, F_{MT}, to decompose a DRR image and obtain both the bone component and the lung mask. Research suggests that transforming images into the LoG domain reduce the domain gap between DRR and CXR [19], facilitating better domain adaptation. Therefore, we initially transform both the DRR images I_D and the CXR images I_X into the LoG domain using the LoG operator. The LoG operator combines the Gaussian and Laplacian filters to enhance edge responses while reducing noise.

18.3.2 CXR Bone Decomposition via Domain Adaptation

To further narrow the gap between the LoG-DRR and LoG-CXR domains, in step-2, we propose to modify the style of LoG-CXR to align it with that of LoG-DRR. This is achieved using CycleGAN [26], to effectively utilize the domain knowledge embedded in the multi-task decomposition network F_{MT} learned in step-1.

In particular, we employ two generators: one for translating LoG-CXR to LoG-DRR (G_D), and another for translating LoG-DRR to LoG-CXR (G_X). Since our CXR and CT datasets are unpaired, CycleGAN is configured in an unpaired mode. This configuration prevents the use of a reconstruction loss between the generated image and its paired ground-truth. Instead, we incorporate discriminators to differentiate between the generated LoG-DRR and the real LoG-DRR (D_D), as well as between the generated LoG-CXR and the real LoG-CXR (D_X). The two generators and their corresponding discriminators are trained adversarially, following the standard CycleGAN procedure [26].

After the training of the generators is complete, domain adaptation at the data level can be achieved by transforming each LoG-CXR $\Delta_g I_X$ into $\Delta_g I_{fakeD}$ using the generator G_D. The pretrained multi-task decomposition network F_{MT} can then be directly applied to $\Delta_g I_{fakeD}$ to obtain the low-resolution bone decomposition and lung mask results:

$$\Delta_g I_{fakeD} = G_D(\Delta_g I_X), \tag{18.9}$$

$$I_{predMT} = F_{MT}(\Delta_g I_{fakeD}) = [\Delta_g I_{predbone}; M_{predlung}], \tag{18.10}$$

where $\Delta_g I_{fakeD}$ is the domain adaptation result of CXR I_X, $\Delta_g I_{predbone}$ and $M_{predlung}$ are the low-resolution bone decomposition result.

18.3.3 High-Resolution Bone Decomposition

In step 3, we aim to perform CXR bone suppression at high resolution. This process consists of two primary sub-steps: low-resolution bone upsampling and high-resolution CXR intensity normalization.

Low-Resolution Bone Upsampling The low-resolution bone image $\Delta I_{predbone}$ and lung mask $M_{predlung}$, generated by the multi-task decomposition network F_{MT}, are upsampled to high resolution (e.g., 1024 × 1024) as follows:

$$\Delta_g I^h_{lungbone} = \Delta I^h_{predbone} \times M^h_{predlung}, \tag{18.11}$$

where the superscript ‘h’ in $\Delta_g I^h_{lungbone}$, $\Delta I^h_{predbone}$, and $M^h_{predlung}$ indicates that the images are at the target high-resolution size.

Next, we convert $\Delta_g I^h_{lungbone}$ into a bone mask $M^h_{lungbone}$ by applying a thresholding function $\mathcal{T}$, where intensities below the mean intensity of $\Delta_g I^h_{lungbone}$ are set to 0 and those above the mean are set to 1. We then multiply the original high-resolution CXR I^h_X by this bone mask $M^h_{lungbone}$ to obtain a coarse high-resolution bone image within the lung mask $M^h_{lungbone}$. This can be represented as:

$$M^h_{lungbone} = \mathcal{T}(\Delta_g I^h_{lungbone}), I^h_{Xcoabone} = I^h_X \times M^h_{lungbone}. \tag{18.12}$$

The coarse bone result, denoted as $I^h_{Xcoabone}$, does not accurately reflect the true bone distribution, as it still includes the intensities of lung and soft tissue regions. To address this issue, we calculate the mean intensity I_{b10} within the bone's neighboring regions (within a 10-pixel radius) as an approximation of the lung and soft tissue intensities. We then subtract this value from $I^h_{Xcoabone}$ to more accurately estimate the real bone structure in the CXR:$I^h_{Xbone} = I^h_{Xcoabone} - I_{b10}$.

High-Resolution CXR Intensity Histogram Matching Histogram matching is a technique that preserves the fine details of the original image while aligning the intensity distribution with that of a target image. As illustrated in Fig. 18.4, we use the histogram of the estimated bone image I^h_{Xbone} from the CXR as the reference for the bone intensity distribution. The intensity distribution of the LoG-CXR bone component $\Delta_g I^h_{lungbone}$ is then adjusted by matching its histogram to the reference distribution, resulting in the final bone component $I^h_{finalbone}$, expressed as:

$$I^h_{finalbone} = HM(\Delta_g I^h_{lungbone}, D^h_{Xbone}), \tag{18.13}$$

where HM is histogram matching, D^h_{Xbone} is the target bone intensity distribution of I^h_{Xbone}.

18.3.4 High-Resolution CXR Bone Suppression

In step-4, we finally subtract the rectified bone component $I^h_{finalbone}$ from the original CXR to generate the final bone suppression result $I^h_{BS} = I_X - I^h_{finalbone}$, where I^h_{BS} represents the final high-resolution bone-suppressed CXR.

18.3.5 Experiments of HRCS

18.3.5.1 Datasets

We evaluate our method on three publicly available datasets. A total of 246 CT volumes from LIDC-IDRI [1] are used as unpaired CT structural priors to train F_{MT} in the first stage. The datasets consist of 662 CXRs with a resolution of 1024×1024 from the Shenzhen hospital dataset [9] and 112,120 CXRs with resolutions of approximately 3000×3000 from the Chest-14 dataset [22].

18.3.5.2 HRCS Bone-Suppressed CXRs for Automatic Disease Classification

To further demonstrate the effectiveness of our method for lung disease diagnosis, we fed our bone-suppressed results from both datasets into a lung disease prediction system based on DenseNet-121 [7]. We concatenate two original CXR images and one bone-suppressed CXR image from our method to create a three-channel input. This three-channel image is then used as input to the DenseNet-121 [7].

The DenseNet-121 [7] models in both tests utilize three convolutional layers with full padding, using 3×3 convolutional kernels and 64 filters. The Shenzhen hospital dataset [9] is classified into two categories (normal vs. abnormal), while the Chest-14 dataset [22] is classified into 14 categories. Both X-ray datasets are split according to their official splits [9, 22]. The data augmentation and training strategies follow those described in previous work [17].

The quantitative prediction results for both datasets are summarized in Tables 18.1 and 18.2, along with the results of other methods evaluated on the official splits. Our method achieves state-of-the-art performance for lung disease classification on both datasets.

Lung diseases such as pneumothorax, edema, and fibrosis can cause subtle changes in lung textures, which may be difficult to detect, especially when occluded by ribs. We hypothesize that bone suppression can improve the accuracy of automatic disease classification, and this is supported by the results in Table 18.1.

For the Shenzhen hospital dataset, our method improves the AUC by 0.050 and accuracy by 0.054. The false-positive rate also drops from 20.9% to 12.2%. Notably, these performance improvements were achieved in an unpaired training setting,

Table 18.1 Area under the curve (AUC) for the prediction of 14 lung diseases on the ChestX-ray14 dataset

Method	Wang et al. [22]	Yao et al. [24]	DenseNet-121 [7, 17]	DenseNet-121 + DecGAN[12]	DenseNet-121 + Our method
Atelectasis	0.700	0.733	0.777	**0.781**	0.776
Cardiomegaly	0.810	0.858	0.879	0.881	**0.908**
Effusion	0.759	0.806	0.825	0.827	**0.842**
Infiltration	0.661	0.675	0.696	0.703	**0.711**
Mass	0.693	0.727	0.835	0.835	**0.836**
Nodule	0.669	0.773	0.773	**0.778**	0.750
Pneumonia	0.658	0.690	0.730	0.737	**0.742**
Pneumothorax	0.799	0.805	0.842	0.843	**0.863**
Consolidation	0.703	0.717	0.761	**0.762**	0.758
Edema	0.805	0.806	0.847	0.851	**0.854**
Emphysema	0.833	0.842	**0.920**	0.917	0.918
Fibrosis	0.786	0.757	0.823	0.837	**0.847**
Pleura Thicken	0.684	0.724	0.779	0.783	**0.793**
Hernia	0.872	0.824	**0.938**	0.929	0.930
Average	0.745	0.767	0.816	0.819	**0.824**

Table 18.2 The area under the curve (AUC), accuracy (ACC), true positive rate (TP), and true negative rate (TN) for predicting normal versus abnormal cases on the Shenzhen Hospital dataset. The test set consists of 68 abnormal CXRs and 67 normal CXRs

Method	DenseNet-121 [7]	DecGAN [12]	Ours (1-channel)	Ours (3-channel)
AUC	0.895	0.910	0.906	**0.915**
ACC	0.752	0.822	0.814	**0.876**
TP	60.6% (40)	79.1% (53)	86.7% (57)	**87.8% (58)**
TN	**91.0% (61)**	85.7% (58)	77.6% (52)	88.0% (59)

and we believe the improvements could be even more pronounced with supervised training data.

18.3.5.3 HRCS Bone-Suppressed CXRs for Clinical Diagnosis

To assess whether our bone suppression results are beneficial for clinical diagnosis, we conducted a series of experiments involving two radiologists with varying levels of experience. More details are available in the original papers.

18.3.5.4 Bone-Suppression Visualization Results of HRCS

We selected three CXRs (one normal, one with pulmonary calcification, and one with tuberculosis) from the Shenzhen hospital dataset [9] to visually compare bone

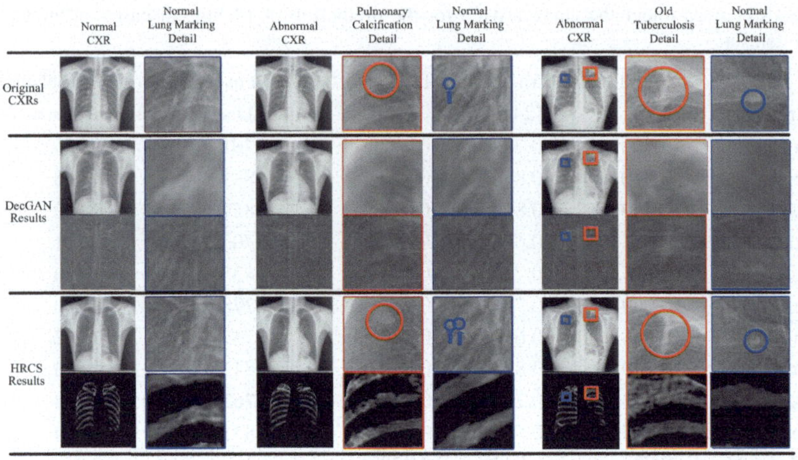

Fig. 18.5 Each bone-suppression method is represented by two rows and eight columns. The top row displays the bone-suppressed images, while the bottom row shows the result of subtracting these images from their corresponding original CXRs. The first two columns present normal CXR results generated by various methods, while the last six columns contain two abnormal CXRs (one with pulmonary calcification and one with old tuberculosis). The images within blue boxes highlight normal detail regions, whereas red boxes indicate abnormal regions

suppression results from different methods. As shown in Fig. 18.5, our method has three advantages: (1) Our bone-suppressed results are more visually pleasing. (2) Our method can retain large nodules (e.g., calcifications in the fourth column and old tuberculosis in the seventh column) as well as small details (e.g., small vascular sections in the fifth and last columns). (3) The shapes and details are clearer in our results compared to others, as seen in the lung markings in the second, fifth, and last columns, and in the nodules in the fourth and seventh columns. These advantages help reduce reading difficulty and the risk of misdiagnosis.

18.3.6 Discussion

From the above results, we conclude: (1) Our method produces superior image quality after bone suppression compared to state-of-the-art approaches. (2) Our bone-suppressed images enhance lung disease classification accuracy and outperform existing methods. (3) Bone-suppressed images help reduce clinical misdiagnosis, especially false negatives. (4) Our approach aids in reducing reading difficulty and the likelihood of misdiagnosis.

18.3.7 Conclusion of HRCS

In this section, we presented a method for automatically obtaining bone-suppressed CXRs. Our approach integrates learning-based and physical model-based methods, combining the advantages of both: automation and high-resolution results with low computational cost. Specifically, we proposed an unsupervised bone suppression method using structural priors derived from unpaired CT images. We applied LoG transformation and domain adaptation to reduce the domain gap between DRRs and CXRs, leveraging CT domain knowledge. We then used a multi-task decomposition network and histogram matching to generate high-resolution bone images. Experiments and clinical evaluations on two benchmark CXR datasets demonstrate that bone-suppressed images enhance both clinical diagnosis and automatic lung disease classification.

A limitation of our approach is that the diversity of the generated DRR images is limited and may not accurately reflect the imaging conditions of all CXRs, particularly in extreme cases. For example, our method may not perform well for CXRs without bones or with bones of very low contrast.

However, generating the bone image first and then subtracting it from the original CXR proves to be an effective approach for producing high-resolution, high-quality bone-suppressed CXRs. In addition to the previously discussed advantage that HRCS places lower demands on the quality of the generated bone itself, another key reason is that bones are generally easier to generate than soft tissues. Therefore, we want to identify more tasks that benefit from having the bone image directly, rather than a fully bone-suppressed image. Pelvic X-ray bone extraction serves as an ideal task that directly benefits from having access to the bone image itself.

18.4 PELvis Extraction (PELE)

Pelvic X-rays (PXRs) are commonly utilized in clinical decision-making for conditions involving the pelvis, the lower section of the trunk that provides structural support and stability. Specifically, PXR-based landmark detection aids in downstream analyses and supports computer-assisted diagnosis and treatment planning for pelvic disorders. While PXRs have advantages such as lower radiation exposure and reduced cost compared to computed tomography (CT), they pose a challenge due to the overlay of soft tissues, such as the intestines and bladder, which can obscure the underlying pelvic bone structures. This overlap may affect the accuracy of landmark detection in certain cases. Existing deep learning-based landmark detection methods typically address this issue indirectly by focusing on network architecture improvements. However, approaches that explicitly tackle soft tissue obstruction in PXRs remain relatively uncommon.

In this section, we present the PELE module, designed to extract pelvic structures from PXRs, thereby enhancing downstream analyses such as landmark detection.

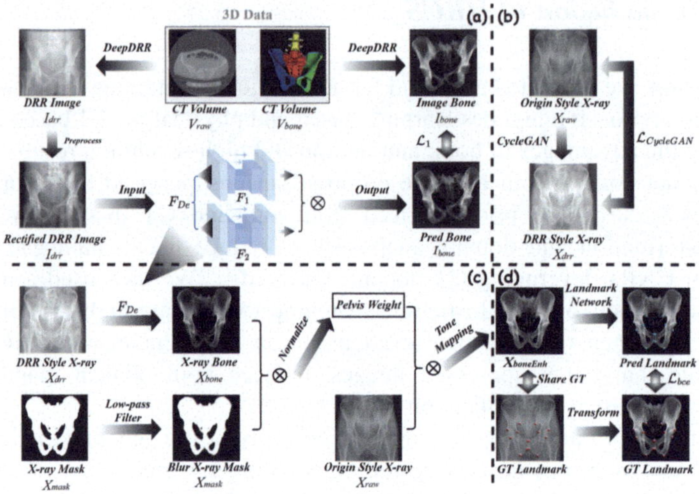

Fig. 18.6 (**a**) and (**b**) The diagram of the proposed PELvis Extraction (PELE) module. (**c**) The enhancement module. (**d**) The landmark detection flow

As shown in Fig. 18.6, the PELE module consists of two stages: (a) image decomposition via F_{DE} and (b) domain adaptation through F_{DA}.

Image Decomposition The goal is to decompose a 2D PXR X_{raw} into a pelvis-only image X_{bone} and a tissue-only image X_{tissue}, i.e., $X_{raw} \rightarrow (X_{bone}, X_{tissue})$, using a learned deep network. However, it is challenging due to the lack of pelvis-only images paired with 2D PXRs. Inspired by previous work [2, 6, 10, 13], we leverage 3D prior knowledge from CT and use a 2D digitally reconstructed radiograph (DRR) as a bridge between 3D CT and 2D PXRs.

From a 3D CT volume V_{raw} and its isolated pelvis portion V_{bone}, we generate 2D DRR images of V_{raw} and V_{bone}, denoted as I_{raw} and I_{bone}, respectively, using the DeepDRR [20] algorithm. We then train a deep neural network F_{DE} to perform DRR-based decomposition: $I_{bone} = F_{DE}(I_{raw})$.

To improve the performance of F_{DE}, we also introduce bone mask segmentation as an auxiliary task. Specifically, given a CT volume V_{raw} and its bone mask annotation V_{mask}, the bone portion is obtained via $V_{bone} = V_{raw} \odot V_{mask}$, where $\odot$ denotes element-wise multiplication. We project the 3D V_{mask} to create the 2D mask image I_{mask} using DeepDRR. The training process consists of two steps: (i) First, two networks are trained: a nnU-Net F_1 for predicting I_{mask} and a U-Net F_2 for predicting I_{bone}; (ii) Then, the product $I_{mask} \odot I_{bone}$ is used as the final bone prediction $\hat{I}_{bone}$:

$$I_{mask} = F_1(I_{raw});\ I_{bone} = F_2(I_{raw});\ \hat{I}_{bone} = F_{DE}(I_{raw}) = I_{mask} \odot I_{bone}. \tag{18.14}$$

Domain Adaptation Although DRR images share the same dimensions as PXRs, there still exists a domain gap between them. Therefore, the decomposition model F_{DE} cannot be directly applied to PXR X_{raw}. To bridge this gap, we employ domain adaptation (DA) using CycleGAN [26] as the backbone. CycleGAN learns a forward mapping network F_{DA} from PXR to DRR, as well as an inverse mapping $I_{raw} = F_{DA}(X_{raw})$. The predicted pelvis for X_{raw}, denoted as X_{bone}, is then given by:

$$X_{bone} = F_{DE}(I_{raw}) = F_{DE}(F_{DA}(X_{raw})). \tag{18.15}$$

18.4.1 Pelvis Enhancement

The extracted pelvis image X_{bone} sometimes contains artifacts, especially in poorly penetrated areas such as the hip bones, sacrum, and tailbone, which can affect diagnosis. To address this, we propose an enhancement module to generate the final output, $X_{boneEnh}$, as shown in Fig. 18.6c. We smooth and normalize the pelvic contour edge in X_{bone} to obtain a processed pelvic bone image $X_{bonePre}$, using a Gaussian filter for smooth transitions:

$$X_{bonePre} = \mathcal{N}[\mathcal{G}(X_{mask}) \odot X_{bone}], \tag{18.16}$$

where X_{mask} is the binary bone mask, $\mathcal{N}$ denotes the normalization operator, and $\mathcal{G}$ is a low-pass filter (e.g., Gaussian filter). Next, we multiply $X_{bonePre}$ with X_{raw} to incorporate PXR details and apply tone mapping (e.g., Gamma correction) to enhance dark areas and reveal finer details. The final enhanced image is $X_{boneEnh}$.

18.4.2 Pelvic Landmark Detection

As depicted in Fig. 18.6d, we use the enhanced pelvis image $X_{boneEnh}$ to train a landmark detection network Φ. Landmark annotations on X_{raw} are used to generate ground truth (GT) heatmaps H_{gt}. For a given landmark position (x_0, y_0), the GT heatmap $H_{gt}(x, y)$ is defined as:

$$H_{gt}(x, y) = \frac{1}{\sqrt{2\pi}\sigma} \exp\left\{-\frac{(x - x_0)^2 + (y - y_0)^2}{2\sigma^2}\right\}, \tag{18.17}$$

where σ is the standard deviation of the Gaussian distribution. The detection network is trained using $X_{boneEnh}$ and supervised by the GT heatmaps H_{gt}. As $X_{boneEnh}$ and X_{raw} share the same spatial grid, the predicted landmarks can be directly mapped onto X_{raw}. We evaluate two baseline landmark detection models: U-Net [18] and GU2Net [25]. U-Net is a popular model in medical analysis, while

GU2Net is a universal landmark detection model that combines local features with global context.

18.4.3 Experiment of PELE

18.4.3.1 Datasets

For the CT dataset, we use the publicly available CTPelvic1K dataset [16], which consists of 1184 volumes (over 320K slices). DRR images are generated using the DeepDRR [20] algorithm and resized to 512 × 512 via bilinear interpolation. In total, 919 DRR images are generated to train F_{DA}, and 200 high-quality images are selected to train F_{DE}. For PXRs, we curate 850 images from three different sources: Dataset1 consists of 400 high-resolution PXRs from the open-source CGMH-PelvisSeg dataset, provided by CGMHai Lab. Dataset2 includes 150 images from an open-source dataset provided by [3]. Dataset3 is an in-house dataset comprising 300 PXRs, retrospectively collected from cooperative hospitals under institutional review board (IRB) policies.

18.4.3.2 PELE Bone-Suppressed CXR for Landmark Detection

We selected 14 corresponding landmarks based on the CE Angle, acetabular index, H-line, and Perkin quadrant [14, 15, 23], which are commonly used in clinical auxiliary diagnosis. All images were annotated by a pelvic surgeon with over ten years of experience and subsequently reviewed by D2, who focused on verifying the locations forming the CE Angle, acetabular index, and H-line, and made corrections where necessary after consulting with D1.

For evaluation, we utilize mean radial error (MRE) to quantify the Euclidean distance between ground truth and predicted landmarks, along with successful detection rate (SDR) at four radii: 3, 4, 6, and 9 pixels (px), as shown in Table 18.3.

Table 18.3 presents the quantitative performance of various baselines before and after incorporating the PELE module. Notably, when trained with only 107 PXRs (12.5% of all PXRs), the MRE improvement is particularly pronounced, with a gain of over 200% compared to the baseline. This suggests that PELE offers a substantial advantage for small datasets. With 50% of the data (i.e., 425 PXRs), our method achieves an MRE of 1.83 and an SDR of 94.41% within a 9px radius. Furthermore, PELE demonstrates good generalization by working effectively with different baselines (i.e., U-Net, GU2Net), indicating that it can be applied to a range of models.

As illustrated in Fig. 18.7, the red points represent the ground truth, while the blue points denote the predicted landmarks. It is evident that the localization of the detected landmarks has significantly improved after applying the PELE module, as the visual distance between the predicted and actual points has noticeably decreased.

Table 18.3 Performance of various landmark detection models with and without the PELE module. The highest scores are highlighted in **bold**, while the second-best results are underlined

Models	Training data	MRE (px)	STD (px)	SDR (%) 3px	4px	6px	9px
GU2Net [25]	107	11.64	30.79	52.40	67.34	82.84	90.50
GU2Net with PELE	107	4.85	**12.95**	**53.43**	**67.40**	**83.40**	91.30
U-Net [18]	107	10.70	30.99	51.12	66.13	81.82	90.07
U-Net with PELE	107	**4.74**	14.33	52.79	66.42	83.17	**91.52**
GU2Net [25]	213	6.66	23.44	54.30	70.00	85.97	92.26
GU2Net with PELE	213	**4.39**	11.12	**54.53**	**70.71**	**85.99**	**93.04**
U-Net [18]	213	6.98	22.01	52.30	68.05	83.45	91.30
U-Net with PELE	213	4.72	**10.65**	53.70	69.27	84.51	92.24
GU2Net [25]	425	3.81	20.53	56.54	73.10	87.04	93.35
GU2Net with PELE	425	2.01	9.75	**56.89**	**73.49**	**88.14**	**94.41**
U-Net [18]	425	3.41	19.48	55.17	72.63	86.65	92.70
U-Net with PELE	425	**1.83**	**9.32**	55.49	73.18	87.33	93.38

18.4.4 Conclusion of PELE

The design of the PELE module significantly improves the accuracy of pelvic landmark detection across various baseline models. By explicitly addressing the overlay of soft tissues, such as the intestines and bladder, which can obscure the underlying pelvic bone structures in PXR images, the module isolates the pelvis, thereby enhancing the reliability of landmark positioning and the identification of critical structures. This improvement facilitates more accurate diagnosis and treatment planning for downstream clinical tasks.

18.5 Conclusion

DecGAN directly decomposes CXRs into bone CXR images, lung CXR images, and other soft-tissue CXR images, thereby generating a bone-suppressed CXR by removing the bone component. These decomposed CXRs are highly effective for deep learning models, such as CXR disease classification. However, radiologists may have concerns about the quality of the generated CXRs. For instance, they might worry about the introduction of artificial artifacts and find the resolution too low for clinical use, which significantly reduces the clinical value of DecGAN.

HRCS adopts an alternative approach to bone suppression. It only generates a bone CXR image and subtracts this bone image from the original CXR to obtain a bone-suppressed CXR. This method has higher clinical value because it can produce high-resolution bone-suppressed CXRs without introducing artificial artifacts. This is because HRCS subtracts the generated bone CXR from the original CXR, rather

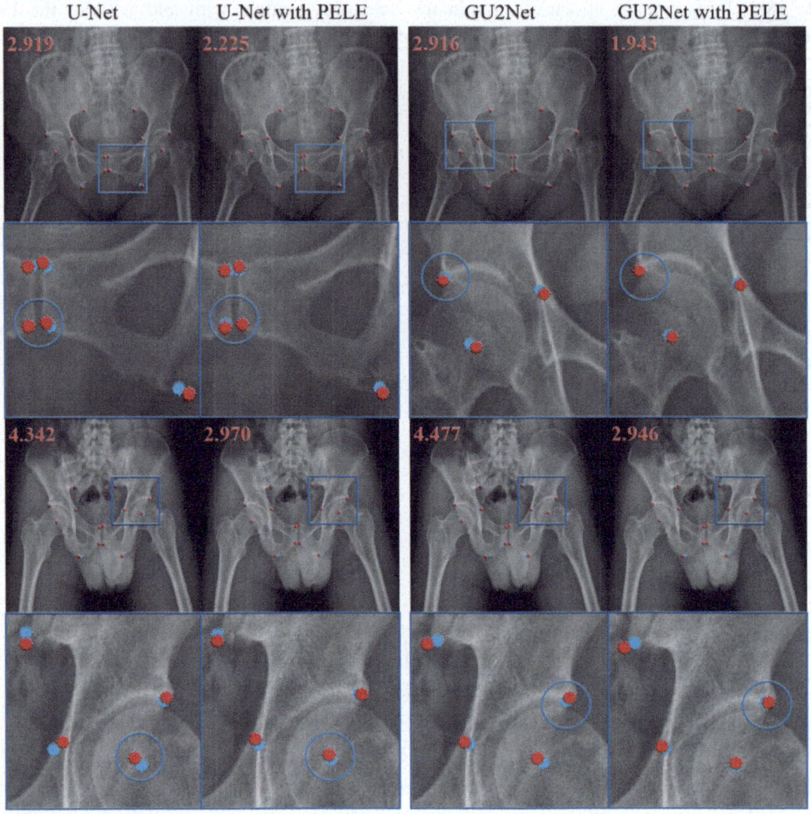

Fig. 18.7 Visualizations of various methods under the 213 training data setting. Blue points indicate the predicted landmarks, while red points correspond to the ground truth labels. The following row presents close-up views of local details to better illustrate the results. The MRE value is shown in the top left corner for comparison. The blue circles are just for reference

than directly generating a bone-suppressed CXR, which reduces the difficulty of the task. Besides, HRCS can generate a low-resolution bone CXR, which is then resized to high resolution, just ensuring that no critical details are lost in the final bone-suppressed CXR (no artifacts are added in the low-resolution bone CXR).

PELE follows the approach of HRCS but benefits from using the generated pelvic bone image directly, rather than relying on a fully bone-suppressed image. Pelvic X-ray bone extraction is an ideal task that directly benefits from having access to the bone image itself.

All three of the introduced methods embed 3D CT priors into 2D X-ray imaging using GANs to extract bone structures from X-ray images. Using GANs to directly generate specific CXRs, such as bone-only or bone-suppressed CXRs, is a straightforward idea borrowed from natural image computer vision tasks. However, when adapting methods from natural image tasks, it is crucial to consider the clinical value. In most cases, medical AI methods should serve as an aid for radiologists rather than making decisions independently. The methods should be highly interpretable, and the generated results should assist radiologists in their decision-making process.

There are several promising directions for **further research.** First, leveraging large foundational models for modality transfer presents a valuable opportunity. These large-scale networks are capable of extracting more robust and nuanced features, which could significantly enhance the performance of medical imaging tasks, including bone suppression. Second, expanding the decomposition beyond the current focus on bones is an intriguing direction. Currently, bones are the primary target because their density is much higher than that of other tissues, making them easier to isolate and suppress. However, incorporating additional components, such as soft tissues and organs, could lead to a more comprehensive approach to CXR decomposition. This could improve the utility of bone-suppressed images and help address a broader range of clinical needs.

References

1. Armato III SG, McLennan G, Bidaut L, McNitt-Gray MF, Meyer CR, Reeves AP, Zhao B, Aberle DR, Henschke CI, Hoffman EA, et al (2011) The lung image database consortium (LIDC) and image database resource initiative (IDRI): a completed reference database of lung nodules on ct scans. Med Phys 38(2):915–931
2. Aubert B, Cresson T, De Guise J, Vazquez C (2022) X-ray to DRR images translation for efficient multiple objects similarity measures in deformable model 3D/2D registration. IEEE Trans Med Imag 42(4):897–909
3. Cheng CT, Wang Y, Chen HW, Hsiao PM, Yeh CN, Hsieh CH, Miao S, Xiao J, Liao CH, Lu L (2021) A scalable physician-level deep learning algorithm detects universal trauma on pelvic radiographs. Nat Commun 12(1):1066
4. Ergun DL, Mistretta CA, Brown DE, Bystrianyk R, Sze KW, Kelcz F, Naidich PD (1990) Single-exposure dual-energy computed radiography: improved detection and processing. Radiology 174(1):243–249
5. Han H, Li J, Jain AK, Shan S, Chen X (2019) Tattoo image search at scale: joint detection and compact representation learning. IEEE Trans Pattern Anal Mach Intell 41(10):2333–2348
6. Han L, Lyu Y, Peng C, Zhou SK (2022) GAN-based disentanglement learning for chest x-ray rib suppression. Med Image Anal 77:102369
7. Huang G, Liu Z, L VDM, Weinberger KQ (2017) Densely connected convolutional networks. In: IEEE CVPR, vol 1, pp 2261–2269
8. Huang Z, Li H, Shao S, Zhu H, Hu H, Cheng Z, Wang J, K Zhou S (2024) Pele scores: pelvic x-ray landmark detection with pelvis extraction and enhancement. IJCAS 19(5):939–950
9. Jaeger S, Candemir S, Antani S, Wáng YXJ, Lu P, Thoma G (2014) Two public chest x-ray datasets for computer-aided screening of pulmonary diseases. Quant Imaging Med Surg 4(6):475
10. Kasten Y, Doktofsky D, Kovler I (2020) End-to-end convolutional neural network for 3D reconstruction of knee bones from bi-planar X-ray images. In: MICCAI workshop. Springer, Berlin, pp 123–133
11. Keserci B, Yoshida H (2002) Computerized detection of pulmonary nodules in chest radiographs based on morphological features and wavelet snake model. Med Image Anal 6(4):431–447

12. Li Z, Li H, Han H, Shi G, Wang J, K Zhou S (2019) Encoding CT anatomy knowledge for unpaired chest x-ray image decomposition. In: MICCAI. Elsevier, Amsterdam, pp 275–283
13. Li H, Han H, Li Z, Wang L, Wu Z, Lu J, Zhou SK (2020) High-resolution chest x-ray bone suppression using unpaired ct structural priors. IEEE Trans Med Imag 39(10):3053–3063
14. Liu C, Xie H, Zhang S, Xu J, Sun J, Zhang Y (2019) Misshapen pelvis landmark detection by spatial local correlation mining for diagnosing developmental dysplasia of the hip. In: MICCAI. Springer, Berlin, pp 441–449
15. Liu C, Xie H, Zhang S, Mao Z, Zhang Y (2020) Misshapen pelvis landmark detection with local-global feature learning for diagnosing developmental dysplasia of the hip. IEEE Trans Med Imag PP(99):1
16. Liu P, Han H, Du Y, Zhu H, Li Y, Gu F, Xiao H, Li J, Zhao C, Xiao L, Wu X, Zhou S (2021) Deep learning to segment pelvic bones: large-scale ct datasets and baseline models. Int J Comput Assist Radiol Surg 16:749–756
17. Rajpurkar P, Irvin J, Zhu K, Yang B, Mehta H, Duan T, Ding D, Bagul A, Langlotz C, Shpanskaya K, et al (2017) Chexnet: radiologist-level pneumonia detection on chest x-rays with deep learning. arXiv preprint arXiv:171105225
18. Ronneberger O, Fischer P, Brox T (2015) U-net: convolutional networks for biomedical image segmentation. In: MICCAI. Springer, Berlin, pp 234–241
19. Shi Z, Zhao M, He L, Wang Y (2011) A combinational filtering method for enhancing suspicious structures in chest x-rays. J Inform Comput Sci 8(7):997–1005
20. Unberath M, Zaech J, Lee SC, Bier B, Fotouhi J, Armand M, Navab N (2018) Deepdrr–a catalyst for machine learning in fluoroscopy-guided procedures. In: MICCAI
21. Wang F, Han H, Shan S, Chen X (2017) Deep multi-task learning for joint prediction of heterogeneous face attributes. In: Proc. FG, pp 173–179
22. Wang X, Peng Y, Lu L, Lu Z, Bagheri M, Summers RM (2017) Chestx-ray8: hospital-scale chest x-ray database and benchmarks on weakly-supervised classification and localization of common thorax diseases. In: IEEE CVPR, pp 3462–3471
23. Wang Y, Lu L, Cheng C, Jin D, Harrison AP, Xiao J, Liao C, Miao S (2019) Weakly supervised universal fracture detection in pelvic x-rays. In: MICCAI. Springer, Berlin, pp 459–467
24. Yao L, Prosky J, Poblenz E, Covington B, Lyman K (2018) Weakly supervised medical diagnosis and localization from multiple resolutions. arXiv preprint arXiv:180307703
25. Zhu H, Yao Q, Xiao L, Zhou SK (2021) You only learn once: universal anatomical landmark detection. In: MICCAI. Springer, Berlin, pp 85–95
26. Zhu J, Park T, Isola P, Efros AA (2017) Unpaired image-to-image translation using cycle-consistent adversarial networks. In: IEEE ICCV, pp 2242–2251

The manufacturer's authorised representative in the EU is Springer Nature Customer Service Centre GmbH, Europaplatz 3, 69115 Heidelberg, Germany. If you have any concerns regarding our products, please contact ProductSafety@springernature.com

Printed and bound by CPI Group (UK) Ltd, Croydon, CR0 4YY
30/09/2026
02225600-0013